i never knew i had a
choice

explorations in personal growth

Gerald Corey
California State University
Diplomate in Counseling Psychology
American Board of Professional Psychology

Marianne Schneider Corey
Consultant

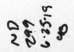

i never knew i had a

choice

explorations in personal growth

Gerald Corey
California State University
Diplomate in Counseling Psychology
American Board of Professional Psychology

Marianne Schneider Corey
Consultant

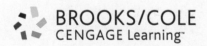

BROOKS/COLE
CENGAGE Learning™

Australia • Brazil • Japan • Korea • Mexico • Singapore • Spain • United Kingdom • United States

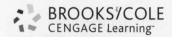
BROOKS/COLE
CENGAGE Learning™

I Never Knew I Had a Choice: Explorations in Personal Growth, Tenth Edition
Gerald Corey, Marianne Schneider Corey

Executive Editor: Jon-David Hague

Developmental Editor: Julie Martinez

Assistant Editor: Naomi Dreyer

Editorial Assistant: Amelia Blevins

Media Editor: Elizabeth Momb

Content Project Manager: Rita Jaramillo

Senior Brand Manager: Elisabeth Rhoden

Market Development Manager: Kara Parsons

Art Director: Caryl Gorska

Manufacturing Planner: Judy Inouye

Rights Acquisitions Specialist:
   Roberta Broyer

Production and Composition: Cenveo

Photo Researcher: Heidi Jo Corey

Photo Vendor: Bill Smith Group

Text Researcher: Premedia Global

Copy Editor: Kay Mikel

Text and Cover Design: Ingalls Design

Cover Image: Visuals Unlimited, Inc. /
   Patrick Smith

Library of Congress Control Number: 2012937548

For product information and technology assistance, contact us at **Cengage Learning Customer & Sales Support, 1-800-354-9706.**

For permission to use material from this text or product, submit all requests online at **www.cengage.com/permissions.** Further permissions questions can be e-mailed to **permissionrequest@cengage.com.**

Student Edition:
ISBN-13: 978-1-285-06768-1
ISBN-10: 1-285-06768-1

Loose-leaf Edition:
ISBN-13: 978-1-285-08935-5
ISBN-10: 1-285-08935-9

Brooks/Cole
20 Davis Drive
Belmont, CA 94002-3098
USA

Cengage Learning is a leading provider of customized learning solutions with office locations around the globe, including Singapore, the United Kingdom, Australia, Mexico, Brazil, and Japan. Locate your local office at **www.cengage.com/global.**

Cengage Learning products are represented in Canada by Nelson Education, Ltd.

To learn more about Brooks/Cole, visit **www.cengage.com/brookscole** Purchase any of our products at your local college store or at our preferred online store www.CengageBrain.com.

Printed in China
3 4 5 6 7 17 16 15 14

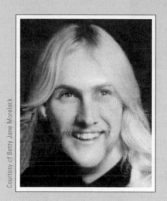

In memory of our friend Jim Morelock, a searcher who lived and died with dignity and self-respect, who struggled and questioned, who made the choice to live his days fully until time ran out on him at age 25.

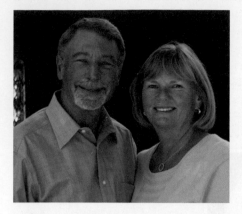

GERALD COREY is a Professor Emeritus of Human Services and Counseling at California State University at Fullerton. He received his doctorate in counseling from the University of Southern California. He is a Diplomate in Counseling Psychology, American Board of Professional Psychology; a licensed psychologist; a National Certified Counselor; a Fellow of the American Psychological Association (APA, Counseling Psychology); a Fellow of the American Counseling Association (ACA); and a Fellow of the Association for Specialists in Group Work (ASGW). Along with Marianne Schneider Corey, Jerry received the Lifetime Achievement Award from the American Mental Health Counselors Association in 2011 and the Eminent Career Award from ASGW in 2001. He was the recipient of the Outstanding Professor of the Year Award from California State University at Fullerton in 1991. He regularly teaches both undergraduate and graduate courses in group counseling and ethics in counseling. He is the author or coauthor of 16 textbooks in counseling currently in print, along with numerous journal articles. His book, *Theory and Practice of Counseling and Psychotherapy*, has been translated into Arabic, Indonesian, Portuguese, Korean, Turkish, and Chinese. *Theory and Practice of Group Counseling* has been translated into Korean, Chinese, Spanish, and Russian.

Jerry and Marianne Schneider Corey often present workshops in group counseling. In the past 35 years the Coreys have conducted group counseling training workshops for mental health professionals at many universities in the United States as well as in Canada, Mexico, China, Hong Kong, Korea, Germany, Belgium, Scotland, England, and Ireland. In his leisure time, Jerry likes to travel, hike and bicycle in the mountains and the desert, and drive his 1931 Model A Ford. The Coreys have been married for 48 years; they have two adult daughters and three grandchildren.

Recent publications by Jerry Corey, all with Brooks/Cole, Cengage Learning, most having been translated into various languages, include:

▶ *Groups Process and Practice*, Ninth Edition (2014, with Marianne Schneider Corey and Cindy Corey)

▶ *Theory and Practice of Counseling and Psychotherapy*, Ninth Edition (and *Student Manual*) (2013)

▶ *Case Approach to Counseling and Psychotherapy*, Eighth Edition (2013)

▶ *The Art of Integrative Counseling*, Third Edition (2013)

▶ *Theory and Practice of Group Counseling*, Eighth Edition, (and *Student Manual*) (2012)

▶ *Issues and Ethics in the Helping Professions*, Eighth Edition (2011, with Marianne Schneider Corey and Patrick Callanan)

▶ *Becoming a Helper*, Sixth Edition (2011, with Marianne Schneider Corey)

▶ *Group Techniques,* Third Edition (2004, with Marianne Schneider Corey, Patrick Callanan, and J. Michael Russell)

Jerry is coauthor (with Barbara Herlihy) of *Boundary Issues in Counseling: Multiple Roles and Responsibilities*, Second Edition (2006) and *ACA Ethical Standards Casebook*, Sixth Edition (2006); he is coauthor (with Robert Haynes, Patrice Moulton, and Michelle Muratori) of *Clinical Supervision in the Helping Professions: A Practical Guide*, Second Edition (2010); he is the author of *Creating Your Professional Path: Lessons From My Journey* (2010). All four of these books are published by the American Counseling Association.

Jerry has made several educational DVD and video programs on various aspects of counseling practice: (1) *Groups in Action: Evolution and Challenges—DVD and Workbook* (2014, with Marianne Schneider Corey and Robert Haynes); (2) *DVD for Theory and Practice of Counseling and Psychotherapy: The Case of Stan and Lecturettes* (2013); (3) *DVD for Integrative Counseling: The Case of Ruth and Lecturettes* (2013, with Robert Haynes); (4) *DVD for Theory and Practice of Group Counseling* (2012); and (5) *Ethics in Action: CD-ROM* (2003, with Marianne Schneider Corey and Robert Haynes). All of these programs are available through Brooks/Cole, Cengage Learning.

MARIANNE SCHNEIDER COREY is a licensed marriage and family therapist in California and is a National Certified Counselor. She received her master's degree in marriage, family, and child counseling from Chapman College. She is a Fellow of the Association for Specialists in Group Work (ASGW) and was the recipient of this organization's Eminent Career Award in 2001. She received the Lifetime Achievement Award from the American Mental Health Counselors Association in 2011. She also holds memberships in the American Counseling Association, the Association for Specialists in Group Work, the American Group Psychotherapy Association, the American Mental Health Counselors Association, the Association for Counselor Education and Supervision, the Association for Multicultural Counseling and Development, and the Western Association for Counselor Education and Supervision.

Marianne has been involved in leading groups for different populations, providing training and supervision workshops in group process, facilitating self-exploration groups for graduate students in counseling, and co-facilitating training groups for group counselors and weeklong residential workshops in personal growth. Both Marianne and Jerry Corey have conducted training workshops, continuing education seminars, and personal growth groups in the United States, Germany, Ireland, Belgium, Mexico, Hong Kong, China, and Korea. She sees groups as the most effective format in which to work with clients and finds it the most rewarding for her personally.

Marianne has coauthored the following books with Brooks/Cole, Cengage Learning, all of which have been translated into various languages:

▸ *Groups Process and Practice*, Ninth Edition (2014, with Gerald Corey and Cindy Corey)

▸ *Issues and Ethics in the Helping Professions*, Eighth Edition (2011, with Gerald Corey, and Patrick Callanan)

▸ *Becoming a Helper*, Sixth Edition (2011, with Gerald Corey)

▸ *Group Techniques*, Third Edition (2004, with Gerald Corey, Patrick Callanan, and Michael Russell)

Marianne has made educational video programs (with accompanying student workbooks) for Brooks/Cole, Cengage Learning: *Groups in Action: Evolution and Challenges—DVD and Workbook* (2014, with Gerald Corey and Robert Haynes); and *Ethics in Action*: CD-ROM (2003, with Gerald Corey and Robert Haynes).

Marianne and Jerry have been married since 1964. They have two adult daughters (Heidi and Cindy), two granddaughters (Kyla and Keegan), and one grandson (Corey). Marianne grew up in Germany and has kept in close contact with her family and friends there. In her free time, she enjoys traveling, reading, visiting with friends, bike riding, and hiking.

brief contents

1 Invitation to Personal Learning and Growth 2

2 Reviewing Your Childhood and Adolescence 38

3 Adulthood and Autonomy 72

4 Your Body and Wellness 110

5 Managing Stress 136

6 Love 176

7 Relationships 200

8 Becoming the Woman or Man You Want to Be 234

9 Sexuality 260

10 Work and Recreation 282

11 Loneliness and Solitude 316

12 Death and Loss 340

13 Meaning and Values 370

14 Pathways to Personal Growth 402

contents

ABOUT THE AUTHORS vi

BRIEF CONTENTS ix

CONTENTS xi

PREFACE xvii

1 Invitation to Personal Learning and Growth 2

Where Am I Now? 3

Choice and Change 4

Models for Personal Growth 7

Are You an Active Learner? 24

Multiple Intelligences and Multiple Learning Styles 25

Fixed Versus Growth Mindsets 29

Getting the Most from This Book: Suggestions for Personal Learning 31

Summary 33

Where Can I Go From Here? 33

Website Resources 34

2 Reviewing Your Childhood and Adolescence 38

Where Am I Now? 39

Stages of Personality Development: A Preview 40

Infancy 44

Early Childhood 48

Impact of the First Six Years of Life 51

Middle Childhood 56

Pubescence 60

Adolescence 61

Summary 67

Where Can I Go From Here? 67

Website Resources 68

3 Adulthood and Autonomy 72

Where Am I Now? 73`

The Path Toward Autonomy and Interdependence 74

Stages of Adulthood 88

Early Adulthood 90

Middle Adulthood 93

Late Middle Age 97

Late Adulthood 99

Summary 104

Where Can I Go From Here? 105

Website Resources 106

4 Your Body and Wellness 110

Where Am I Now? 111

Wellness and Life Choices 112

Maintaining Sound Health Practices 117

Your Bodily Identity 125

Summary 131

Where Can I Go From Here? 132

Website Resources 132

5 Managing Stress 136

Where Am I Now? 137

Sources of Stress 138

Effects of Stress 141

Ineffective Reactions to Stress 144

Posttraumatic Stress Disorders 149

Sexual Exploitation 151

Vicarious Traumatization 157

Constructive Responses to Stress 158

Time Management 160

Meditation 162

Mindfulness 164

Deep Relaxation 165

Yoga 166

Therapeutic Massage 167

Summary 169

Where Can I Go From Here? 170

Website Resources 171

CONTENTS

6 Love 176

Where Am I Now? 177

Love Makes a Difference 178

Learning to Love and Appreciate Ourselves 180

Authentic and Inauthentic Love 181

Theories of Love 185

Barriers to Loving and Being Loved 187

Love in a Changing World 192

Is It Worth It to Love? 193

Summary 195

Where Can I Go From Here? 195

Website Resources 196

7 Relationships 200

Where Am I Now? 201

Types of Intimacy 202

Meaningful Relationships: A Personal View 204

Anger and Conflict in Relationships 209

Dealing With Communication Barriers 214

Relationships in a Changing World 218

Gay and Lesbian Relationships 220

Separation and Divorce 225

Summary 229

Where Can I Go From Here? 229

Website Resources 230

8 Becoming the Woman or Man You Want to Be 234

Where Am I Now? 235

Male Roles 236

Female Roles 244

Alternatives to Rigid Gender-Role Expectations 252

Summary 255

Where Can I Go From Here? 255

Website Resources 256

9 Sexuality 260

Where Am I Now? 261

Learning to Talk Openly About Sexual Issues 262

Developing Your Sexual Values 264

Guilt and Misconceptions About Sex 267

Learning to Enjoy Sensuality and Sexuality 269

The Healthy Dimensions of Sexuality 271

Sex and Intimacy 272

The Controversy Over Sexual Addiction 274

The Hazards of Unprotected Sex 275

Summary 277

Where Can I Go From Here? 278

Website Resources 278

10 Work and Recreation 282

Where Am I Now? 283

Higher Education as Your Work 285

Choosing an Occupation or Career 286

The Process of Deciding on a Career 294

Choices at Work 297

Changing Careers in Midlife 301

Retirement 302

The Place of Recreation in Your Life 305

Summary 309

Where Can I Go From Here? 310

Website Resources 311

11 Loneliness and Solitude 316

Where Am I Now? 317

The Value of Solitude 318

The Experience of Loneliness 320

Learning to Confront the Fear of Loneliness 321

Creating Our Own Loneliness Through Shyness 323

Loneliness and Our Life Stages 328

Time Alone as a Source of Strength 335

Summary 335

Where Can I Go From Here? 336

Website Resources 336

12 Death and Loss 340

Where Am I Now? 341
Our Fears of Death 343
Death and the Meaning of Life 344
Suicide: Ultimate Choice, Ultimate Surrender, or Ultimate Tragedy? 349
Freedom in Dying 352
The Hospice Movement 354
The Stages of Death and Loss 356
Grieving Over Death, Separation, and Other Losses 360
Summary 365
Where Can I Go From Here? 365
Website Resources 366

13 Meaning and Values 370

Where Am I Now? 371
Our Quest for Identity 372
People Who Live With Passion and Purpose 374
When Good People Do Bad Things: The Lucifer Effect 375
When Ordinary People Do Extraordinary Things 376
Our Search for Meaning and Purpose 377
Religion/Spirituality and Meaning 381
Our Values in Action 384
Embracing Diversity 386
Making a Difference 393
Summary 396
Where Can I Go From Here? 397
Website Resources 398

14 Pathways to Personal Growth 402

Where Am I Now? 403
Self-Assessment as a Key to Personal Growth 404
Overcoming Barriers, Opening Doors 407
Pathways for Continued Self-Exploration 409
Counseling as a Path to Self-Understanding 409
Dreams as a Path to Self-Understanding 412
Concluding Comments 414
Where Can I Go From Here? 415
Website Resources 416

REFERENCES AND SUGGESTED READINGS 421
INDEX 441

I Never Knew I Had a Choice is intended for college students of any age and for all others who wish to expand their self-awareness and explore the choices available to them in significant areas of their lives. The topics discussed include choosing a personal style of learning; reviewing childhood and adolescence and the effects of these experiences on current behavior and choices; meeting the challenges of adulthood and autonomy; maintaining a healthy body and wellness; managing stress; appreciating the significance of love, intimate relationships, gender roles, and sexuality; work and recreation; dealing creatively with loneliness and solitude; understanding and accepting death and loss; choosing one's values and meaning in life; embracing diversity; and pathways to personal growth.

This is a personal book in which we describe our own experiences and values with regard to many of the issues we raise. In addition, we encourage readers to examine the choices they have made and how these choices affect their present level of satisfaction. Each chapter begins with a self-inventory—Where Am I Now?—that gives readers the opportunity to focus on their present beliefs and attitudes. Within the chapters, Take Time to Reflect exercises encourage readers to pause and reflect on the issues raised. Additional activities and exercises (Where Can I Go From Here?) are suggested at the end of each chapter for use in the classroom or outside of class. We want to stress that this is an unfinished book; readers are encouraged to become coauthors by writing about their own reactions in the book and in the journal pages provided at the end of each chapter.

Throughout the book we have updated material to reflect current thinking, but the underlying themes we focus on are timeless. The introductory chapter addresses the importance of self-exploration and invites students to consider the value in learning about themselves, others, and personal growth. Social concerns must balance self-interests, however, and we maintain that self-fulfillment can occur only when individuals have a sense of social consciousness.

WHAT'S NEW IN THE TENTH EDITION?

This edition provides the most up-to-date developments in the field, and we have added new topics, expanded and revised existing topics, abbreviated the discussion of some topics, and updated the References and Suggested Readings at the end of the book. General features that have been revised throughout include new personal stories illustrating key themes, current research findings relevant to original and new topics for each chapter, updated Take Time to Reflect exercises, and new Where Can I Go From Here? activities at the end of each chapter. The chapter-by-chapter overview that follows highlights the changes in this 10th edition.

Chapter 1 (Invitation to Personal Learning and Growth) presents several models of personal growth. The chapter includes some revision of the choices leading to change and updated material on what constitutes happiness. Also added is a discussion of the stages of change and an individual's readiness for making changes. Increased coverage is devoted to positive psychology and attaining a sense of well-being. We have updated the discussion of multiple intelligences and learning styles, with an expanded discussion of emotional intelligence. We present a new discussion on the topic of fixed versus growth mindsets, address the advantages of a growth mindset, and clarify how our mindsets are shaped by messages we receive about success and failure.

Chapter 2 (Reviewing Your Childhood and Adolescence) contains an expanded discussion of the role of early childhood experiences on later personality development. This chapter continues to feature Erikson's psychosocial model and the self-in-context theories as they deal with development throughout the life span. There is a new discussion of the concept of emotional and social competence, and new material on social networking as a way of connecting with peers in adolescence, the impact of cyberbullying on adolescents, and the benefits and drawbacks of social networking. Increased attention is given to resiliency in childhood as well.

In Chapter 3 (Adulthood and Autonomy) we continue the discussion of the life-span perspective by focusing on the psychosocial theory and the self-in-context perspective. This chapter has been streamlined to highlight choices we can make at each of the phases of life and the unique challenges facing the individual at each stage. Increased coverage on common cognitive distortions and learning how to critically evaluate our self-defeating thinking have been added to this chapter.

Chapter 4 (Your Body and Wellness) has a revised discussion of wellness and life choices. There is some minor updating of these topics: sleep, exercise, eating, and spirituality. We continue to invite readers to examine their lifestyle choices and how these decisions can enhance their health. Positive health patterns are highlighted.

Chapter 5 (Managing Stress) examines the impact of stress on the body, causes of stress, ineffective and constructive reactions to stress, and stress and the healthy personality. Revisions have been made to the role of culture in our perception of stress, environmental sources of stress, the power of resilience in coping with stress, and a range of constructive practices for managing stress. Recent research has been included on meditation, mindfulness, yoga, and massage. The section on posttraumatic stress disorder has been significantly updated and expanded, and a new section on vicarious traumatization has been added.

Chapter 6 (Love) deals with the many facets of love, the meaning of love, and our fears of loving and being loved. There is a new section on theories of love, with an emphasis on the importance of early bonding and attachment styles as a foundation for later relationships. Another new section on love in a changing world addresses ways that technological advances can either enhance our relationships or become a barrier to connection with people.

Chapter 7 (Relationships) contains guidelines for meaningful interpersonal relationships, including friendships, couple relationships, and family relationships. The section on gay and lesbian relationships has been updated and expanded, and we have added a discussion regarding hate crimes and sexual orientation. A new section on intimate partner violence and abuse and one on relationships in a changing world, which addresses how technological advances are affecting relationships, have been added. We discuss social networking, online dating, and infidelity in cyberspace and look at both the advantages and disadvantages of social networking with respect to relationships.

Chapter 8 (Becoming the Woman or Man You Want to Be) contains numerous new resources to update the discussion of male roles, female roles, gender-role conflict, gender-role socialization, women and work choices, and challenging traditional gender roles. Increased attention is given to factors related to gender-role socialization.

Chapter 9 (Sexuality) has been substantially revised to emphasize the positive, healthy aspects of sexuality. We look more in-depth at the messages we receive about sexuality from the media and from society. New sections include enjoying sexual intimacy in later life, the controversy over sexual addiction, and the importance of personal choices in preventing sexually transmitted illnesses.

Chapter 10 (Work and Recreation) contains a revised section on occupational fields associated with various personality types. New material has been added on the dynamics of discontent at work, toxic working conditions, abusive supervision, the relationship between self-esteem and work, and forced retirement. Reflecting the realities of today, we include a discussion of choices in the context of difficult economic times and employment cutbacks.

Chapter 11 (Loneliness and Solitude) discusses the creative dimensions of solitude, along with increased coverage on the different kinds of loneliness we face. We briefly examine the social fitness model as a way to deal with shyness and have updated our discussion of shyness.

Chapter 12 (Death and Loss) contains a revised discussion of the models for understanding the process of death and dying. The section on suicide has been updated and expanded. Coverage on the importance of grieving our losses and cultural variations in the mourning process have also been revised.

Chapter 13 (Meaning and Values) addresses the meaning of life, and we have provided many more examples of people who live with passion and purpose in their quest for a meaningful existence. New sections highlight Professor Philip Zimbardo's research on why good people do bad things as well as what makes ordinary people perform exceptional heroic acts. We have added a discussion on making a difference and the steps each of us can take in making the world a better place.

Chapter 14 (Pathways to Personal Growth) encourages students to think about where they will choose to go from here. The main question is, "Do you like the person you are today?" Readers are reminded that their journey toward personal growth is only beginning. The importance of self-assessment as a key to personal growth is highlighted, and readers are guided in reviewing salient topics throughout the book. A variety of avenues for growth are suggested that readers may wish to pursue now and in the future in making changes in the way they are living.

Fundamentally, our approach in *I Never Knew I Had a Choice* is humanistic and personal; that is, we stress the healthy and effective personality and the common struggles most of us experience in becoming mature adults. We especially emphasize accepting personal responsibility for the choices we make and consciously deciding whether and how we want to change our lives. There are multiple approaches to the study of personal adjustment and growth. We emphasize the existential and humanistic approach because to us it best sheds light on the role of choice and responsibility in creating a meaningful life for ourselves. We also include other theoretical perspectives in many of the chapters, a few of which are choice theory and reality therapy, transactional analysis, cognitive behavior therapy, feminist theory, self-in-relation theory, and the psychosocial approach to development.

Although our own approach can be broadly characterized as humanistic and existential, our aim has been to challenge readers to recognize and assess their own choices, beliefs, and values rather than to accept our particular point of view. Our basic premise is that a commitment to self-exploration creates new potentials for choice. Many of the college students and counseling clients with whom we work are relatively well-functioning people who desire more from life and who want to recognize and remove barriers to their personal creativity and freedom.

The experiences of those who have read and used earlier editions of *I Never Knew I Had a Choice* reveal that the themes explored have application to a diversity of ages and backgrounds. Readers who have taken the time to write us about their reactions say that the book encouraged them to take an honest look at their lives and resulted in them making certain changes.

I Never Knew I Had a Choice was developed for a variety of self-exploration courses, including Introduction to Counseling, Therapeutic Group, Psychology of Personal Growth, Personal Development, Personal Growth in Human Relationships, Personality and Adjustment, Interpersonal Relations, Human Potential Seminar, and Psychology of Personal Well-Being. *Choice* has also been adopted in courses ranging from the psychology of personal growth on the undergraduate level to graduate courses for training teachers and counselors. Courses that make use of an interactive approach will find *Choice* a useful tool for discussion.

We have written this book to facilitate interaction—between student and instructor, among the students within a class, between students and significant people in their lives, between the reader and us as authors—but most important of all, our aim is to provide the reader with an avenue for thoughtful reflection.

An updated *Instructor's Resource Manual* accompanies this textbook. It includes test items, both multiple-choice and essay, for each chapter; a student study guide covering all chapters; suggested reading; questions for thought and discussion; numerous activities and exercises for classroom participation; guidelines for using the book and teaching the course; examples of various formats of personal-growth classes; guidelines for maximizing personal learning and for reviewing and integrating the course; PowerPoint presentations; additional websites; and a student evaluation instrument to assess the impact of the course on readers.

Acknowledgments

We would like to express our deep appreciation for the insightful suggestions given to us by friends, associates, reviewers, students, and readers.

The reviewers of the entire manuscript of this 10th edition of *Choice* provided us with many useful ideas for the refinement of this book, and many of their suggestions have been incorporated in the present edition. They are:

Paul Blisard, Missouri State University;

Amanda Connell, graduate student, California State University, Fullerton;

Jacquelyn Fargano, National University;

Melinda Gonzales-Backen, Arizona State University;

Sandy Holbrook, Southeast Kentucky Community and Technical College;

Mary Livingston, Louisiana Tech University;

Tommy Lopez, Central Piedmont Community College;

Wendy McNeeley, Howard Payne University;

Michael Paviak, Ursuline College;

Linda Petroff, Central Community College;

Candace Shivers, Mount Wachusett Community College;

Glynis Strause, Costal Bend College; and

Shane Williamson, Lindenwood University.

Reviewers who contributed ideas for the revision of selected chapters for the 10th edition include Caroline Bailey, California State University, Fullerton (Chapters 2 and 3); Bernardo Carducci, Shyness Research Institute, Indiana University Southeast (Chapter 11); and William Blau, Copper Mountain College, Joshua Tree, California (Chapter 12).

Finally, as is true of all our books, *I Never Knew I Had a Choice* continues to develop as a result of a team effort, which includes the combined efforts of several people at Brooks/Cole, Cengage Learning. We thank Seth Dobrin, editor of social work and sociology; Jon-David Hague, executive editor and publisher; Julie Martinez, consulting editor, who monitored the review process; Caryl Gorska, for her superb work on the interior design and cover of this book; Elizabeth Momb, media editor; Naomi Dreyers, supplemental materials for the book; and Rita Jaramillo, project manager. We appreciate the work of Heidi Jo Corey in researching and selecting the photographs for this edition. We thank Ben Kolstad of Cenveo Publisher Services, who coordinated the production of this book. Special recognition goes to Kay Mikel, the manuscript editor of this edition, whose exceptional editorial talents continue to keep this book reader friendly. We appreciate Susan Cunningham's work in preparing the index.

Special recognition goes to Michelle Muratori, Johns Hopkins University, who consulted with us in revising this 10th edition. She assisted in the revision of all chapters, looked up current research on selected topics, revised and added personal stories for most of the chapters, updated the website resources, and made suggestions for integrating new topics. In addition, we recognize Michelle for her work on updating the *Instructor's Resource Manual* and assisting in developing the other supplements.

The efforts and dedication of all of these people have contributed to the high quality of this edition.

Gerald Corey and Marianne Schneider Corey

the review process, Caryl Gorska, for her expert work on the interior design and cover of the book, Elizabeth Momb, media editor, Naomi Dreyer, supplemental materials for the book, and Fara Tabatabai, project manager. We appreciate the work of Hiedi Jo Corey, research, and selecting the photographs for this edition. We thank Ken Karsted of Cengage Publisher Services, who coordinated the production of this book. Special recognition goes to Kay Mikel, the manuscript editor of this edition, whose exceptional editorial talents continue to keep this book reader friendly. We appreciate Susan Cunningham's work in preparing the index.

Special recognition goes to Michelle Muratori, Johns Hopkins University, who consulted with us in revising this 10th edition. She assisted in the revision of all chapters, looked into current research on selected topics, revised and added personal stories for most of the chapters, and aided the website resources, and made suggestions for invigorating new topics. In addition, we recognize Mik Belle for her work updating the Instructor's Resource Manual and assisting in developing the other supplements.

The effort and dedication of all of these people have contributed to the high quality of this edition.

Gerald Corey and Marianne Schneider Corey

i never knew i had a

choice

explorations in personal growth

Gerald Corey

California State University
Diplomate in Counseling Psychology
American Board of Professional Psychology

Marianne Schneider Corey

Consultant

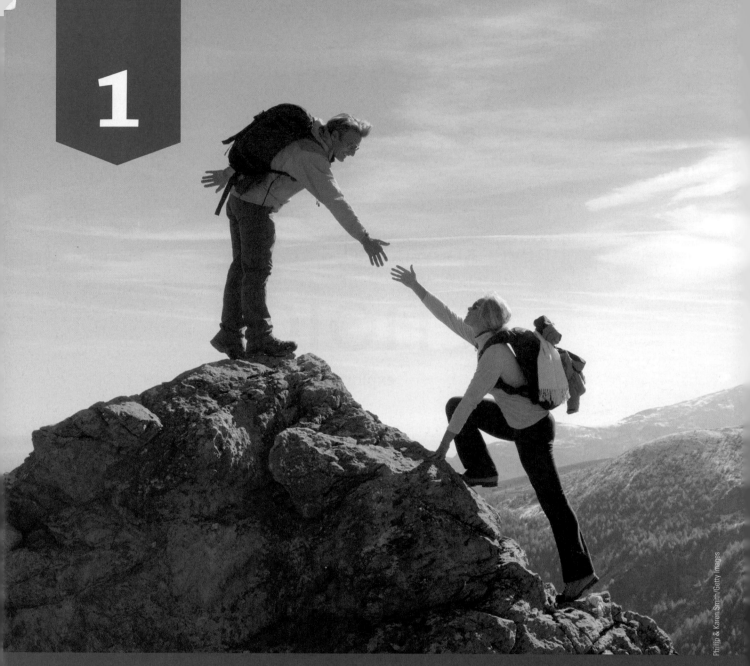
Phillip & Karen Smith/Getty Images

1

INVITATION TO PERSONAL LEARNING AND GROWTH

› Where Am I Now?

› Choice and Change

› Models for Personal Growth

› Are You an Active Learner?

› Multiple Intelligences and Multiple Learning Styles

› Fixed Versus Growth Mindsets

› Getting the Most From This Book: Suggestions for Personal Learning

› Summary

› Where Can I Go From Here?

› Website Resources

> *The unexamined life is not worth living.*
>
> —SOCRATES

WHERE AM I NOW?

Each chapter begins with a self-inventory designed to assess your attitudes and beliefs regarding a particular topic. Think about each question. By answering these questions as honestly as you can, you will increase your awareness and clarify your personal views on a range of subjects.

Use this scale to respond to these statements:

4 = I *strongly agree* with this statement.
3 = I *agree* with this statement.
2 = I *disagree* with this statement.
1 = I *strongly disagree* with this statement.

1. I believe I influence the course of my life through my choices.

2. I have a good sense of the areas in my life that I can change and those aspects that I cannot change.

3. Generally, I have been willing to pay the price for taking the personal risks involved in choosing for myself.

4. I believe it is within my power to change even if others around me do not change.

5. I think happiness and success are largely related to a sense of belonging and to social connectedness.

6. I try to strike a balance between meeting my own needs and meeting the needs of others.

7. At their deepest core, I think people are good and can be trusted to move forward in a positive way.

8. I am an active learner.

9. I feel ready to make changes in my life that will result in personal growth even if the process is painful at times.

10. I am willing to challenge myself to examine my life in an honest way.

Personal growth involves a commitment to change. Whether you change your beliefs, your attitudes, or your behaviors, the process through which change occurs can be intimidating, if not overwhelming. It is natural to wonder whether the changes involved in personal growth are worth the effort they require. Whether you choose it or not, change is an inevitable part of life, and it is just one of the many compelling reasons to embark on this journey of personal learning and growth.

When contemplating changes in your life, you first need to assess where you are now. Is your life satisfying? Are you getting what you want out of life? Do you sense a need to make changes in your daily life? Do you have an understanding of how your actions affect others? Perhaps even more fundamental is whether you believe you have the capacity to change. As you read this book, it is our hope that you will increase your awareness about who you are, how you relate to the world, and the choices open to you about ways to experience personal growth. We hope you will feel inspired to make the changes that are likely to result in a more fulfilling life.

CHOICE AND CHANGE

We Do Have Choices!

It is exciting for us when we see students and clients discover that they can be more in charge of their own lives than they ever dreamed possible. As one counseling client put it:"One thing I can see now that I didn't see before is that I can change my life if I want to. *I never knew I had a choice!*" This remark captures the central message of this book: we can make choices, and we do have the power to re-create ourselves through our choices. Although you may wonder whether doing what it takes to bring about change is worth the effort, we hope you do not stop at this point.

Reflect on the quality of your life and consider whether you want to change, and if so in which ways. Realize that the process of changing your attitudes and behaviors can be unsettling. Challenge your fears rather than being stopped by them. Socrates, in his wisdom, said,"The unexamined life is not worth living." Examine your values and your behavior. What crises have you faced? How did these crises affect your life? Did they represent a significant turning point for you? As you engage yourself in this book, consider ways to use any challenging life situations as opportunities for discovering choices and making changes.

What Brings Us Happiness?

Making choices for yourself and having self-control are important ingredients in happiness. However, Buddhists teach us that trying to control what cannot be controlled will not lead to fulfillment. Identify changes that are within your power to make and those that are not within your power. In considering what leads to happiness, remember that many of your decisions will be influenced by your relationships with significant people in your life; we are all social beings. Character strengths that build connections to people and purposes larger than the self predict future well-being (Gillham et al., 2011). Making a commitment to examine your life does not mean becoming wrapped up in yourself to the exclusion of everyone else. Unless you know and care about yourself, however, you will struggle to connect with others in a meaningful way.

Philip Hwang (2000) asserts that happiness entails possessing a healthy balance of both self-esteem and other-esteem. Rather than searching for ways to enhance self-esteem, Hwang makes a strong case for promoting personal and social responsibility. **Other-esteem** involves respect, acceptance, caring, valuing, and promoting others, without reservation. We need to strive to understand others who may think, feel, and act differently from us. American culture stresses the self, independence, and self-sufficiency, but a meaningful life includes connections to others in love, work, and community. Hwang suggests that our challenge is to learn to see the world anew by reexamining our attitudes, values, and beliefs and developing a *balance* between caring for self and showing high esteem for others. It is not a matter of self-interests versus interest in others, for we can care for both ourselves and others. Caring for others can be rewarding in itself; in addition, others are likely to reciprocate in positive ways when we demonstrate concern for them.

Weiten, Dunn, and Hammer (2012) examined empirical studies on what constitutes happiness and found that happiness is more a subjective matter than an objective state. A number of factors contribute to determining our subjective well-being, or happiness. The following factors are *relatively unimportant* in determining our general happiness: money, age, gender, parenthood, intelligence, and physical attractiveness. Factors that are *somewhat important* in determining our subjective well-being include health, social activity, culture, and religion. These are moderately good predictors of happiness. Research indicates that a few factors are *very important* ingredients for overall happiness: love and intimate relationships, work, genetics, and personality.

Weiten and his colleagues (2012) suggest caution in making conclusions about happiness based on research alone. However, they point out that the research on happiness does not seem to support popular notions about what makes us happy. Our level of happiness does not depend on our positive and negative experiences as much as some believe. Instead, how we feel about our experiences and how we perceive what we have in life are crucial in bringing us happiness.

Much of this book is devoted to addressing factors that relate to your general level of happiness and subjective well-being. You will be invited to explore your choices in key areas of life such as personality, health, managing stress, love, intimate relationships, gender, sexuality, work, recreation, solitude, spirituality/religion, and meaning in life. Happiness is not simply something that automatically comes our way; we believe happiness is largely a function of the choices we make in each of these areas of living.

Are You Ready to Change?

Deciding to change is not a simple matter. You may have entertained some of these thoughts when you contemplated making a change in your life:

▶ I don't know if I want to rock the boat.

▶ Things aren't all that bad in my life.

▶ I'm fairly secure, and I don't want to take the chance of losing this security.

▶ I'm afraid that if I start to think too much I might overwhelm myself.

It is common to have doubts and fears about making changes. In fact, it is a mark of courage to acknowledge your hesitations to change and your anxiety over accepting greater responsibility for your life.

It is no easy matter to take an honest look at your life. Those who are close to you may not approve of or like your changes. They may put up barriers to your efforts. Your cultural background may be in conflict with the cultural values of the society in which you live. These factors can increase your anxiety as you contemplate making your own choices rather than allowing others to choose for you.

What is the best way to bring about change? The process of change begins when you are able to recognize and accept certain facets of yourself, even though you may not want to acknowledge some personal characteristic. Sometimes it is not possible to make a desired change, but even in these cases you have power over your attitude. You can choose how you perceive, interpret, and react to your situation. The Serenity Prayer* outlines the sphere of our responsibility:

> God, grant me the serenity to accept the things I cannot change, courage to change the things I can, and wisdom to know the difference.

The **paradoxical theory of change** holds that personal change tends to occur when we become aware of *what we are* as opposed to trying to become *what we are not* (Beisser, 1970). The more we attempt to deny some aspect of our being, the more we remain the same. Thus, if you desire change in some area of your life, you first need to accept who and what you are. If you live in denial, it is difficult to make changes. Recognizing who you are at the present time is the starting point for making changes.

Change is not facilitated by being critical of yourself. Change occurs when you are able to view yourself as you are and treat yourself kindly and respectfully. Once you are able to identify and acknowledge those aspects of yourself that you tend to deny, you increase your choices and open yourself to possibilities for changing. Start with small steps in the direction you want to move. It helps to remember that perfection is a direction, not a goal that you arrive at once and for all. Wanting to be different is a key first step.

The Stages of Change

Change is rarely easy, and most of the time we are ambivalent about making significant changes. Reluctance to change is a normal and expected part of the growth process. It is so common, in fact, that Prochaska and Norcross (2010) developed a framework for a change model that describes five identifiable stages. In the *precontemplation stage*, the individual has no intention of changing a behavior pattern in the near future. In the *contemplation stage*, the person is aware of a problem and is considering overcoming it, but the individual has not yet made a commitment to take action to bring about the change. In the *preparation stage*, the person intends to take action immediately and reports some small behavioral changes. In the *action stage*, the individual is taking steps to modify his or her behavior to solve a problem. During the *maintenance stage*, the individual works to consolidate the gains made and to prevent relapse.

*Attributed to Friedrich Oetinger (1702–1782) and Reinhold Niebuhr, "The Serenity Prayer" (1934).

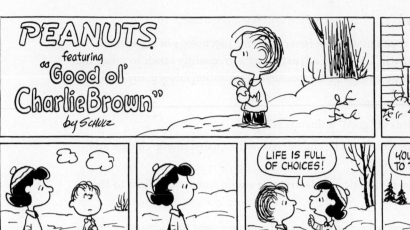
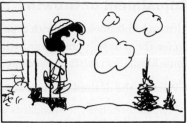
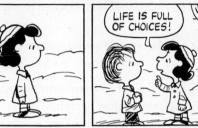
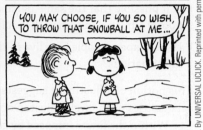
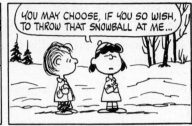
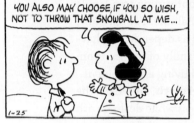
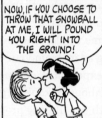
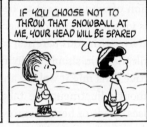
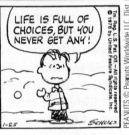

People do not pass neatly through these five stages in linear fashion, and an individual's readiness can fluctuate throughout the change process. If change is initially unsuccessful, individuals may return to an earlier stage. You may want to change certain patterns because they are no longer serving you, yet you cling to these familiar patterns either because you are afraid to leave what is known or because the costs of changing are too high. Although you may see advantages to making life changes, you may have many concerns and fears about changing. It is important to find an inner source of motivation that will enable you to challenge your fear and make life-affirming choices.

Self-exploration—being honest with yourself and others, thinking for yourself, deciding to acquire new ways of being, and making a commitment to live by your choices—requires concerted effort. A degree of discomfort and even fear may be associated with discovering more about yourself. When you are considering making life changes or acting in new ways, ask yourself this question: "What is the cost, and is it worth the price?" Change is a proactive process, and only *you* can decide what you want to change and how much change is right for you.

MODELS FOR PERSONAL GROWTH

Changing your life exposes you to new experiences. But just what does personal growth entail? In this section we contrast the idea of growth with that of adjustment and offer a humanistic model of what ideal growth can be.

Adjustment or Growth?

Although this book deals with topics in what is often called "the psychology of adjustment," we prefer the phrase "personal growth." The term **adjustment** is frequently taken to mean that some ideal norm exists by which people should be measured. This notion raises many questions:

▶ What is the desired norm of adjustment?

▶ Who determines the standards of "good" adjustment?

▶ Is it possible that the same person could be considered well adjusted in one culture and poorly adjusted in some other culture?

▶ Do we expect people who live in chaotic and destructive environments to adjust to their life situations?

This notion of adjustment suggests a single standard of measurement that identifies universal qualities of the well-adjusted or psychologically healthy person.

Within the limits imposed by genetic and environmental factors, we see the possibilities for creating our own vision of who we want to become rather than conforming to a single standard. In forming this vision, cultural values and norms play a crucial role. For example, if you are in your 20s and live with your parents, some would view this as dependent behavior on your part and think that you should be living apart from your family of origin. From another cultural perspective, this might well be an expected or desired living arrangement.

Instead of talking about adjustment, we talk about **personal growth**, in which the individual defines and assesses his or her own growth in a lifelong process while dealing with numerous crises at various stages of life. These crises can be seen as challenges to change, giving life new meaning. Growth also encompasses a relationship with significant others, the community, and the world. You do not grow in a vacuum but through your engagement with other people. To continue to grow, you have to be willing to let go of some old ways of thinking and acting so new dimensions can develop. When reading and studying, think about the ways you may have restricted your choices and the degree to which you are willing to exercise new choices and take action to bring about change. Ask yourself these questions:

▶ What do I want for myself, for others, and from others?

▶ What do I like about my life?

▶ What am I having difficulty with in my life?

▶ How would I like to be different?

▶ What are possible consequences if I do or do not change?

▶ How will my changes affect others in my life?

▶ What choices are open to me at this time in my life?

▶ How does my culture influence the choices I make?

▶ Do my cultural values enhance or inhibit my ability to make changes?

A Humanistic Approach to Personal Growth

I Never Knew I Had a Choice is based on a humanistic view of people. A central concept of this approach to personal growth is **self-actualization**. Striving for self-actualization means working toward fulfilling our potential, toward becoming all that we are capable of becoming. **Humanistic psychology**, which emphasizes the constructive and positive side of human experience, is based on the premise that the striving for growth exists in each of us but is not an automatic process. Because growth often involves pain and turmoil, many of us experience a constant struggle between our desire for security, or dependence, and our desire to experience the delights of growth.

A related approach is known as **positive psychology**, the study of positive emotions and positive character traits (Seligman, Steen, Park, & Peterson, 2005). Psychologists have given more attention to negative emotions than positive emotions, and there has been a historical focus on studying pathology, weaknesses, and suffering. The advocates of positive psychology call for increased study of hope, courage, contentment, happiness, well-being, perseverance, resilience, tolerance, and personal resources. The humanistic emphasis on optimism, growth, and health laid the foundation for the development of the positive psychology movement, which is increasingly influencing the field of contemporary psychology (Weiten et al., 2012).

Positive psychology is not synonymous with positive thinking. There are three important distinctions:

> First, positive psychology is grounded in empirical and replicable scientific study. Second, positive thinking urges positivity on us for all times and places, but positive psychology does not. Positive psychology recognizes that in spite of the advantages of positive thinking, there are times when negative or realistic thinking is appropriate....
> The third distinction . . . is that many scholars of positive psychology have spent decades working on the "negative" side of things—depression, anxiety, trauma, etc. [Positive psychologists] do not view positive psychology as a replacement for traditional psychology, but merely as a supplement to the hard-won gains of traditional psychology. (Positive Psychology Center, 2007)

Both humanistic psychology and positive psychology are based on common principles. Humanistic psychology focuses on a set of philosophical assumptions about what makes life meaningful. Positive psychologists explore factors that make people happy and focuses on human strengths and how people can flourish and be successful in daily life. Seligman (2002), the founder of positive psychology, identified three distinct pathways considered necessary to living a full life: experiencing pleasure and positive emotions, pursuing engagement, and achieving meaning. More recently, Schueller and Seligman (2010) explored the relationship between the pursuit of these pathways and their effect on well-being. **Subjective well-being** involves the experience of positive emotions and a lack of negative emotions as well as a cognitive evaluation of one's life as good. **Objective well-being** involves educational and occupational success. In their study, participants with an orientation toward engagement and meaning reported higher levels of both types of well-being than did individuals with an orientation toward pleasure.

Key Figures in Development of the Humanistic Approach

Many people have made significant contributions to humanistic psychology, and in this section we introduce you to some of the pioneers in the evolution of the humanistic approach. We focus on seven key people who have devoted much of their professional careers to the promotion of psychological growth and the self-actualization process. As you read, note the close parallels between the struggles and life experiences of these individuals in early childhood and the focus of their adult investigations. Based on a set of life experiences, these individuals made choices that influenced the development of their theories and their treatment modalities. If you are interested in learning more about these theorists after this brief introduction, we recommend *Theories of Personality* (Schultz & Schultz, 2013).

Alfred Adler's Social Orientation **Alfred Adler** (1958, 1964, 1969), a contemporary of Sigmund Freud, was a forerunner of the humanistic movement in psychology. In opposition to Freud's deterministic views of the person, Adler's theory stresses self-determination. Adler's early childhood was not a happy time; his experiences were characterized by a struggle to overcome weaknesses and feelings of inferiority, and the basic concepts of his theory grew out of his willingness to deal with his personal problems. His brother died while a very young boy, in the bed next to Alfred's. Indeed, Adler was sickly and very much aware of illness and death, and at the age of 4 he almost died of pneumonia. He heard the doctor tell his father, "Alfred is lost." Adler associated this particular time with his decision to become a physician. He felt inferior to his older brother, who was vigorous and healthy, and also felt inferior to other neighborhood children, who were healthier and could engage in athletics. Adler saw feelings of inferiority as the wellsprings of creativity, and he challenged his fears and doubts throughout his life. He is a good example of a person who shaped his own life as opposed to having it determined by fate.

Adlerian psychologists contend that we are not the victims of fate but are creative, active, choice-making beings whose every action has purpose and meaning. Adlerians talk of people being discouraged rather than being "psychologically sick." Adlerian therapists view their work as providing encouragement so people can grow to become what they were meant to be. They teach people better ways to meet the challenges of life tasks, provide direction, help people change unrealistic assumptions and beliefs, and offer encouragement to those who are discouraged.

Adler's basic concepts include community feeling and social interest. Adler equates **community feeling** with belonging to the ongoing development of humankind; **social interest** is being at least as interested in the well-being of others as we are with ourselves. Happiness comes from being of use to others and establishing meaningful relationships in a community. Adler asserted that only when we feel united with others can we act with courage in facing and dealing with life's problems. Because we are embedded in a society, we cannot be understood in isolation from our social context. Self-actualization is thus not an individual matter; it is only within the group that we can actualize our potential. Adler maintained that the degree to which we successfully share with others and are concerned with their welfare is a measure of our maturity. Social interest becomes the standard by which to judge psychological health.

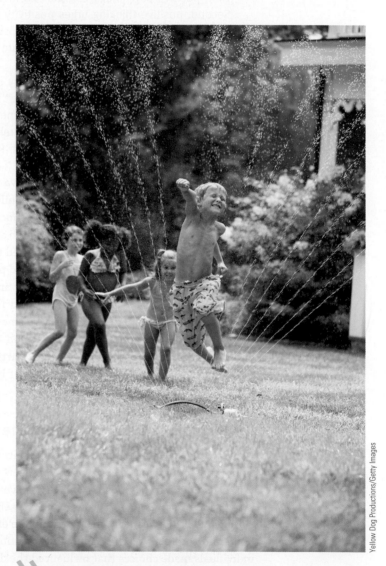

Yellow Dog Productions/Getty Images

》 Social interest begins developing at an early age.

Adler had a passionate concern for the common person and was outspoken about child-rearing practices and school reforms. He spoke and wrote in simple, nontechnical language so everyone could understand and apply the principles of his approach in a practical way to meet the challenges of daily life. Although Adler had an overly crowded work schedule most of his professional life, he still took some time to sing, enjoy music, and be with friends.

Carl Jung's Depth Psychology Perspective
Carl Jung (1961), a contemporary of Adler, made a monumental contribution to the depth of understanding of the human personality. His pioneering work sheds light on human development, particularly during middle age. Jung's personal life paved the way for the expansion of his theoretical notions. His loneliness as a child is reflected in his personality theory, which focuses on the inner world of the individual. Jung's emotional distance from his parents contributed to his feeling of being cut off from the external world of conscious reality. Jung had a difficult and unhappy childhood marked by deaths, funerals, neurotic parents in a failing marriage, religious doubts and conflicts, and bizarre dreams and visions. Largely as a way of escaping the difficulties of his childhood and the marital tensions between his parents, Jung turned inward and became preoccupied with pursuing his unconscious experiences as reflected in his dreams, visions, and fantasies. This preoccupation with his inner subjective world guided Jung throughout his life and influenced the development of his theory of personality (Schultz & Schultz, 2013). At age 81 he wrote about his recollections in his autobiography, *Memories, Dreams, Reflections* (Jung, 1961).

According to Jung, humans are not merely shaped by past events but strive for growth as well. Our present personality is determined both by who and what we have been and also by the person we hope to become. The process of growth and self-determination is oriented toward the future. Jung's theory is based on the assumption that humans tend to move toward the fulfillment or realization of all their capabilities. Achieving **individuation**—a fully harmonious and integrated personality—is a primary goal. To reach this goal, we must become aware of and accept the full range of our being. The public self we present is only a small part of who and what we are. For Jung, both constructive and destructive forces coexist in the human psyche, and to become integrated we must accept the **shadow side** of our nature with our primitive impulses such as selfishness and greed. If we deny the shadow aspects of our personality, they are more likely to control us and have a negative influence on our behavior. For example, if we chronically deny any feelings of anger, these feelings are likely to be expressed in some way through bodily symptoms and depression. Acceptance does not mean being dominated by this shadow dimension of our being, but simply recognizing that this is a *part* of our nature.

Carl Rogers's Person-Centered Approach
Carl Rogers (1980), a major figure in the development of humanistic psychology, founded what is known as the person-centered approach. He was perhaps one of the most influential figures in revolutionizing the direction of counseling theory and practice. He focused on the importance of nonjudgmental listening and acceptance as a condition for people to feel free enough to change. Rogers's emphasis on the value of autonomy seems to have grown, in part, out of his own struggles to become independent from his parents. Rogers grew up fearing his mother's critical judgment. In an interview, Rogers mentioned that he could not imagine talking to his mother about anything of significance because he was sure she would have some negative judgment. He also grew up in a home where strict religious standards governed behavior. In his early years, while at a seminary studying to be a minister, Rogers made a critical choice that influenced his personal life and the focus of his theory. Realizing that he could no longer go

along with the religious thinking of his parents, Rogers questioned the religious dogma he was being taught, which led to his emancipation and his psychological independence. As a college student, he took the risk of writing a letter to his parents telling them that his views were changing from fundamentalist to liberal and that he was developing his own philosophy of life. Even though he knew that his departure from the values of his parents would be difficult for them, he felt that such a move was necessary for his own intellectual and psychological freedom. He showed a questioning stance toward life, a genuine openness to change, and demonstrated the courage to pursue unknown paths in both his personal and professional life.

Rogers built his entire theory and practice of psychotherapy on the concept of the **fully functioning person**. Fully functioning people tend to reflect and ask basic questions: "Who am I?" "How can I discover my real self?" "How can I become what I deeply wish to become?" "How can I get out from behind my facade and become myself?" Rogers maintained that when people give up their facade and accept themselves they move in the direction of being open to experience (that is, they begin to see reality without distorting it). They trust themselves and look to themselves for the answers to their problems, and they no longer attempt to become fixed entities or products, realizing instead that growth is a continual process. Such fully functioning people, Rogers wrote, are in a fluid process of challenging and revisiting their perceptions and beliefs as they open themselves to new experiences.

In contrast to those who assume that we are by nature irrational and destructive unless we are socialized, Rogers exhibited a deep faith in human beings. In his view people are naturally social and forward-moving, strive to function fully, and have at their deepest core a positive goodness. In short, people are to be trusted, and because they are basically cooperative and constructive, there is no need to control their aggressive impulses.

During the last 15 years of his life, Rogers applied the person-centered approach to world peace by training policymakers, leaders, and groups in conflict. Perhaps his greatest passion was directed toward the reduction of interracial tensions and the effort to achieve world peace, for which he was nominated for the Nobel Peace Prize. He earned recognition around the world for his pioneering achievements in developing a theory and practice of humanistic psychotherapy.

Natalie Rogers's Person-Centered Expressive Arts Therapy **Natalie Rogers** is a pioneer in the field of expressive arts therapy. Expressive arts employs a variety of forms—movement, painting, sculpting, music, writing, and improvisation—in a supportive setting to facilitate growth and healing. Natalie expanded on her father's (Carl Rogers) theory of creativity by using the expressive arts to enhance personal growth for individuals and groups. Her approach, known as **person-centered expressive arts therapy**, extends person-centered theory by helping individuals access their feelings through spontaneous creative expressions. This creative expression can be through symbols, color, movement, sound, or drama. Using the arts in a safe, person-centered environment enables the individual to express deep emotions and feelings often inaccessible through words. Personal integration of mind, body, emotion, and spirit may result from this method of release, insight, self-discovery, and self-empowerment.

Just as her father's work was influenced by his upbringing and departures from his parents' views, so did Natalie's work evolve from what she felt was lacking in her father's theory. Carl Rogers seldom openly expressed anger at home or in relation to his colleagues (except in letter writing). As a woman growing up in an era when females were meant to be accommodating to men, Natalie eventually discovered her underlying anger at being a second-class citizen. Her art was one vehicle to express and gain insight into this injustice. She also expressed her anger at her father because he was unknowingly a part of the patriarchal system. He was surprised, but willing to hear about the role he and other men played in holding women back.

In *The Creative Connection: Expressive Arts as Healing*, Natalie Rogers (1993) outlines some of the humanistic principles that underlie the expressive arts approach:

▸ All people have an innate ability to be creative.

▸ The creative process is transformative and healing.

▸ Personal growth and higher states of consciousness are achieved through self-awareness, self-understanding, and insight.

▸ Self-awareness, understanding, and insight are achieved by delving into our feelings of grief, anger, pain, fear, joy, and ecstasy. Our feelings are an energy source.

▸ A connection exists between our life force—our inner core, or soul—and the essence of all beings.

▸ As we journey inward to discover our essence or wholeness, we discover our relatedness to the outer world, and the inner and outer become one.

The various art modes interrelate in what Natalie Rogers (1993, 2011) calls the *creative connection*. When we move, it affects how we write or paint. When we write or paint, it affects how we feel and think. Natalie believes that the tendency toward actualization and reaching one's full potential, including one's innate creativity, is undervalued, discounted, and frequently squashed in our society because traditional educational institutions tend to promote conformity rather than original thinking and the creative process. Natalie's deep faith in the individual's innate drive to become fully oneself is basic to the work in person-centered expressive arts. Individuals have a tremendous capacity for self-healing through creativity in a supportive environment created by counselors who are genuine, warm, empathic, open, and honest. When one feels appreciated, trusted, and given support to use individuality to develop a plan, create a project, write a paper, or to be authentic, the challenge is exciting, stimulating, and provides a sense of personal expansion.

Today, at 83 years of age, Natalie Rogers continues to find ways to bring meaning to her personal and professional life. Just this past year she taught and facilitated workshops in England, Spain, and South Korea, and she continues to teach a 6-week expressive arts program in California.

Zerka T. Moreno and Psychodrama Zerka Toeman Moreno is a pioneer in the development of psychodrama, which is a humanistic approach to understanding people (see Horvatin & Schreiber 2006; Moreno, Blomkvist, & Rutzel, 2000). **Psychodrama**, founded by the psychiatrist Jacob L. Moreno, is primarily humanistic and is an action approach to group therapy in which people explore their problems through role playing, enacting situations using various dramatic ways of gaining insight, discovering their own creativity, and developing behavioral skills. Psychodrama encourages us to rework our lives as if they were dramatic situations and we were the playwrights. Those who participate in a psychodrama do not merely talk about their problems—they bring their past, present, and future concerns to life by enacting scenarios. Rather than telling people about their problems, they show others in the psychodrama group how significant life events are affecting them in the present moment. Participants use a number of action-oriented methods when expressing their feelings and thoughts about a particular problem, and these action methods are important tools for bringing about healing. For a more detailed introductory discussion of psychodrama, see Corey (2012, chap. 8).

Zerka Moreno, the co-creator of psychodrama, has contributed much to the theory and practice of psychodrama. We asked her to write a piece about her own process of getting involved in the field of psychodrama, her relationship and work with her husband J. L. Moreno, and highlights of her personal journey. Here is what she wrote:

> What I should most like people to remember about me is that I was fortunate to be in awe of life in its multiple dimensions. Meeting J. L. Moreno when I brought my psychotic older sister to him for treatment was a major turning point in my life. Moreno dealt with people who were psychotic because he fully grasped what they were experiencing and coping with, and it was his desire to accompany them in their healing process and to assist them in finding new meaning in life. His humility in dealing with them was touching. He also opened up entire horizons for me that I could not begin to imagine. Most of all, he saw something in me and believed in me in a way no other human being had. This made a huge impact on me, both personally and professionally.

I became Moreno's student at the end of 1941, after my sister was discharged in a functioning state. I had been an art student with the idea of becoming a fashion designer. As a recent immigrant from England, I needed to earn a living, so I became a secretary. When Moreno offered me a scholarship to study with him, I insisted that I wanted to use my skills to assist him in working on his manuscripts, magazines, and books. When he opened his New York City Institute in March 1942, Moreno appointed me as his research assistant. I was totally unschooled in psychiatry, except for witnessing my sister's recurring illness. I was able to learn about psychodrama from my 7 years of apprenticeship from this master. Along with Moreno's encouragement and constant support, I came to believe that I could be a director of psychodrama. He began to include me in his treatment decisions with patients. I learned a great deal about psychodrama by participating in them with Moreno, especially in my roles as an auxiliary ego as a double (techniques in psychodrama), as well as doing research and writing about our work. During our partnership over a period of 33 years, the influence of our work spread internationally.

One of my contributions to the field was the fact that I could do psychodrama work in my own way. I learned that I did not need to have J. L.'s special charisma to effectively facilitate a psychodrama and that I could develop my own unique therapeutic style by using my own gifts of spontaneity and creativity. Since Moreno's death in 1974, I have been able to continue to bring our work to countries around the globe. What I have learned from working in various countries is that these diverse cultures do indeed color the psychodramas in which people become involved. For instance, in Japan in the 1980s I was conducting a psychodrama and my suggestion to present a family photograph did not succeed, for doing this would go against the participants' culture. In Korea, the overriding problem presented by professional women was their relationship to their mothers-in-law. In Turkey, I expected the group members to work on their experiences of the recent earthquakes. Instead, the group participants presented family problems for exploration, much as one would find in the United States. The one universal theme seems to be this: Suffering wears the same face everywhere, no matter what its source.

I have been pleased to be involved in writing about psychodrama and bringing this therapeutic approach to many people. I am presently working on completing my memoirs. Although I have cut back on my travels, people are still coming to me for weekend workshops, some from abroad. Today, in my 95th year, I can truly say with Edith Piaff: "Non, je ne regrette rien." Not only are there no regrets, but rather profound gratitude for what my life has been.

Virginia Satir's Experiential Family Therapy* **Virginia Satir** was one of the pioneers in family therapy, and she was influenced by the philosophy of Carl Rogers; the "here-and-now" focus of the Gestalt therapists; and the process orientation of systems therapists. She was very person-centered and humanistic in her approach to working with individuals and families. When Satir was 5 years old, she remembers her parents talking and that she wanted to know what they were up to. She often mentioned in her workshops that this was when she decided to be a "detective on parents." Later she viewed herself as a detective who sought out and listened for the reflections of self-esteem with her clients. Her therapeutic work convinced her of the value of a strong, nurturing relationship based on interest and fascination with those in her care.

In 1937 Satir began both graduate school and a teaching career. She made a point of meeting the families of her students in their own homes. Satir was extremely good at making contact with families and winning them over. Through her connecting efforts, discipline problems disappeared, and whenever she needed parental support, she always had it.

Satir completed her master's degree in 1948 at the University of Chicago. Throughout her graduate education, she received the discrimination that most married women endured: She was not supposed to be at university; she was supposed to be home and in service to her husband. The male faculty made that abundantly clear in both their grading of her work and their communications with her in classes and advising. Satir had amazing perseverance to overcome the sexism she faced alone. She provided a role model for strong women who have a dream and are willing to pursue it against the odds.

Satir started clinical practice as a social worker in an agency but quickly formed a private practice. She often told the story of meeting and working with a young woman for some time. After a while, it dawned on her that maybe this teenager had a mother. When the mother was invited in, the young woman regressed to a previous state. Bringing the father into therapy was another step. Each time, Satir focused on the development of self-esteem in the family members and helped them to communicate directly and openly with each other. Her goal became one of facilitating emotional honesty. This was the start of her work in family practice as well as the foundation for what she would soon call *conjoint family therapy* (see Satir, 1983). Later Satir (1988) wrote *The New Peoplemaking*, which described the processes of nurturing families and was published in more than 25 languages.

During her career, Satir worked with more than 5,000 families, conducting workshops in every part of the world and with every culture. Over her lifetime as a family therapist, Satir gained international fame and developed many innovative interventions. She was highly intuitive and believed spontaneity, creativity, humor, self-disclosure, risk-taking, and personal touch were central to family therapy.

In the early summer of 1988, after returning from a month-long training in the Soviet Union, she told many people that change was on the way there and that she wanted to be a part of it. She encouraged other counselors and therapists to join her there in trying to make a difference. In June, however, she began to feel sick, and she was rushed to a hospital in Colorado where she was diagnosed with cancer. On September 10, 1988, at the age of 72, she died at home in the company of friends and family.

Abraham Maslow's Humanistic Psychology **Abraham Maslow** (1970), like Adler and Jung, had a difficult childhood. Maslow experienced his family as a miserable one, viewed his father as aloof and unhappy, and saw his mother as a horrible creature. As a child, Maslow saw himself as being different from others. He was embarrassed by his scrawny physique and

---

*This section was written by one of our colleagues, Dr. James Bitter of East Tennessee State University. He worked closely with Virginia Satir and received much of his training in family therapy with her.

large nose, and he remembered feeling extremely inferior to others during his adolescent years. As a way of compensating for his feelings of inferiority, he turned to reading books. Maslow eventually distinguished himself as a leader in the humanistic psychology movement. During the time he was at the peak of his career, Maslow developed various illnesses including depression, stomach disorders, insomnia, and heart disease (Schultz & Schultz, 2013).

Maslow was one of the most influential psychologists to contribute to our understanding of self-actualizing individuals. He built on Adler's and Jung's works in some significant ways, yet he distinguished himself in discovering a psychology of health. Maslow was concerned with taking care of basic survival needs, and his theory stresses a hierarchy of needs, with satisfaction of physiological and safety needs as a prerequisite to being concerned about actualizing one's potentials. Self-actualization became the central theme of the work of Abraham Maslow (1968, 1970, 1971). Maslow uses the phrase "the psychopathology of the average" to highlight his contention that merely "normal" people may never extend themselves to become what they are capable of becoming. Further, he criticized Freudian psychology for what he saw as its preoccupation with the sick and negative side of human nature. If our findings are based on observations of a sick population, Maslow reasoned, a sick psychology will emerge. Maslow believed that too much research was being conducted on anxiety, hostility, and neuroses and too little into joy, creativity, and self-fulfillment.

In his quest to create a humanistic psychology that would focus on our potential, Maslow studied what he called self-actualizing people and found that they differed in important ways from so-called normals. Some of the characteristics Maslow found in these people included a capacity to tolerate and even welcome uncertainty in their lives, acceptance of themselves and others, spontaneity and creativity, a need for privacy and solitude, autonomy, a capacity for deep and intense interpersonal relationships, a genuine caring for others, a sense of humor, an inner-directedness (as opposed to the tendency to live by others' expectations), and the absence of artificial dichotomies within themselves (such as work/play, love/hate, and weak/strong). Maslow's theory of self-actualization is presented next along with its implications for the humanistic approach to psychology.

Overview of Maslow's Self-Actualization Theory

Maslow postulated a **hierarchy of needs** as a source of motivation. The most basic are the physiological needs. If we are hungry and thirsty, our attention is riveted on meeting these basic needs. Next are the safety needs, which include a sense of security and stability. Once our physical and safety needs are fulfilled, we become concerned with meeting our needs for belonging and love, followed by working on our need for esteem, both from self and others. We are able to strive toward self-actualization only after these four basic needs are met: physiological, safety, love, and esteem.

Maslow emphasized that people are not motivated by all five needs at the same time. The key factor determining which need is dominant at a given time is the degree to which those below it are satisfied. Some people come to the erroneous conclusion that if they were "bright" enough or "good" enough they would be further down the road of self-actualization. The truth may be that in their particular cultural, environmental, and societal circumstances these people are motivated to work toward physical and psychological survival, which keeps them functioning at the lower end of the hierarchy. Keep in mind that an individual is not much concerned with actualization, nor is a society focused on the development of culture, if the basic needs are not met.

We can summarize some of the basic ideas of the humanistic approach by means of Maslow's model of the self-actualizing person (Figure 1.1). He describes self-actualization in *Motivation and Personality* (Maslow, 1970), and he also treats this concept in his other

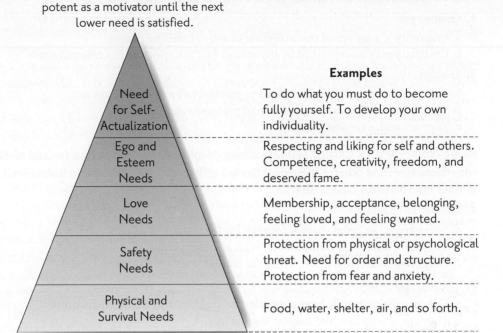

Each higher need does not become
potent as a motivator until the next
lower need is satisfied.

Examples

Need for Self-Actualization — To do what you must do to become fully yourself. To develop your own individuality.

Ego and Esteem Needs — Respecting and liking for self and others. Competence, creativity, freedom, and deserved fame.

Love Needs — Membership, acceptance, belonging, feeling loved, and feeling wanted.

Safety Needs — Protection from physical or psychological threat. Need for order and structure. Protection from fear and anxiety.

Physical and Survival Needs — Food, water, shelter, air, and so forth.

From *Motivation and Personality* by Abraham H. Maslow. Copyright 1987. Reprinted by permission of Prentice-Hall, Inc., Upper Saddle River, N.J.

books (Maslow, 1968, 1971). Some core characteristics of self-actualizing people are self-awareness, freedom, basic honesty and caring, and trust and autonomy.

Self-Awareness Self-actualizing people are aware of themselves, of others, and of reality. Specifically, they demonstrate the following behavior and traits:

1. *Efficient perception of reality*

    a. Self-actualizing people see reality as it is.
    b. They have an ability to detect inconsistencies.
    c. They avoid seeing things in preconceived categories.

2. *Ethical awareness*

    a. Self-actualizing people display a knowledge of what is right and wrong for them.
    b. They have a sense of inner direction.
    c. They avoid being pressured by others and living by others' standards.

3. *Freshness of appreciation.* Like children, self-actualizing people have an ability to perceive life in a fresh way.

4. *Peak moments*

    a. Self-actualizing people experience times of being one with the universe; they experience moments of joy.
    b. They have the ability to be changed by such moments.

Freedom Self-actualizing people are willing to make choices for themselves, and they are free to reach their potential. This freedom entails a sense of detachment and a need for privacy, creativity, and spontaneity, and an ability to accept responsibility for choices.

1. *Detachment*

    a. For self-actualizing people, the need for privacy is crucial.

    b. They have a need for solitude to put things in perspective.

2. *Creativity*

    a. Creativity is a universal characteristic of self-actualizing people.

    b. Creativity may be expressed in any area of life; it shows itself as inventiveness.

3. *Spontaneity*

    a. Self-actualizing people do not need to pretend to be what they are not.

    b. They display a naturalness and lack of pretentiousness.

    c. They act with ease and grace.

Basic Honesty and Caring Self-actualizing people show a deep caring for and honesty with themselves and others. These qualities are reflected in their interest in humankind and in their interpersonal relationships.

1. *Sense of social interest*

    a. Self-actualizing people have a concern for the welfare of others.

    b. They have a sense of communality with all other people.

    c. They have an interest in bettering the world.

2. *Interpersonal relationships*

    a. Self-actualizing people have a capacity for real love and fusion with another.

    b. They are able to love and respect themselves.

    c. They are able to go outside themselves in a mature love.

    d. They are motivated by the urge to grow in their relationships.

3. *Sense of humor*

    a. Self-actualizing people can laugh at themselves.

    b. They can laugh at the human condition.

    c. Their humor is not hostile.

Trust and Autonomy Self-actualizing people exhibit faith in themselves and others; they are independent; they accept themselves as valuable persons; and their lives have meaning.

1. *Search for purpose and meaning*

    a. Self-actualizing people have a sense of mission, of a calling in which their potential can be fulfilled.

    b. They are engaged in a search for identity, often through work that is a deeply significant part of their lives.

2. *Autonomy and independence*

    a. Self-actualizing people have the ability to be independent.

    b. They resist blind conformity.

    c. They are not tradition-bound in making decisions.

3. *Acceptance of self and others*

    a. Self-actualizing people avoid fighting reality.

    b. They accept nature as it is.

    c. They are comfortable with the world.[*]

---

*From Motivation and Personality *by Abraham H. Maslow. Copyright © 1987. Reprinted by permission of Prentice-Hall, Inc., Upper Saddle River, N.J.*

This profile is best thought of as an ideal rather than a final state that we reach once and for all. Thus it is more appropriate to speak about the self-actualizing process rather than becoming a self-actualized person.

Self-actualization is a Western concept grounded in **individualism**; it affirms the uniqueness, autonomy, freedom, and intrinsic worth of the individual and emphasizes personal responsibility for our behavior and well-being. The ultimate aim of this orientation is the growth of the individual in becoming all that he or she can be. By contrast, Eastern philosophy is based on **collectivism**, which affirms the value of preserving and enhancing the well-being of the group. The collective orientation emphasizes unity, unification, integration, and fusion. Rather than viewing self-actualization as the ultimate good, the collective orientation emphasizes cooperation, harmony, interdependence, achievement of socially oriented and group goals, and collective responsibility. When we consider personal growth and encourage individuals striving toward self-actualization, we need to keep in mind both Western and Eastern perspectives. Individualism and collectivism are not polar opposites but lie along a continuum. Characteristics from both perspectives can be integrated in a creative synthesis.

MAYA ANGELOU

An Example of a Self-Actualizing Person

A good example of a person on the path of self-actualizing is Maya Angelou, a well-known writer and poet. She has written many books that continue to have an impact on her readers and is a frequent speaker to various groups. Maya Angelou embodies many of the characteristics Maslow describes. In *Maya Angelou: The Poetry of Living*, Margaret Courtney-Clarke (1999) uses 10 words to describe Maya Angelou: joy, giving, learning, perseverance, creativity, courage, self-respect, spirituality, love, and taking risks. Various contributors expanded on these themes and gave brief personal reactions to this woman whom they view as very special.

JOY Maya's message to young children is: "Laugh as much as you can! Take every opportunity to rejoice. Find the humor in life at every opportunity." (Defoy Glenn, p. 19)

GIVING "You cannot give what you don't have. Maya has this reservoir of love for people and that's why they love her, because it's like a mirror image." (Louise Meriwether, p. 28)

LEARNING "She has an absolute rapacious desire to know; she really wants to know about everything. . . ." (Connie Sutton, p. 40)

PERSEVERANCE "Maya has come to believe that troubles are a blessing. They force you to change, to believe." (Andrew Young, p. 62)

CREATIVITY "The human brain is capable of more things than we can imagine, and if one dreams it—and believes it—one certainly should try it. As Maya says, 'The human mind is a vast storehouse, there is no limit to it.'" (Defoy Glenn, p. 69)

COURAGE "Maya speaks with courage all the time. She talks about courage as a virtue. In most of her presentations she uses this. She has the courage to say, 'We are more alike than we are unalike.'" (Velma Gibson Watts, p. 76)

SELF-RESPECT "Maya often says, 'I am a human being and nothing human can be alien to me, and if a human did it, I can do it. I possess the capacity to do it.'" (Defoy Glenn, p. 90)

SPIRITUALITY "A phenomenal woman! She embraces us with her great love, informs us with her profound wisdom, and inspires us with her poetic and artistic genius. A person of uncommon dignity, rare courage, undaunted faith, dogged determination, grace, integrity, and finally, matchless generosity—Maya Angelou is an international treasure." (Coretta Scott King, p. 108)

LOVE "If you want to see a miracle in the twentieth century look at Maya Angelou. The spirit is always moving. It moves to far ends of the earth. A spirit of love, of care, of liberation. . . . Maya Angelou's spirit liberates." (Rev. Cecil Williams, p. 110)

TAKING RISKS "The process of decay starts the moment things are created. So, to hold on too tightly prevents one from getting things, because one's hands are so full one cannot take on anything else." (Defoy Glenn, p. 126)

Think of some ways you can engage in the self-actualizing process. The activities at the end of each chapter and the Take Time to Reflect sections scattered throughout the book can help you begin this lifelong quest.

Choice Theory Approach to Personal Growth

Although this book is based largely on the humanistic approach in psychology, we draw from other psychological schools in exploring key topics. One of these approaches is **reality therapy**, which is based on a cognitive behavioral model. Reality therapy teaches people how to make effective choices and satisfy their basic needs. Choice theory underlies the practice of reality therapy, which was founded by the psychiatrist William Glasser. **Choice theory** posits that everything we do can be explained in terms of our attempts to satisfy our basic needs: *survival, love and belonging, power or achievement, freedom or independence,* and *fun.* We all have these five needs, but they vary in strength. For example, we all have a need for love and belonging, but some of us need more love than others. Choice theory is based on the premise that because we are by nature social creatures we need to both receive and give love. Choice theory posits that the need to *love and to belong* is the primary need because we need people to satisfy our other needs.

Glasser (1998, 2000) has written a great deal about taking an active stance toward controlling our destiny. He believes that many people are unhappy because they are not satisfying their needs and thus they are not in control of how they are living. He suggests that we can gain a sense of control by accepting responsibility and becoming active. Rather than accepting passive statements such as "I am depressed," Glasser helps his psychotherapy clients realize their active role in *depressing, angering, headaching,* or *anxietying* themselves. He emphasizes that people choose these behaviors in an attempt to meet their needs and wants, and people have some control over what they continue to choose to do. Although it may be difficult to directly control your feelings and thoughts, Glasser maintains that you do have control over what you are *doing.* If you change what you are doing, you increase the chances that your feelings and thoughts will also change. For instance, if you are depressing over failing an exam, it may be difficult to directly control your feelings of disappointment. You could spend much energy berating yourself; however, you could also use that same energy to reflect on ways to prevent this situation from occurring in the future. By engaging in a new way of thinking and behaving, it is likely that you will eventually begin to feel differently about this situation.

Choice theory explains that our "total behavior" is always our best attempt to get what we want to satisfy our needs. **Total behavior** teaches that all behavior is made up of four inseparable but distinct components—*acting, thinking, feeling,* and *physiology*—that necessarily accompany all of our actions, thoughts, and feelings. Behavior is purposeful because it is designed to close the gap between what we want and what we perceive we are getting. Specific behaviors are always generated from this discrepancy. Our behaviors come from the inside, and thus we choose our destiny.

Robert Wubbolding (2000, 2011), a reality therapist, describes the key procedures used in the practice of reality therapy using an acronym, **WDEP.** Each of the letters refers to a cluster of strategies: W = wants and needs; D = direction and doing; E = self-evaluation; and P = planning. These strategies are designed to promote change, which we will return to as we discuss many of the topics in the remaining chapters. Let's look at each of these strategies in more detail.

Wants (Exploring Wants, Needs, and Perceptions) A critical question that we frequently raise in this book is, "What do you want?" Here are some useful questions to help you answer this question:

▸ If you could be all that you want to be, what kind of person would you be?

▸ How would you be different if you were living as you want to?

▸ What are you most missing in life?

▸ What stops you from making the changes you would like to make?

Direction and Doing Reality therapy stresses current behavior and is concerned with past events only insofar as they influence how clients are behaving now. Even though problems may be rooted in the past, we need to learn how to deal with them in the present by learning better ways of getting what we want. Problems must be solved either in the present or through a plan for the future. The key question is, "What are you doing?"

Evaluation The core of reality therapy is to invite individuals to make the following self-evaluation: "Does your present behavior have a reasonable chance of getting you what you want now, and will it take you in the direction you want to go?" Ultimately, it is up to you to evaluate your present actions. You are not likely to change until you first decide that a change is advantageous. Making this choice hinges on first making an honest self-assessment. Wubbolding (2000, 2011) suggests questions like these:

▸ Is what you are doing helping or hurting you?

▸ Is what you are doing now what you want to be doing?

▸ Is your behavior working for you?

▸ Does it help you to look at it that way?

▸ Is what you want realistic or attainable?

▸ After you carefully examine what you want, does it appear to be in your best interests and in the best interest of others?

Planning and Action Making behavioral changes involves identifying specific ways to fulfill your wants and needs. Once clients determine what they want to change, they are generally ready to explore other possible behaviors and formulate an action plan. The key question is, "What is your plan?" The process of creating and carrying out plans enables people to begin to gain effective control over their lives. Once you determine what you want to change, the next step is to formulate an action plan. A plan gives you a starting point, but plans can be modified as needed. Although planning is important, it is effective only if we have made a self-evaluation and determined that we want to change a behavior.

Wubbolding (2000, 2011) discusses the central role of planning and commitment in the change process. He uses the acronym SAMIC[3] to capture the essence of a good plan: simple, attainable, measurable, immediate, involved, controlled by the planner, committed to, and continuously done. Here are some of the characteristics of an effective plan:

▶ It is important for an action plan to be realistic. A question to ask is, "What plans could you make now that would result in a more satisfying life?"

▶ Good plans are simple and easy to understand. Plans need to be specific, concrete, and measurable, yet they also should be flexible and open to revision.

▶ The plan involves a positive course of action, and it is stated in terms of what you are willing to do. Even small plans can help you take significant steps toward your desired changes.

▶ Plans that you can carry out independently of what others do are the best plans.

▶ Effective plans are repetitive and, ideally, are performed daily.

▶ Plans are carried out as soon as possible: "What are you willing to do today to begin to change your life?"

▶ Before you carry out your plan, evaluate it with someone you trust to determine whether it is realistic and attainable. It is useful to evaluate it again and make any revisions that may be necessary.

As you study the topics in this book, think about areas of your life you want to change, develop an action plan, and find ways to commit to implementing your plan. Include this exploration in your journal writing in the pages provided at the end of each chapter.

TAKE TIME TO REFLECT

These sections in this book provide an opportunity for you to pause and reflect on your own experiences as they relate to the topic being discussed. There are no "right" and "wrong" answers; rather, answer the questions in a way that makes sense to you and has personal meaning. You may have to make a conscious effort to look within yourself for the response or answer that makes sense to you rather than searching for the expected response that is external to you.

1. To what degree do you have a healthy and positive view of yourself? Do you appreciate yourself, or do you discount your own worth? Respond to these statements using the following code:

3 = This statement is true of me *most* of the time.
2 = This statement is true of me *some* of the time.
1 = This statement is true of me *almost none* of the time.

_____ I think and choose for myself.
_____ I like myself.
_____ I know what I want in life.
_____ I am able to ask for what I want.
_____ I feel a sense of personal power.
_____ I am open to change.
_____ I feel equal to others.

_____ I am sensitive to the needs of others.

_____ I care about others.

_____ I can act in accordance with my own judgment without feeling guilty if others disapprove of me.

_____ I do not expect others to make me feel good about myself.

_____ I can accept responsibility for my own actions.

_____ I am able to give compliments to others.

_____ I am able to accept compliments.

_____ I can give affection.

_____ I can receive affection.

_____ I am loyal to my family.

_____ I am a contributing member of society.

_____ I am a positive influence in my community.

_____ I am generally accepted by others.

_____ I can give myself credit for what I do well.

_____ I can enjoy my own company.

_____ I am capable of forming meaningful relationships.

_____ I live in the here and now and am not preoccupied with the past or the future.

_____ I feel a sense of significance.

_____ I am not diminished when I am with those I respect.

_____ I believe in my ability to succeed in projects that are meaningful to me.

_____ I am open to learning from others, including my elders.

_____ I feel comfortable with my ability to speak in social situations.

_____ I feel comfortable with my ability to speak in professional and work-related situations.

_____ I am not devastated by my imperfections.

Now go back over this inventory and identify not more than five areas that keep you from being as self-accepting as you might be. What can you do to increase your awareness of situations in which you do not fully accept yourself? For example, if you have trouble giving yourself credit for things you do well, how can you become aware of times when you discount yourself? When you do become conscious of situations in which you put yourself down, think of alternatives.

2. Take a few minutes to review Maslow's theory of self-actualization and then consider these questions as they apply to you:

▸ Which of these qualities do you find most appealing? Why?

▸ Which would you like to cultivate in yourself?

▸ Which of Maslow's ideal qualities do you most associate with living a full and meaningful life?

▸ Who in your life comes closest to meeting Maslow's criteria for self-actualizing people?

3. We recommend that later in the course you review your answers to this exercise and take this inventory again. Compare your answers and note any changes that you may have made in your thinking or behavior.

ARE YOU AN ACTIVE LEARNER?

The self-actualization process implies that you will be an **active learner:** that is, you assume responsibility for your education, you question what is presented to you, and you apply what you learn in a personally meaningful way. Your schooling experiences may not have encouraged you to learn actively. Review your school experiences and assess whether you are an active learner.

What do you want out of college or out of life in general? Identifying, clarifying, and reaching goals must be an active process related to your values. Getting a clear sense of your values is no easy task. Many people have trouble deciding what they really want. If this is true for you, a first step you can take in sorting out what you want from college is to ask yourself these questions:

▸ Am I doing now what I want to be doing?

▸ Do my actions reflect my values?

▸ Do I believe I have the right to make my own choices?

▸ Am I finding meaning in what I am doing?

▸ What would I rather be doing?

Use the idea of what you would rather be doing as a catalyst for changing. What will it take for you to say "I am doing what I really want to be doing right now"? You may redefine many of your values at various points in your college or work career and throughout your life. But your goals will be much more meaningful if you define them for yourself rather than allow others to set goals for you.

We think you will get a great deal more from your college education if you spend time now reflecting on your past experiences. Think about how your present values and beliefs are related to your experiences in school. Recall a particularly positive school experience. How might it be affecting you today? Consider your educational experiences up to this point and think about your attitudes and behaviors as a student. What kinds of experiences have you had as a student so far, and how might these experiences influence the kind of learner you are today? If you like the kind of learner you are now, or if you have had mostly good experiences with school, you can build on that positive framework as you approach this course. You can continue to find ways to involve yourself with the material you will read, study, and discuss. Once you become aware of particular aspects of your education that you do not like, you can decide to change your style of learning. In what ways do you want to become a different learner now than you have been in the past? We hope you will find ways to bring meaning to your learning by being active in the process. You can get the most out of your courses if you develop a style of learning in which you raise questions and search for answers within yourself.

One way to begin to become an active learner is to think about your reasons for taking this course and your expectations concerning what you will learn. We invite you to make the choice to be actively engaged by applying the themes in this book in your life. The following Take Time to Reflect exercise will help you clarify what you want from this course.

TAKE TIME TO REFLECT

1. What are your main reasons for taking this course, and what do you most want to accomplish? _____

_____

2. What do you expect this course to be like? Check all the comments that apply.

_____ I expect to talk openly about issues that matter to me.

_____ I expect to get answers to certain problems in my life.

_____ I expect the course to help me become a happier person.

_____ I expect to reduce my fear of expressing my feelings and ideas.

_____ I expect to be challenged on why I am the way I am.

_____ I expect to learn more about how other people function.

_____ I expect to better understand myself by the end of the course.

3. What are you willing to do to become actively involved in your learning? Check the appropriate comments.

_____ I am willing to participate in class discussions.

_____ I am willing to read the material and think about how it applies to me.

_____ I am willing to question my assumptions and look at my values.

_____ I am willing to spend some time most days reflecting on the issues raised in this course.

_____ I am willing to keep a journal, recording my reactions to what I read and experience and assessing my progress on meeting my goals and commitments.

Other commitments to become an active learner include:_____

_____

_____

MULTIPLE INTELLIGENCES AND MULTIPLE LEARNING STYLES

Earlier we talked about personal growth and self-actualization, which depend on self-awareness and your ability to learn from life experiences. The kind of growth that is involved in the self-actualization model cannot be captured by the traditional view of intelligence, which emphasizes the verbal-linguistic domain. The expanded model of multiple intelligences discussed in this section can be used to explain the talents and skills people use to achieve growth. We explore the many facets of the concept of multiple intelligences and show the diversity of ways we learn and, at the same time, grow. There is no single best way to learn; by exploring our own abilities, we can capitalize on developing a learning style that suits us.

To get the most out of your education, you need to know where your talents lie and how you learn. People differ in how they learn best and in what kinds of knowledge they tend to learn most easily. For example, auditory learners tend to understand and retain ideas better from hearing them spoken, whereas visual learners tend to learn more effectively when they can literally see what they are learning. By learning as much as you can about your own learning style, you can maximize your success in college regardless of your field of study.

Behind differences in learning styles may lie basic differences in intelligence. Intelligence is not a single, easily measured ability but a group of complex, multidimensional abilities, and learners may find that they have strengths in several different areas. The theory of multiple intelligences was developed in 1983 by Howard Gardner (1983, 1993, 2000), a professor of

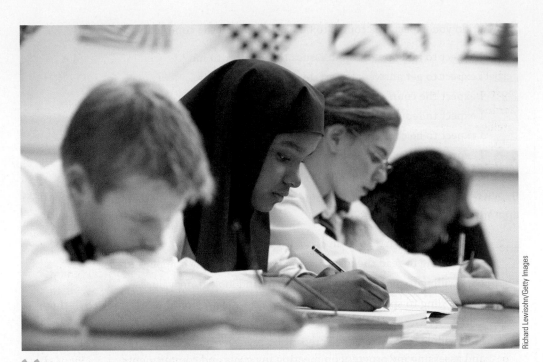

Richard Lewisohn/Getty Images

» Intelligence is not an easily measured ability, but rather a complex multidimensional ability and strengths.

education at Harvard University. He discovered that we are capable of eight different types of intelligence and learning:

▸ Verbal-linguistic

▸ Musical-rhythmic

▸ Logical-mathematical

▸ Visual-spatial

▸ Bodily-kinesthetic

▸ Intrapersonal

▸ Interpersonal

▸ Naturalistic

To this list, Daniel Goleman (2006) adds *emotional intelligence* as a critical aspect of intelligence with definite implications for personal learning. Emotional intelligence pertains to the ability to control impulses, empathize with others, form responsible interpersonal relationships, develop cooperative attitudes and behaviors, and develop intimate relationships. When emotional competencies are lacking, Goleman believes this results in disconnection, which, in turn, leads to prejudice, self-involvement, aggressive behavior, depression, addictive behavior, and an inability to manage emotions. In *The Brain and Emotional Intelligence: New Insights* (2011) Goleman draws from the field of affective neuroscience to deepen our understanding of emotional intelligence. Compelling evidence from neural imaging and lesion studies suggests that emotional intelligence resides in brain regions that are distinct from those involved in mathematical, verbal, and spatial intelligence. Emotional intelligence is certainly basic to learning interpersonal skills, yet this domain tends not to be emphasized in the educational programs of our schools and colleges. Goleman (2006, 2007) suggests that school programs must include developing essential human competencies such as empathy, curiosity, compassion, self-control, and a sense of cooperation.

According to Gardner (1983, 1993, 2000), most attention in the schools is given to the verbal-linguistic and logical-mathematic abilities, what we generally refer to as IQ. However, most of the other forms of intelligence and learning are equally vital to success in life. Gardner believes that increased attention should be given to those people who have other intelligences such as naturalists, musicians, architects, artists, designers, dancers, entrepreneurs, and therapists. Armstrong (1993, 1994) believes that the most remarkable feature of the theory of multiple intelligences is a framework for understanding eight different potential pathways to learning. For students who have difficulty with the more traditional linguistic or logical ways of learning, the theory of multiple intelligences suggests other effective ways to teach and learn.

Let's examine the specific characteristics of each of these kinds of intellectual abilities and then consider the implications for college learning.

▶ If you are a **verbal-linguistic learner**, you have highly developed auditory skills, enjoy reading and writing, like to play word games, and have a good memory for names, dates, and places; you like to tell stories; and you are good at getting your point across. You learn best by saying and hearing words. Your learning is facilitated by opportunities to listen and to speak. You prefer to learn by listening to lectures or audiotapes, and by discussing what you have heard. You will probably profit more from reading after you have heard about the material you are to read. You may learn best by taping lectures and listening to them again or by listening to your textbook on audiotape. Reciting information and teaching others what you know are useful ways for you to learn. People whose dominant intelligence is in the verbal linguistic area include poets, authors, speakers, attorneys, politicians, lecturers, and teachers.

▶ If you are a **musical-rhythmic learner**, you are sensitive to the sounds in your environment, enjoy music, and prefer listening to music when you study or read. You appreciate pitch and rhythm. You probably like singing to yourself. You learn best through melody and music. Musical intelligence is obviously demonstrated by singers, conductors, and composers, but also by those who enjoy, understand, and use various elements of music.

▶ If you are more a **logical-mathematical learner**, you probably like to explore patterns and relationships, and you enjoy doing activities in sequential order. You are likely to enjoy mathematics, and you like to experiment with things you do not understand. You like to work with numbers, ask questions, and explore patterns and relationships. You may find it challenging to solve problems and to use logical reasoning. You learn best by classifying information, engaging in abstract thinking, and looking for common basic principles. People with well-developed logical-mathematical abilities include mathematicians, biologists, medical technologists, geologists, engineers, physicists, researchers, and other scientists.

▶ If you are a **visual-spatial learner**, you prefer to learn by reading, watching videotapes, and observing demonstrations. You will learn better by seeing pictures and graphically mapping out material to learn rather than relying mainly on listening to lectures. You tend to think in images and pictures. You are likely to get more from a lecture *after* you have read the material. Besides the printed word, you may learn well by seeing pictures and forming images of what is to be learned. You learn by looking at pictures, watching movies, and seeing slides. You may rely on word processors, books, and other visual devices for learning and recall. People with well-developed visual-spatial abilities are found in professions such as sculpting, painting, surgery, and engineering.

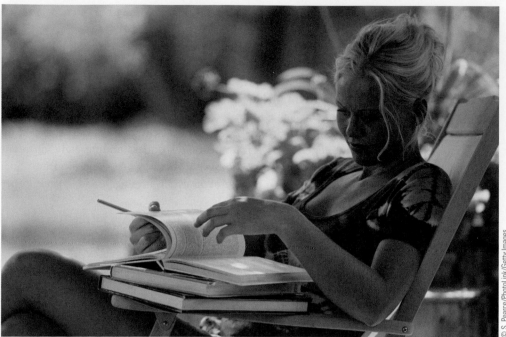

There are multiple intelligences and multiple learning styles.

▶ If you are a **bodily-kinesthetic learner**, you process knowledge through bodily
   sensations and use your body in skilled ways. You have good balance and coordination;
   you are good with your hands. You need opportunities to move and act things out.
   You tend to respond best in classrooms that provide physical activities and hands-on
   learning experiences. You prefer to learn by doing, by getting physically involved through
   movement and action. You tend to learn best by experimenting and figuring out ways
   of solving a problem. People who have highly developed bodily-kinesthetic abilities
   include carpenters, television and stereo repairpersons, mechanics, dancers, gymnasts,
   swimmers, and jugglers.

▶ If you are an **intrapersonal learner**, you prefer your own inner world, you like to be
   alone, and you are aware of your own strengths, weaknesses, and feelings. You tend to
   be a creative and independent thinker; you like to reflect on ideas. You probably possess
   independence, self-confidence, determination, and are highly motivated. You may
   respond with strong opinions when controversial topics are discussed. You learn best by
   engaging in independent study projects rather than working on group projects. Pacing
   your own instruction is important to you. People with intrapersonal abilities include
   entrepreneurs, philosophers, and psychologists.

▶ If you are an **interpersonal learner**, you enjoy being around people, like talking to
   people, have many friends, and engage in social experiences. You learn best by relating,
   sharing, and participating in cooperative group environments. People with strong
   interpersonal abilities are found in sales, consulting, community organizing, counseling,
   teaching, or one of the helping professions.

▶ If you are a **naturalist learner**, you have ability in observing patterns in nature,
   identifying and classifying objects, and understanding natural and human-made systems.
   Skilled naturalists include farmers, botanists, hunters, ecologists, and landscapers.

▶ If you are an **emotional learner**, you have competence in the emotional realm: empathy, concern for others, curiosity, self-control, cooperation, the ability to resolve conflicts, the ability to listen well, communication skills, and connections with others. You are interested in cultivating matters of your heart as much as those of your head, and you are interested in the interdependence of people at least as much as you are in developing your own independence. Emotional learners promote cooperative and collaborative learning, reach out to others, and apply what they know to making the world a better place to live.

The model of **multiple intelligences** is best used as a tool to help you identify areas you may want to pursue. Consider what the possible kinds of intelligences and learning styles are and then decide where your strengths lie and which particular pathways interest you the most. Although you may have a preference for one of these pathways to learning, remain open to incorporating elements from some of the other styles as well. In a course such as this, it can benefit you if you look for ways to blend the emotional domain with the other forms of intelligence and learning styles. You are likely to find that you learn best by integrating many pathways, rather than by depending exclusively on one avenue in your educational journey. The more you can view college as a place to use all your talents and improve your learning abilities in all respects, the more meaningful and successful your college journey will be.

As you will see in Chapter 10, other factors besides ability (or intelligence) need to be considered in deciding on a field of study or a career. For further reading on this topic, we recommend 7 Kinds of Smart: Identifying and Developing Your Many Intelligences by Thomas Armstrong (1993).

FIXED VERSUS GROWTH MINDSETS

One goal of this chapter is to help you to prepare for success in your journey of self-exploration and personal growth. As you embark on this journey, reflect on what success means to you. Is it about validating your abilities and proving to yourself and others that you are bright, talented, and capable? If so, it is likely that you have a **fixed mindset**. Or do you define success as striving to learn something new and stretching yourself even at the risk of encountering struggle and setbacks? If so, it is likely that you have a **growth mindset**. In the next Take Time to Reflect, you can test your mindset.

In *Mindset: The New Psychology of Success*, renowned Stanford University psychologist Carol S. Dweck (2006) explains how your mindset can determine whether you become the person you want to be and live up to your potential. If you believe that your qualities are etched in stone (a *fixed mindset*), you will have to prove yourself over and over again. If you operate from the premise that you "have only a certain amount of intelligence, a certain personality, and a certain moral character—well, then you'd better prove that you have a healthy dose of them. It simply wouldn't do to look or feel deficient in these most basic characteristics" (p. 6). By contrast, if you have a *growth mindset*, you can cultivate your basic qualities through your own efforts. In Dweck's words, "The passion for stretching yourself and sticking to it, even (or especially) when it's not going well, is the hallmark of the growth mindset. This is the mindset that allows people to thrive during some of the most challenging times in their lives" (p. 7).

We have been shaped by the messages about success and failure we have received since childhood (perhaps from well-intentioned adults), but we can choose to change these messages if they are holding us back. Of course, letting go of a fixed mindset is not easy. To let go of traits that have been the main source of your self-esteem and embrace challenge, struggle, criticism, and setbacks is understandably unsettling to just about anyone. As Dweck (2006) states, "It may feel as though the fixed mindset gave you your ambition, your edge, your individuality. Maybe you fear you'll become a bland cog in the wheel just like everyone else. Ordinary. But opening yourself up to growth makes you more yourself, not less" (p. 226).

As you reflect on changes that you would like to make in your life, consider how you might approach this from a growth mindset orientation. How can you stretch yourself? What risks might be worth taking to get the desired results? If you encounter roadblocks or setbacks along the way, how can you deal with them constructively? Visualize a concrete plan in vivid detail for carrying out the tasks involved in reaching your goal and, most important of all, follow through.

TAKE TIME TO REFLECT

Test your mindset by taking this brief version of the *Mindset* quiz.*

Instructions: Show how much you agree or disagree with each statement by selecting the option that best corresponds to your opinion.

SA = Strongly agree
A = Agree
MA = Mostly agree
MD = Mostly disagree
D = Disagree
SD = Strongly disagree

_____ 1. You have a certain amount of intelligence, and you can't really do much to change it.

_____ 2. Your intelligence is something about you that you can't change very much.

_____ 3. No matter who you are, you can significantly change your intelligence level.

_____ 4. To be honest, you can't really change how intelligent you are.

_____ 5. You can always substantially change how intelligent you are.

_____ 6. You can learn new things, but you can't really change your basic intelligence.

_____ 7. No matter how much intelligence you have, you can always change it quite a bit.

_____ 8. You can change even your basic intelligence level considerably.

_____ 9. You have a certain amount of talent, and you can't really do much to change it.

_____ 10. Your talent in an area is something about you that you can't change very much.

_____ 11. No matter who you are, you can significantly change your level of talent.

_____ 12. To be honest, you can't really change how much talent you have.

_____ 13. You can always substantially change how much talent you have.

_____ 14. You can learn new things, but you can't really change your basic level of talent.

_____ 15. No matter how much talent you have, you can always change it quite a bit.

_____ 16. You can change even your basic level of talent considerably.

Some of the statements reflect a fixed mindset (1, 2, 4, 6, 9, 10, 12, and 14); others reflect a growth mindset (3, 5, 7, 8, 11, 13, 15, and 16). There are no right or wrong answers. The purpose of the quiz is to help you to assess whether you lean more toward having a fixed or growth mindset.

*Adapted from the full quiz, which can be found on the official website of *Mindset* at http://www.mindsetonline.com/testyourmindset.

*We appreciate the information provided by Janet Delesanti in updating this section on multiple intelligences.

GETTING THE MOST FROM THIS BOOK: SUGGESTIONS FOR PERSONAL LEARNING

Throughout this book, we both write in a personal style and share with you how we arrived at our beliefs and values. We hope that knowing our assumptions, values, and biases will help you evaluate your own position more clearly. We are not suggesting that you adopt our philosophy of life, but that you use the material in this book as a catalyst for your own reflection. There are no simple answers to complex life issues, and each person's life is unique. We have concerns about the kind of self-help books that give an abundance of advice or attempt to offer easy answers. Information and even suggestions can be useful at the right time, but rarely can an individual's problems be resolved by uncritically accepting others' advice or directives. Although giving advice may be of benefit in the short term, it often does not teach people how to deal with the range of present and future problems they may face.

In the chapters that follow, we offer a great deal of personal information for you to reflect on and to use as a basis for making better choices. Our aim is to raise questions that lead to thoughtful reflection on your part and to meaningful dialogue with others. We encourage you to develop the practice of examining questions that engage you and have meaning in your life. Instead of looking for simple solutions to your problems, consider making time for personal reflection as a way to clarify your options in many areas of your life. Listen to others and consider what they say, but even more important, learn to listen to your own voice within for direction. This book can become a personal companion; use it to enhance your reflection on questions that are personally significant to you.

This course is likely to be different from many of the courses you have taken. Few courses deal primarily with you as the subject matter. Most college courses challenge you intellectually, but this book is geared toward integrating intellectual and personal learning. To a large degree, what you get from this course will depend on what you are willing to invest of yourself. It is important that you clarify your goals and identify the steps you can take to reach them. The following guidelines will help you become active and involved in personal learning as you read the book and participate in your class.

1. **PREPARING.** Read this book for your personal benefit, and make use of the *Take Time to Reflect* and the *Where Can I Go From Here?* sections. Considerations such as your age, life experiences, and cultural background will have a bearing on the meaning and importance of certain topics to you. We have written this book from our own cultural framework, but the topics we address are common to all of us. In our work with people from various cultures, we continue to find that these human themes transcend culture and unite us in our life struggles.

2. **DEALING WITH FEARS.** It is natural to experience some fear about participating personally and actively in the class. We encourage you to challenge yourself to talk openly about your possible fear of sharing personal concerns and about establishing boundaries that will work for you. How you deal with your fears is more important than trying to eliminate your anxieties. Facing your fears takes courage and a genuine desire to increase your self-awareness. It is a first big step toward expanding the range of your choices.

3. **ESTABLISHING TRUST.** You can choose to take the initiative in establishing the trust necessary for you to participate in this course in a meaningful way, rather than wait for others to create a climate of trust. One way to establish trust is to talk with your instructor outside of class.

4. PRACTICING SELF-DISCLOSURE. Disclosing yourself to others is one way to come to know yourself more fully. Sometimes participants in self-awareness courses or experiential groups fear that they must give up their privacy to be active participants. However, you can be open and at the same time retain your privacy by deciding how much you will disclose and when it is appropriate to do so.

5. LISTENING. Work on developing the skill of really listening to what others are saying without thinking of what you will say in reply. Active listening requires remaining open and carefully considering what others say instead of too quickly giving reasons and explanations.

6. MAINTAINING AN OPEN ATTITUDE. Strive to keep a sense of openness, with both yourself and others in the class. As you listen to others and read, reflect on ways you might question some of your beliefs and assumptions.

7. AVOIDING SELF-FULFILLING PROPHECIES. You can increase your ability to change by letting go of ways you have categorized yourself or been categorized by others. If you start off with the assumption that you are stupid, helpless, or boring, you will probably convince others as well.

8. PRACTICING OUTSIDE OF CLASS. One important way to get the maximum benefit from a class dealing with personal learning is to think about ways of applying what you learn in class to your everyday life. Make specific contracts with yourself (as part of your action plan described early in this chapter) by identifying what you are willing to do to achieve the changes you want to make.

9. EMBRACING THE IDEA THAT EVERY STEP COUNTS. Small changes can ripple into larger changes and provide hope for people who want to make changes in daily living. Effective solutions are not always directly related to our problems. Sometimes one small change leads to larger and more significant changes. It is important to recognize, appreciate, and credit yourself with the small changes you are making.

10. KEEPING A JOURNAL. In one sense this is an *unfinished* book. You are invited to become a coauthor by completing the writing of this book in ways that are meaningful to you. Throughout the book we suggest that you keep a journal. There are pages provided at the end of each chapter for you to write your journal entries. It is important that you decide what to put in it and how to use it. Reviewing your journal will help you identify some of your critical choices and areas of conflict. Consider writing about some of these topics:

▸ What I learned about others and myself through today's class session

▸ The topics that were of most interest to me (and why)

▸ The topics that held the least interest for me (and why)

▸ The topics I wanted to talk about

▸ The topics I avoided talking about

▸ Particular sections (or issues) in the chapter that had the greatest impact on me (and why)

▸ Some specific things I am doing in everyday life as a result of this class

▸ Some concrete changes in my attitudes, values, and behavior that I find myself most wanting to make

▸ What I am willing to do to make these changes

▸ Some obstacles I encounter in making the changes I want to make

It is best to write what first comes to mind. Spontaneous reactions tend to tell you more about yourself than well-thought-out comments.

SUMMARY

We do not have to live by the plans that others have designed for us. With awareness we can begin to design our own blueprints and make significant choices. Taking a stand in life by making choices can result in both gains and losses. Changing long-standing patterns is not easy, and there are many obstacles to overcome. Yet exercising your freedom has many rewards. One of these benefits is personal growth, which involves a lifelong process of expanding self-awareness and accepting new challenges. It does not mean disregard for others but rather implies fulfilling more of our potential, including our ability to care for others. Keep in mind that until our basic needs have been met we are not really much concerned about becoming fully functioning persons. Self-actualization is not something that we do in isolation; rather, it is through meaningful relationships with others and through social interest that we discover and become the persons we are capable of becoming. Paradoxically, we find ourselves when we are secure enough to go beyond a preoccupation with our self-interests and become involved in the world with selected people.

Striving for self-actualization does not cease at a particular age but is an ongoing process. Rather than speaking of self-actualization as a final end point that we attain, it is best to consider the process of becoming a *self-actualizing* person. Four basic characteristics of self-actualizing people are self-awareness, freedom, basic honesty and caring, and trust and autonomy. This course can be a first step on the journey toward achieving your personal goals and living a self-actualizing existence, while at the same time contributing to making the world a better place.

A major purpose of this chapter is to encourage you to examine your responsibility for making your learning meaningful. Even if your earlier educational experiences have taught you to be a passive learner and to avoid taking risks in your classes, being aware of this influence gives you the power to change your learning style and mindset. We invite you to decide how personally involved you want to be in the course you are about to experience.

Where Can I Go From Here?

At the end of each chapter are additional activities and exercises that we suggest you practice, both in class and out of class. Ultimately, you will be the one to decide which activities you are willing to do. You may find some of the suggested exercises too threatening to do in a class, yet exploring the same activities in a small group in your class could be easier. If small discussion groups are not part of the structure of your class, consider doing the exercises alone or sharing them with a friend. Do not feel compelled to complete all the activities; select those that have the most meaning for you at this time in your life.

1. These are exercises you can do at home or in class in small groups. They are intended to help you focus on specific ways in which you behave. We have drawn the examples from typical fears and concerns often expressed by college students. Study the situations by putting yourself in each one and deciding how you might typically respond. Then keep an account in your journal of actual instances you encounter in your classes.

Situation A: You would like to ask a question in class, but you are afraid that your question will sound dumb and that others will laugh.

Issues: Will you simply refrain from asking questions? If so, is this a pattern you care to continue? Are you willing to practice asking questions, even though you might experience some anxiety? What do you imagine will happen if you ask questions? What would you like to have happen?

Situation B: You feel that you have a problem concerning authority figures. You feel intimidated, afraid to venture your opinions, and even more afraid to state your own point of view.

Issues: Does this description fit you? If it does, do you want to change? Do you ever examine where you picked up your attitudes toward yourself in relation to authority? Do you think they are still appropriate for you?

Situation C: Your instructor seems genuinely interested in the students and the course, and she has extended herself by inviting you to come to her office if you have any problems with the course. You are having real difficulty with some concepts and doing poorly on the tests and assignments. Nevertheless, you keep putting off going to see the instructor to talk about your problems in the class.

Issues: Have you been in this situation before? If so, what kept you from talking with your instructor? If you find yourself in this kind of situation, are you willing to seek help before it is too late?

2. Review Maslow's characteristics of self-actualizing people, and consider the following questions:

    a. To what degree are these characteristics a part of your personality?

    b. Do you think Maslow's ideal of self-actualization fits for individuals of all cultural and ethnic groups? Are any characteristics inappropriate for certain cultures?

3. Identify five changes you would most like to make in your life. Describe your current stage of change for each of these goals or potential changes. What prevents you from advancing to the next stage? How would your life be different if you could make these changes?

4. Explain how you developed your mindset and whether you have a fixed or growth mindset. What messages did you receive in your family about success and failure that may have contributed to your way of thinking? Did other individuals play a role in shaping your mindset? If so, explain.

5. Suggested Readings. At the end of each chapter we provide some suggestions for further reading. For the full bibliographic entry for each of the sources listed, consult the References and Suggested Readings at the back of the book. For a detailed discussion of the key figures associated with the humanistic psychology movement, see Schultz and Schultz (2013). For a book on person-centered expressive arts therapy, see Natalie Rogers (1993). To read about fixed versus growth mindsets, see Dweck (2006).

WEBSITE RESOURCES

Included here are some valuable websites. For access to these websites, video activities, and other supporting materials, visit Cengage Learning's Counseling CourseMate website for *I Never Knew I Had a Choice,* 10th Edition, at **www.cengagebrain.com.**

MENTAL HELP NET
www.mentalhelp.net

Recommended Search Words: "mental help net"

Mental Help Net is an excellent site that explores all aspects of mental health. This site includes daily updated news articles, online support forums, books, and so on. With links to thousands of resources, whatever you are looking for about mental health is probably here.

AMERICAN SELF-HELP GROUP CLEARINGHOUSE
www.selfhelpgroups.org

Recommended Search Words: "American self-help group clearing house"

This site provides contact information for more than 1,100 national, international, model and online self-help support groups.

AMERICAN COUNSELING ASSOCIATION (ACA)
www.counseling.org

Recommended Search Words: "American counseling association"

ACA is the major organization of counselors in the U.S.; the ACA resource catalog provides information on various aspects of the counseling profession. The site provides information about membership, ethics, journals, books, home-study programs, videotapes, and audiotapes. Members have free access to the ACA Podcast Series.

AMERICAN PSYCHOLOGICAL ASSOCIATION (APA)
www.apa.org

Recommended Search Words: "American psychological association"

This is the major professional organization of psychologists in the U.S. This website provides leads for current research and literature on many of the topics in this book.

MINDSET
www.mindsetonline.com

Recommended Search Words: "Mindset"

This website features Dr. Carol Dweck's book *Mindset: The New Psychology of Success*. Visit this site to test your mindset, to learn how to change your mindset, and for links to information about Dweck's work.

POSITIVE PSYCHOLOGY CENTER
www.ppc.sas.upenn.edu

Housed at the University of Pennsylvania, the Positive Psychology Center, founded by Dr. Martin E. P. Seligman, provides a wealth of resources for anyone interested in the study of positive psychology.

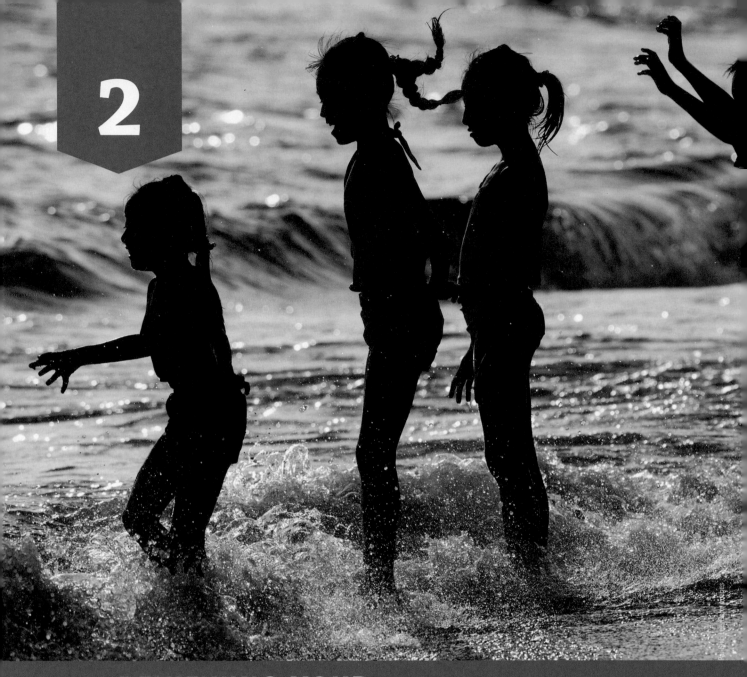

REVIEWING YOUR CHILDHOOD AND ADOLESCENCE

> Where Am I Now?

> Stages of Personality Development: A Preview

> Infancy

> Early Childhood

> Impact of the First Six Years of Life

> Middle Childhood

> Pubescence

> Adolescence

> Summary

> Where Can I Go From Here?

> Website Resources

> What we resist persists.

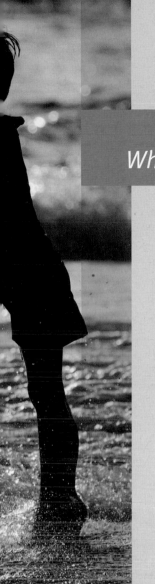

What we resist persists.

WHERE AM I NOW?

Use this scale to respond to these statements:

4 = I *strongly agree* with this statement.
3 = I *agree* with this statement.
2 = I *disagree* with this statement.
1 = I *strongly disagree* with this statement.

1. I am capable of looking at my past decisions and then making new decisions that will significantly change the course of my life.

2. "Shoulds" and "oughts" get in the way of my living my life the way I want.

3. To a large degree I have been shaped by the events of my childhood and adolescent years.

4. When I think of my early childhood years, I remember feeling secure, accepted, and loved.

5. As a child, I was taught that it was acceptable to express feelings such as anger, fear, and jealousy.

6. I had desirable models to pattern my behavior after when I was growing up.

7. In looking back at my early school-age years, I had a positive self-concept and experienced more successes than failures.

8. I went through a stage of rebellion during my adolescent years.

9. My adolescent years were lonely ones.

10. I was greatly influenced by peer group pressure during my adolescence.

This chapter and the next one lay the groundwork for much of the rest of the book by focusing on our lifelong struggle to achieve psychological emancipation, or **autonomy**. The term *autonomy* refers to mature independence and interdependence. As you will recall from the previous chapter, becoming a fully functioning person occurs in the context of relationships with others and with concern for the welfare of others, which is embodied in the concept of interdependence. If you are an autonomous person, you are able to function without constant approval and reassurance, are sensitive to the needs of others, can effectively meet the demands of daily living, are willing to ask for help when it is needed, and can provide support to others. In essence, you have the ability both to *stand alone* and to *stand by* another person. You are at home with both your inner world and your outer world. Although you are concerned with meeting your needs, you do not do so at the expense of those around you. You are aware of the impact your behavior may have on others, and you consider the welfare of others as well as your own self-development. Self-development that occurs at the expense of others will almost inevitably backfire because harm you bring to others will generally result in harm being returned to you. Concern for others is not simply an obligation that requires self-sacrifice; social responsibility can be a route to self-betterment. Healthy relationships involve self-enhancement and attention to the welfare of others.

Achieving personal autonomy is a continuing process of growth and learning. Your attitudes toward gender-role identity, work, your body, love, intimacy, sexuality, loneliness, death, and meaning—themes we discuss in later chapters—were originally influenced by your family of origin and your cultural context and by the decisions you made during your early years. Personality development is a process that occurs throughout the life span. Each stage of life has its own challenges, and you continue to develop and change throughout your life. In this chapter we describe the stages from infancy through adolescence; in Chapter 3 we take up early, middle, and late adulthood.

STAGES OF PERSONALITY DEVELOPMENT: A PREVIEW

Each of the developmental theorists has a somewhat different conceptualization of the stages from infancy to old age. By getting a picture of the challenges at each period of life, you will be able to understand how earlier stages of personality development influence the choices you make later in life. These stages are not precise categories that people fall into neatly, and different theories have slightly different conceptualizations of how long people remain in a given stage of life. In reality there is great variability among individuals within a given developmental phase. Your family of origin, culture, race, gender, and socioeconomic status are factors that have a great deal to do with the manner in which you experience the developmental process. Some people at age 60 are truly old in their appearance, way of thinking, and general health. Yet others at 60 may still retain a great deal of vitality and truly be young. Chronological age is not the only index in considering physical, emotional, and social age. As you will see in this and the following chapter, our beliefs and attitudes have a great deal to do with how vital we are.

There are many theoretical approaches to understanding human development. We cannot address all of these models in this book, but we can establish a foundation from which you will be able to reflect on turning points in your childhood and adolescent years. As you read the detailed descriptions of the life cycle, think about how what is written either fits or does not fit for you. Reflecting on your life experiences will bring enhanced meaning to the discussion of these life stages.

In much of this chapter we describe a model that draws on Erik Erikson's (1963, 1982) theory of human development. We also highlight some major ideas about development from the **self-in-context** approach, which emphasizes the individual life cycle in a systemic perspective (see McGoldrick, Carter, & Garcia Preto, 2011b, for more on this). The **systemic perspective** is grounded on the assumption that how we develop can best be understood through learning about our role and place in our family of origin. The systemic view is that individuals cannot really be understood apart from the family system of which they are a part. We also draw on some basic concepts from Freud's psychoanalytic theory of personality.

Sigmund Freud, the father of **psychoanalysis**, developed one of the most comprehensive theories of personality in the early 1900s. He pioneered new techniques for understanding human behavior, and his efforts resulted in the most comprehensive theory of personality and psychotherapy ever developed. Freud emphasized unconscious psychological processes and stressed the importance of early childhood experiences. According to his viewpoint, our sexual and social development is largely based on the first 6 years of life. During this time, Freud maintained, we go through distinct stages of development. Our later personality development hinges on how well we resolve the demands and conflicts of each stage. Most of the problems people wrestle with in adulthood have some connection with unresolved conflicts dating from early childhood.

Erikson built on and extended Freud's ideas, stressing the psychosocial aspects of development and carrying his own developmental theory beyond childhood. Erikson is often credited with bringing an emphasis on social factors to contemporary psychoanalysis. Although intellectually indebted to Freud, Erikson suggested that we should view human development in a more positive light, focusing on health and growth. Erikson's **psychosocial theory** focuses on the emergence of the self and the ways in which the self develops through our interactions with our social and cultural environment. Later in this chapter we will return to a more detailed discussion about development and protection of the self.

Erikson believes we face the task of establishing equilibrium between ourselves and our social world at each stage of life. Psychosocial theory stresses integration of the biological, psychological, and social aspects of development. This model provides a conceptual framework for understanding trends in development; major developmental tasks at each stage of life; critical needs and their satisfaction or frustration; potentials for choice at each stage of life; critical turning points or developmental crises; and the origins of faulty personality development, which lead to later personality conflicts.

Erikson described human development over the entire life span in terms of eight stages, each marked by a particular crisis to be resolved. For Erikson, a **crisis** is a turning point in life, a moment of transition characterized by the potential to go either forward or backward in development. At these critical turning points, we can achieve successful resolution of our conflicts and move ahead, or we can fail to resolve the conflicts and remain fixated at a transitional period. To a large extent, our lives are the result of the choices we make at each stage of life.

McGoldrick and colleagues (2011b) criticize Erikson's theory of individual development for underplaying the importance of the interpersonal realm and connection to others. In Erikson's individually focused schemes, relational skills and family relationships are not given due recognition. Contextual factors have a critical bearing on our ability to formulate a clear identity as an individual and also to be able to connect to others. The self-in-context perspective takes into account race, socioeconomic class, disability, gender, ethnicity, and culture as central factors that influence the course of development throughout the individual's life cycle. Gender-role socialization can influence development when it comes to

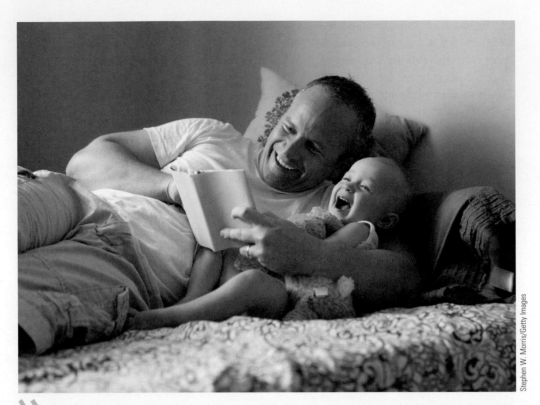

Stephen W. Morris/Getty Images

» A child's basic task in the first year of life is to develop a sense of trust in self, others, and the environment.

choosing a career. Traditional gender boundaries in nursing or construction jobs are being increasingly challenged in today's workforce, but a young man whose goal is to become a nurse may be subtly or overtly challenged about his job choice by gender-biased comments such as "Why a nurse and not a doctor?"

The **feminist perspective**, a systemic approach that emphasizes the social context of behavior and how gender affects behavior, is also critical of the Freudian psychoanalytic approach and Erikson's focus on the individual. During the late 1960s and the early 1970s, feminist writers began to focus on the limitations of traditional psychoanalytic theories and techniques that neglected or misunderstood many aspects of women's experiencing. Feminists began to develop conceptual models and ways of practicing that emphasized going beyond the self and establishing connections with others (Miller & Stiver, 1997). Feminist thought provides a unique perspective on developmental concerns of both women and men and broadens the psychodynamic approach and the psychosocial model of Erikson.

Our approach has been to combine Erikson's psychosocial theory and the self-in-context theory, integrating their separate strengths to provide a meaningful framework for understanding key factors influencing our development throughout the life cycle. The life-span perspective presented in these two chapters relies heavily on concepts borrowed from Erikson's (1982) model and the self-in-context model of McGoldrick and colleagues (2011b). We also rely on the feminist perspective of personality development (see Miller & Stiver, 1997) as this approach applies to the various life stages. In addition, we are indebted to a number of other writers, whom we cite in this chapter.

In *The Human Odyssey: Navigating the Twelve Stages of Life,* Thomas Armstrong (2007) maintains that every stage of life is equally significant and necessary for the welfare of humanity.

Each stage of life has its own unique "gift" to contribute to the world. Armstrong believes that we should take the same attitude toward nurturing the human life cycle as we do toward protecting the environment from global warming. He argues that by supporting each of the developmental stages, we are helping to ensure that people are given care and helped to develop to their fullest potential. Table 2.1 provides an overview of the major turning points in the life-span perspective of human development from infancy through adolescence.

TABLE 2.1	Overview of Developmental Stages From Infancy Through Adolescence		
Life stage	**Self-in-Context View**	**Erikson's Psychosocial View**	**Potential Problems**
Infancy (birth to age 2)	This is a time for the development of empathy and emotional attunement. Some specific tasks include learning to talk, making needs known, developing coordination, recognizing self as a separate person, and trusting others. Infants learn how to sit, stand, walk, run, manipulate objects, and feed themselves. They communicate both frustration and happiness.	*Infancy.* Basic task is to develop a sense of trust in self, others, and the environment. Infants need a sense of being cared for and loved. Absence of a sense of security may lead to suspiciousness and a general sense of mistrust toward human relationships. Core struggle: *trust versus mistrust.* Theme: hope.	Later personality problems that stem from infancy can include greediness and acquisitiveness, the development of a view of the world based on mistrust, fear of reaching out to others, rejection of affection, fear of loving and trusting, low self-esteem, isolation and withdrawal, and inability to form or maintain intimate relationships.
Early childhood (ages 2–6)	The theme of this phase is a growing understanding of interdependence. Great strides in language and motor development are made. A key task is to develop emotional competence, which involves being able to delay gratification. This stage ushers in the awareness of "otherness" in terms of gender, race, and disability. Other tasks include learning cooperative play, being able to share, developing peer relationships, becoming aware of self in relation to the world around us, and increasing our ability to trust others.	*Early childhood.* A time for developing autonomy. Failure to master self-control tasks may lead to shame and doubt about oneself and one's adequacy. Core struggle: *self-reliance versus self-doubt.* Theme: will. *Preschool age.* Characterized by play and by anticipation of roles; a time to establish a sense of competence and initiative. Children who are not allowed to make decisions tend to develop a sense of guilt. Core struggle: *initiative versus guilt.* Theme: purpose.	Children experience many negative feelings such as hostility, rage, destructiveness, anger, and hatred. If these feelings are not accepted, individuals may not be able to accept their feelings later on. Parental attitudes can be communicated verbally and nonverbally. Negative learning experiences tend to lead to feelings of guilt about natural impulses. Strict parental indoctrination can lead to rigidity, severe conflicts, remorse, and self-condemnation.
Middle childhood (ages 6–12)	This is a time when children learn to read, write, and do math. They increase their understanding of self in terms of gender, race, culture, and abilities. There is an increased understanding of self in relation to family, peers, and community. A key task is developing empathy, or being able to take the perspective of others.	*School age.* Central task is to achieve a sense of industry; failure to do so results in a sense of inadequacy. Child needs to expand understanding of the world and continue to develop appropriate gender-role identity. Learning basic skills is essential for school success. Core struggle: *industry versus inferiority.* Theme: competence.	Problems that can originate during middle childhood include negative self-concept, feelings of inferiority in establishing social relationships, conflicts over values, confused gender-role identity, dependency, fear of new challenges, and lack of initiative.

TABLE 2.1	Overview of Developmental Stages From Infancy Through Adolescence		
Life stage	**Self-in-Context View**	**Erikson's Psychosocial View**	**Potential Problems**
Pubescence (ages 11–13 for girls) (ages 12–14 for boys)	A time of finding one's own voice and the beginning of developing a sense of autonomy. Some specific developmental tasks include asserting oneself, developing emotional competence, increasing capacity for moral understanding, coping with dramatic bodily changes, increasing ability to deal with social relationships and work collaboratively, and developing awareness of own and others' sexuality. This is a time of expanded sense of self in relation to peers, family, and community.		
Adolescence (ages 13–20)	The theme of this period is searching for an identity, continuing to find one's voice, and balancing caring of self with caring about others. Key developmental themes include dealing with rapid body changes and body image issues, learning self-management, developing one's sexual identity, developing a philosophy of life and a spiritual identity, learning to deal with intimate relationships, and an expanded understanding of self in relation to others.	*Adolescence.* A critical time for forming a personal identity. Major conflicts center on clarification of self-identity, life goals, and life's meaning. Struggle is over integrating physical and social changes. Pressures include succeeding in school, choosing a job, forming relationships, and preparing for the future. Core struggle: *identity* versus *role confusion*. Theme: fidelity.	A time when an individual may anticipate an *identity crisis*. Caught in the midst of pressures, demands, and turmoil, adolescents often lose a sense of self. If *role confusion* results, the individual may lack sense of purpose in later years. Absence of a stable set of values can prevent mature development of a philosophy to guide one's life.

INFANCY

From birth to age 2 infants become acquainted with their world; this is the period in which experimentation and curiosity begin. Infancy is marked by vitality. The infant is a vibrant and seemingly unlimited source of energy (Armstrong, 2007). Developmental psychologists contend that a child's basic task in the first year of life is to develop a sense of trust in self, others, and the environment. Infants need to count on others; they need to sense that they are cared for and that the world is a secure place. They learn this sense of trust by being held, caressed, and loved.

Infants form a basic conception of the social world during this time, and Erikson (1963) saw their core struggle as **trust versus mistrust**. If the significant other persons in an infant's life provide the needed warmth, cuddling, and attention, the child develops a sense of trust. When these conditions are not present, the child becomes suspicious about interacting with others and acquires a general sense of mistrust toward human relationships. Although neither orientation is fixed in an infant's personality for life, it is clear that well-nurtured infants are in a more favorable position with respect to future personal growth than are their more neglected peers.

Daniel Goleman (2006) believes infancy is the beginning point for establishing emotional intelligence and that timing is a crucial factor in teaching emotional competence, especially in our family of origin and in our culture of origin during infancy. He adds that childhood and adolescence expand on the foundation for learning a range of human competencies. Later development offers critical *windows of opportunity* for acquiring the basic emotional patterns that will govern the rest of our lives.

John Bowlby (1969, 1973, 1980, 1988) studied the importance of attachment, separation, and loss in human development and developed **attachment theory**, an extension of psychoanalytic theory. **Attachment** involves an emotional bonding with another who is perceived as a source of security (Pistole & Arricale, 2003). Bowlby (1988) emphasizes the relationships that the infant has with others, especially the mother (or another "attachment figure"), and proposes that the maintenance of affectional bonds is essential for human survival. Infant attachment relationships can be broadly classified as secure or insecure. The quality of care an infant receives is related to the quality of relationships in later life (Peluso, Peluso, White, & Kern, 2004).

Ainsworth, Blehar, Waters, and Wall (1978) designed an experiment to observe the attachment behavior of young children and, based on these observations, identified three patterns of attachment: secure, anxious-avoidant, and anxious-ambivalent. According to Bowlby (1969, 1973) and Ainsworth et al. (1978), a **secure pattern** is characterized by feelings of intimacy, emotional security, and physical safety when the infant is in the presence of an attachment figure. These infants relate well with others in their world. Infants exhibiting the **anxious-avoidant pattern** experience an insecure attachment relationship because their attachment figures consistently reject them. These infants tend to use some form of disconnection or avoidance as a defense (Bowlby, 1980). Their sense of self is distorted, and their relationships in later life may be impaired. Infants using the anxious-ambivalent pattern exhibit intense distress at their caretaker's departure and an inability to be comforted upon return of the caretaker. Some of the effects of rejection in infancy include tendencies in later childhood to be fearful, insecure, jealous, aggressive, hostile, or isolated. This disconnection with self and others inhibits learning the essential emotional habits that will enable them to care about others, to be compassionate, and to form meaningful connections with others. Both the anxious-avoidant and the anxious-ambivalent patterns of attachment support Bowlby's (1980) contention that children form some style of attachment regardless of the emotional responsiveness from the caregiver.

And what happens beyond infancy? These early experiences with an attachment figure become

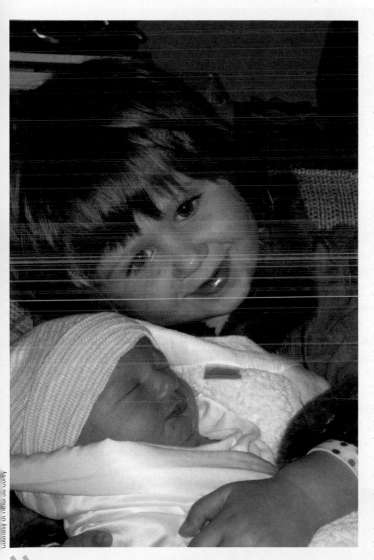

» Infants need to count on others.

internalized by the child, and these patterns serve as the blueprint for future relationships with others (Peluso et al., 2004). Ainsworth and colleagues (1978) have related different kinds of insecure attachments to the caretaker to later childhood and adolescent behavior, which tends to involve emotional detachment, a sense of being alone, uncertainty, and problems in interpersonal relationships. According to Pistole and Arricale (2003), in later relationships secure attachments are characterized by a positive self-image and a positive view of the partner. Adults with secure attachments appropriately rely on the partner as a safe haven and a base for exploration, and they experience satisfying relationships.

A sense of being loved during infancy is the best safeguard against fear, insecurity, and inadequacy. Children who receive love from parents or other attachment figures generally have little difficulty accepting themselves, whereas children who feel unloved and rejected may find it very difficult to accept themselves. In addition, rejected children often learn to mistrust the world and to view it primarily in terms of its ability to do them harm. David's story illustrates the repercussions of emotional deprivation during the early developmental years.

DAVID'S STORY

I learned at an early age that you have to fend for yourself because you can't really trust people. At least, that's how I see it. I was "raised" (if you can call it that) by two alcoholic parents who were never present emotionally—not for me and not for each other. My dad worked late hours, and I spent most of my time with my mother, who was usually drunk by noon. More days than I wish to remember, I was left alone at a playground across the street from a bar that my mother went to while my dad was at work. Sometimes she would get so drunk that she'd forget to take me home. At first, it upset me a lot, but like I said, I got used to it and learned to fend for myself. Somehow I survived my childhood, but not without some scars. I tend to keep people at arm's length, and I haven't been able to have a long-term relationship. As soon as a woman tries to get close to me, I call it quits. I suppose I try to have the upper hand by leaving them before they reject me.

David's case is not so unusual. We have worked with a number of individuals who suffer from the effects of early psychological deprivation, and we have observed that this situation can have lingering adverse effects on a person's level of self-love and the ability to form meaningful relationships later in life. Many people, of all ages, struggle with the issue of trusting others in a loving relationship. They are unable to trust that another can or will love them, they fear being rejected, and they fear even more the possibility of closeness and being accepted and loved. Like David, they may find themselves sabotaging their relationships to avoid being rejected or abandoned by others. Even though their early childhood circumstances vary considerably, if they do not trust themselves or others sufficiently to make themselves vulnerable, they cannot experience love. Ashley was adopted at 2 months of age by parents who were much more supportive than David's, but she encountered her own difficulties later in life.

ASHLEY'S STORY

When I was in my early 20s, I had a yearning to find my birthmother. I get kind of defensive when I discuss this because people automatically assume I was trying to find my biological mother because I was unhappy with my adoptive parents. That is so ludicrous!

I love my parents and wouldn't do anything to hurt them. But despite their best efforts to nurture and care for me, I always felt something was missing—I was like a story that had no beginning. I struggled for years with feeling inadequate—like I wasn't enough. I didn't have a strong sense of who I was, and as a result I had low self-esteem and felt unworthy of love. Being a sensitive and introspective person, I knew I had some "unfinished business" to deal with (a concept I learned in therapy). People would often say to me, "How lucky you are that your parents chose you!" That is true, but it is also true that my first mother decided to give me up. In therapy, I had an opportunity to grieve the loss of a person I didn't even know. Because the actual loss occurred before I had the words to articulate my grief, it took some time in therapy before I could access the emotions associated with being relinquished for adoption. At one point, after much reflection, I decided to search for my birthmother. It may not be the right decision for all adoptees because it is possible to be rejected all over again, but I had to do it to continue my own healing process. Regardless of what I would find, I needed to discover how my story began, and that's exactly what I did.

We have all heard about children who were adopted, perhaps as infants, who are now striving to find their natural parents as Ashley did. Even if they love their adopted parents and view them as having been good parents, these adult children sometimes feel a void and wonder about the circumstances of their adoption. These adult children may feel that their biological mother and father did not want them or that in some way they were defective or at fault for what happened. Many people reexperience their childhood feelings of hurt and rejection during the process of counseling; as a result of healing, they often come to understand that even though they did not feel loved by their parents this does not mean that others find them unlovable now.

The degree of parental nurturance is not the sole predictor of favorable personality development. Children who did not develop secure attachments in infancy may still develop a positive self image and healthy relationships, especially if they are able to garner social support and find a mentor such as a therapist, teacher, or relative some time during their childhood. In addition to social and environmental factors, genetic and biological factors contribute to a person's ability to form good relationships. **Temperament** includes both regulatory and reactive components. As De Pauw and Mervielde (2010) point out, "some children are outgoing, whereas others tend to stay in the background; some are quickly irritated, whereas others are rarely in a bad mood; some children respond aggressively, whereas others have a more gentle nature "(p. 313). The fit between a child's innate traits and characteristics and a parent's temperament and personality certainly affects the quality of their relationship and the child's ability to establish secure attachments and develop positive coping skills. Ganiban and her colleagues (2011) discovered that children's negative emotionality is moderately associated with parent negativity and modestly related to parental warmth. Some children may experience a rocky start in life in part due to the mismatch between their temperament and that of their parents or caregivers. Whatever the cause of their adversity, those who had a difficult infancy or early childhood often manage to rise above it.

Many children exposed to traumatic events demonstrate an ability to adapt to this adversity, which is known as **resiliency**. Pignotti (2011) examined reactive attachment disorder among children who spent time in orphanages and institutions prior to being adopted internationally. Although some of these children developed serious chronic problems, "others have been shown to be resilient in spite of their early history of institutional neglect" (p. 30). Similarly, many children of military personnel who have been deployed are considered to be quite resilient despite being faced with the unique stressor of knowing that their parent is in harm's way and might not return home from war (Lincoln & Sweeten, 2011). Resiliency is a topic of great interest to developmental psychologists because it is not simply something people are born with or without. Numerous innate and environmental factors—including intelligence, temperament, socioeconomic status, and level of parental involvement—work together to influence the extent to which children develop resilience.

Most of us are resilient to some degree, and with support from others and significant choices on our part we can grow in healthy ways despite these negative early experiences. Our present and future existence does not have to be restricted by unfortunate events in our past.

At this point, pause and ask yourself these questions:

▸ How much do I trust others? Myself?

▸ Am I willing to make myself known to a few selected people in my life?

▸ Do I basically accept myself as being OK, or do I seek confirmation outside of myself?

▸ How far will I go in my attempt to be liked? Do I need to be liked and approved of by everyone?

▸ Am I in any way like David or Ashley? Do I know of anyone who has had experiences similar to theirs?

▸ How much do I really know about my early years? What have I heard from my parents and extended family about my infancy and early childhood?

EARLY CHILDHOOD

The tasks children must master in **early childhood** (ages 2–6) include learning independence, accepting personal power, and learning to cope with impulsive and aggressive reactions and behavior. The critical task is to begin the journey toward autonomy by progressing from being taken care of by others to meeting some of their own physical needs. According to Armstrong (2007), the "gift" of this stage of life is *playfulness*. When young children play, they re-create the world anew. They take *what is* and combine it with *what is possible* to fashion new events.

Erikson (1963) identified the core struggle of early childhood, which for him ranges from ages 1 to 3, as the conflict of **autonomy versus shame and doubt**. Children who fail to master the task of establishing some control over themselves and coping with the world around them develop a sense of shame, and they doubt their capabilities. Erikson emphasized that during this time children become aware of their emerging skills and have a drive to try them out. To illustrate this point, I (Marianne) remember when I was feeding one of our daughters during her infancy. Heidi had been a very agreeable child who swallowed all of the food I put into her mouth. One day, much to my surprise, she spit it right back at me! No matter how much I wanted her to continue eating, she refused. This was one way in which Heidi began asserting herself with me. As my children were growing up, I strove to establish a good balance between having them develop their own identity and at the same time providing them with guidance and appropriate limits.

During early childhood, great strides in language and motor development are made. This is a time for the beginning of an increased understanding of what it means to be interdependent. Goleman (2006) points to the importance of developing *emotional competence*, especially learning to regulate and control emotions and to delay gratification. Peer relationships are

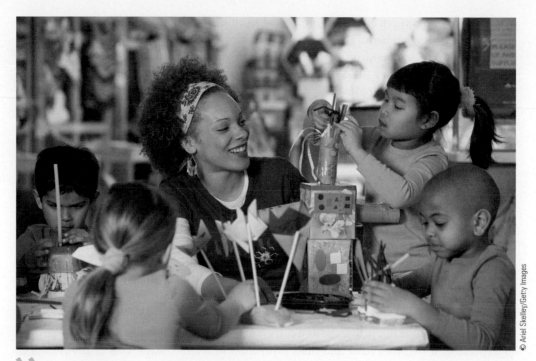

>> In the preschool years, children widen their circle of significant persons and learn more complex social skills.

particularly critical at this time, and children need to acquire a cooperative spirit and the ability to share. This is a time when children begin to become aware of themselves in relation to the world around them. They also become aware of "otherness" in terms of gender, race, and disability (McGoldrick et al., 2011b).

Erikson (1963) identified the preschool years (ages 3–6) as being characterized by play and by anticipation of roles. During this time, children try to find out how much they can do. They imitate others; they begin to develop a sense of right and wrong; they widen their circle of significant persons; they take more initiative; they learn to give and receive love and affection; they identify with their own gender; they begin to learn more complex social skills; they learn basic attitudes regarding sexuality; and they increase their capacity to understand and use language.

According to Erikson, the basic task of these preschool years is to establish a sense of competence and initiative. The core struggle is between **initiative and guilt**. Preschool children begin to initiate many of their own activities as they become physically and psychologically ready to engage in pursuits of their own choosing. If they are allowed realistic freedom to make some of their own decisions, they tend to develop a positive orientation characterized by confidence in their ability to initiate and follow through. If they are unduly restricted or their choices are ridiculed, however, they tend to experience a sense of guilt and ultimately to withdraw from taking an active stance. One middle-aged woman we talked with still finds herself extremely vulnerable to being seen as foolish. She recalls that during her childhood family members laughed at her attempts to perform certain tasks. She incorporated certain messages she received from her family, and these messages greatly influenced her attitudes and actions. Even now she vividly carries these pictures in her head, and to some extent these messages continue to control her life.

Parents who squelch any emerging individuality and who do too much for their children hamper their development. They are saying, however indirectly, "Let us do this for you because you're too clumsy, too slow, or too inept to do things for yourself." Young children need to experiment; they need to be allowed to make mistakes and still feel that they are basically worthwhile. If parents insist on keeping their children dependent on them, the children will begin to doubt their own abilities. If parents do not respect and support their children's efforts, the children may feel ashamed of themselves or become insecure and fearful.

Sometimes children may want to do more than they are capable of doing. For example, the 5-year-old son of a friend of ours went on a hike with his father. At one point the boy asked his father to let him carry a heavy backpack the way the "big people" do. Without saying a word, the father took his backpack off and handed it to his son, who immediately discovered that it was too heavy for him to carry. The boy simply exclaimed, "Dad, it's too heavy for me." He then went happily on his way up the trail. In a safe way the father had allowed his son to discover experientially that he was, indeed, too small. He had also avoided a potential argument with his son.

Young children also must learn to accept the full range of their feelings. They will surely experience anger, and it is important that they know and feel that anger is permissible. Children need to feel loved and accepted with all of their feelings, otherwise they will tend to stifle their anger so as not to lose the love of their parents. When anger cannot be acknowledged or expressed, it becomes toxic and finds expression in indirect ways. One of the results of denying anger is that children may begin to numb their feelings, including joy. Although it is desirable for young children to explore their environment and express themselves, limits and boundaries are key components in teaching children how to manage their feelings and regulate their emotions.

As adults, many of us have difficulty acknowledging our anger, even when it is fully justified. We may swallow our anger and rationalize away other feelings because we learned when we were very young that we were unacceptable when we had such feelings. As children we might have shouted at our parents: "I hate you! I never want to see you again!" Then we may have heard an upset parent reply: "How dare you say such a thing—after all I've done for you! I don't ever want to hear that from you again!" We soon take these messages to mean, "Don't be angry! Never be angry with those you love! Keep control of yourself!" And we do just that, keeping many of our feelings to ourselves, stuffing them in the pit of our stomach and pretending we do not experience them. It is not surprising that so many people suffer from migraine headaches, peptic ulcers, hypertension, and heart disease.

Pause and reflect on some of your own current struggles with these issues:

▶ Am I able to recognize my feelings, particularly if they are "unacceptable" to others?

▶ How was anger expressed in my family?

▶ How do I express anger to those I love?

▶ How was love expressed in my family?

▶ How do I balance depending on others and relying on myself?

▶ Do I let others know what I want? Can I be assertive without being aggressive?

▶ What positive or negative messages did I receive from my parents? Which of these messages did I accept, which did I reject?

▶ Can I recognize when childhood feelings are influencing my choices in relationships and decide to make choices that reflect my current level of emotional awareness instead?

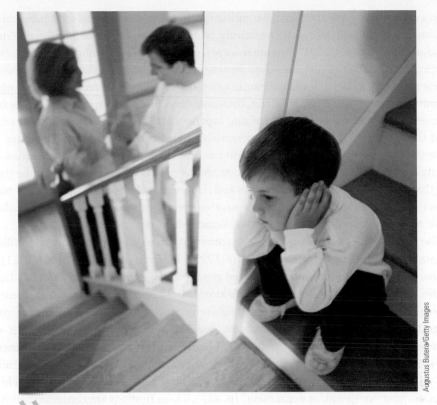

Augustus Butera/Getty Images

» Negative parental interactions can have a lifelong effect on children.

IMPACT OF THE FIRST SIX YEARS OF LIFE

Parenting styles have an impact on early childhood development. Diana Baumrind (1967, 1971, 1978) studied the effects of parenting styles on children's social and intellectual competence. She identified four parenting styles: authoritative, authoritarian, permissive, and neglectful. Authoritative parenting is associated with the most positive behavioral traits in childhood development.

Authoritative parents establish high goals for their children, yet they are accepting and allow their children to explore while maintaining firm limits to help scaffold and structure their children's environment. **Authoritarian parents** are extremely strict, have high demands, and use the threat of physical punishment to control their children. They tend not to allow their children to have input into their world. **Permissive parents** make few demands on their children and tend to indulge their children's desires. **Neglectful parents** are not very accepting of their children, are not greatly involved in their children's lives, but do provide for their children's basic physical needs.

Baumrind found that *authoritative parenting* tends to produce children with self-reliance, self-control, an ability to cope with stress, purposeful behavior, an achievement-orientation, a cooperative attitude, and a curiosity about life. *Authoritarian parenting* tends to result in children with fear, apprehension, passivity, vulnerability to stress, moodiness, and a lack of purpose. *Permissive parenting* tends to produce children with characteristics of rebellion, low self-reliance and self-control, impulsivity, aimlessness, and low achievement. Although parenting styles used during the first 6 years of our life do not determine our adult personality, they are a key factor in how we develop and the kinds of behavioral traits we acquire.

In a recent study, authoritarian parenting was negatively associated with parental legitimacy, and parental legitimacy was negatively associated with future delinquency (Trinkner, Cohn, Rebellon, & Gundy, 2012). In other words, the more parents embraced a philosophy of parenting captured by the sentiment "it's my way or the highway," the less they were perceived by their teenagers as being legitimate authorities. These teens were more likely to engage in delinquent behavior over time. However, these negative childhood experiences can be seen as challenges to address rather than as defining experiences that necessarily limit us as adults.

At times parents may be unduly anxious about wanting to be perfect. They may spend time worrying about "doing the right thing at the right time" and are concerned about their style of parenting and its affect on their children. This chronic anxiety can be the very thing that causes difficulties as their sons and daughters will soon sense that they must be "perfect children." Children can and do survive the mistakes that all parents make, but chronic neglect or overprotection can have negative long-term effects.

The label **helicopter parenting** was coined in reference to parenting the millennial generation (those born between 1982 and 1995). LeMoyne and Buchanon (2011) state that the millennials are "the most protected generation of children in our nation's history" (p. 399). "While earlier generations of children would spend the day riding their bikes and playing outside with friends, completely out of reach of their parents, today's parents use the cell phone, often called *the electronic umbilical cord, . . .* to constantly check on the whereabouts of their children" (p. 400). LeMoyne and Buchanon's research shows that these students feel more negatively about themselves and have lower levels of overall well-being. Moreover, the "[c]hildren of perceived helicopter parents are also more likely to be medicated for anxiety and/or depression" (p. 412). These findings are consistent with Mia's experience as the child of two overprotective parents.

MIA'S STORY

I recently heard the term *helicopter parent* for the first time, and that struck a chord with me. It describes my parents perfectly. I am an only child, and I sometimes wonder what my life would have been like if I had a sibling to share some of the focus. My parents overprotected me to the point that they did everything for me. My mother was a constant worrier as far back as I can remember, and my father was a "doer" and a "fixer"—a real take charge kind of man. They nurtured me, so I hesitate to complain about them, but it felt stifling. As I was growing up, they were so concerned that the school environment was not good enough for me that they pulled me out and homeschooled me starting in second grade. So I was with them all the time (my mom and dad run a small business, so one of them was always overseeing my instruction and monitoring my progress). I had play dates with other kids for "socialization purposes" and had many scheduled activities that my parents "managed." I excelled academically, especially in math, and I think they were concerned that if I made my own decisions and got off track, I would not fulfill my potential. That felt like a lot of pressure.

When I left for college, their over protectiveness continued. I guess I was naïve to think it would just stop. Sure enough, I received phone calls three to four times a day, seven days a week for the first semester. They still call several times a week—well actually, every night, but just once a day. That is an improvement. I am about ready to enter my senior year of college, and although I am academically accomplished, I don't feel confident about making decisions at all. I never really had to, so I didn't get practice being a decision maker. That may sound like a minor problem to whine about, but you have no idea what it is like to grow up being "micromanaged." My parents' intentions were good, so I feel guilty for being angry at them for depriving me of the chance to make my own decisions and to be imperfect. I have started to see a counselor on campus because I have been feeling anxious and depressed. I will graduate from college in a year, but I still feel like a dependent little girl in a lot of ways.

You may be asking yourself why we are emphasizing the events of the first 6 years of development. In our work with clients, we continue to see the influence of these early years on their levels of integration and functioning as adults. Many of these childhood experiences have a profound impact on both the present and the future. If you reached faulty conclusions based on your early life experiences, you may still be operating on the basis of them. If you told yourself as a child, "I can never do enough for my father," then as an adult you may feel that you can never do enough (or be enough) to meet the expectations of those who are significant in your life. Not only is our current functioning influenced by early interpretations, but our future is too. Our goals and purposes have some connection with the way we dealt with emerging issues during the first 6 years of life.

In working in counseling groups with relatively well-functioning adults who have "normal" developmental issues, we find that a new understanding of their early years often entails a certain degree of emotional pain. Yet by understanding these painful events, they have a basis for transcending them and can avoid replaying old self-defeating themes throughout their lifetime. We do not think healthy people are ever really "cured" of their vulnerabilities. For example, during your preschool years, if you felt abandoned by the divorce of your parents, you are still likely to have vestiges of doubts and fears when forming

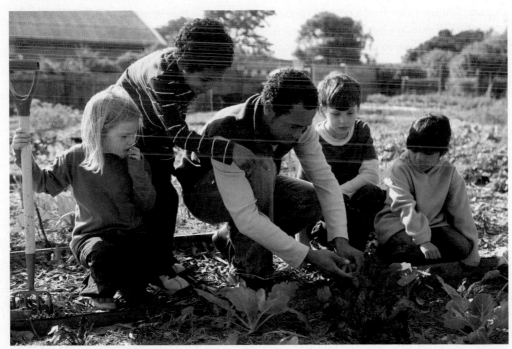

Alistair Berg/Getty Images

》 Our early experiences influence our later development.

54

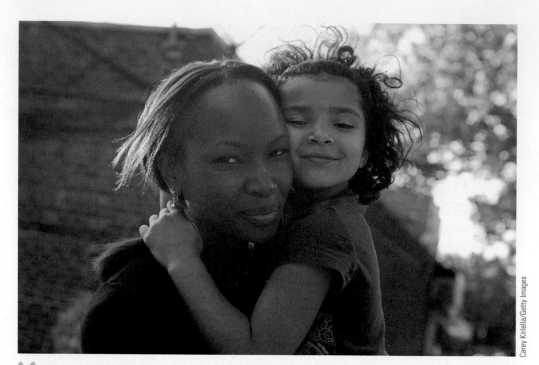

Carey Kirkella/Getty Images

>> A sense of being loved during the early years is the best safeguard against insecurity and inadequacy.

close relationships. You do not have to surrender to these traces of mistrust. Instead, you can gain control of your fears of loving and trusting.

In reviewing your childhood, you may find aspects that you like and do not want to change. You may also find a certain continuity in your life that is meaningful to you. At the same time, if you are honest with yourself, you are likely to become aware of certain revisions you would like to make. This awareness is the first critical step toward change.

Typical problems and conflicts we encounter among people in our therapeutic groups include members' inability to trust themselves and others; an inability to freely accept and give love; difficulty recognizing and expressing the full range of their feelings; guilt over feelings of anger toward loved ones; difficulty in accepting their role as a woman or a man; and problems concerning a lack of meaning or purpose in life or a clear sense of personal identity and aspirations. These adult problems are directly related to the turning points and tasks of the early developmental years. The effects of early learning are reversible in most cases, but these experiences, whether favorable or unfavorable, do influence how we interpret both present and future critical periods in our lives.

Some people learn new values, come to accept new feelings and attitudes, and overcome much of their past negative conditioning. Other people hang on to the past. We cannot change in a positive direction unless we stop blaming others for the way we are now. Statements that begin "If it hadn't been for..." are too often used to justify our fear of change. Blaming others for our present struggles ultimately keeps us trapped. When we become aware of pointing a finger at someone else, it is good to look at our other fingers—pointing back at us! Once we are able to see in ourselves the very traits that we accuse others of, we are able to take charge of our own life. It is imperative that we eventually reclaim the power we have given to others. When we recognize and exercise the power we now have, we increase our choices to move in new directions.

1. Close your eyes and reflect for a moment on your memories of your first 6 years. Attempt to identify your earliest concrete single memory—something you actually remember that happened to you, not something you were told about. Spend a few minutes recalling the details and reexperiencing the feelings associated with this early event.

   ▶ Write down your earliest recollection. _My dad hugging me as he _
   _waited for a good scary 20 seconds before _
   calming down.

   ▶ What is your main memory of each family member? _Mom being loving and _
   a medicine cabinet full of medicine.
   _____

2. Reflect on the events that most stand out for you during your first 6 years of life. In particular, think about your place in your family, your family's reaction to you, and your reactions to each person in your family. What connections do you see between how it felt to be in your family as a child and how you now feel in various social situations? What speculations do you have concerning the impact your family had then and the effect that these experiences continue to have on your current personality? _____
   _____
   _____

3. Take the following self-inventory. Respond quickly, marking "T" if you believe the statement is more true than false for you as a young child and "F" if it tends not to fit your early childhood experiences.

   _____ As a young child, I felt loved and accepted.
   _____ I basically trusted the world.
   _____ I felt that I was an acceptable and valuable person.
   _____ I felt I needed to work for others' approval.
   _____ I experienced a great deal of shame and self-doubt as a child.
   _____ I felt that it was not OK for me to express anger.
   _____ I was trusted to do things for myself.
   _____ I believe I developed a natural and healthy concept of my body and my gender-role identity.
   _____ I had very few friends as a young child.
   _____ I felt that I could talk to significant people about my problems.

Look over your responses. What do they tell you about the person you now are? If you could live your childhood over again, how would you like it to be? How do you think your early childhood experiences have shaped your views about what you consider to be effective parenting? From what you have read in this chapter so far, how does this information challenge or redefine some of your thinking about the role of the first 6 years of life on your personality development? Record your responses in the journal pages provided at the end of the chapter.

MIDDLE CHILDHOOD

During **middle childhood** (ages 6–12), children face these key developmental tasks: engage in social activities; expand their knowledge and understanding of the physical and social worlds; continue to learn and expand their concepts of femininity and masculinity (and gender identity); develop a sense of values; learn new communication skills; learn how to read, write, and calculate; learn to give and take; learn how to accept people who are culturally different; learn to tolerate ambiguity; and learn physical skills. According to Armstrong (2007), imagination is a key "gift" during the first half of this stage. The sense of an inner subjective self develops, and this sense of self is alive with images taken from the environment. During the second half of this stage, ingenuity is a key characteristic. Older children acquire a range of social and technical skills that enables them to deal with the increasing pressure they are facing.

Issues of industry, mastery, achievement, social skills, and interpersonal sensitivity are all key themes during this stage. The achievements of middle childhood contribute in significant ways to our ability to cope with the demands of later periods of development (Newman & Newman, 2012). McGoldrick and colleagues (2011b) point out that during middle childhood there is an increased understanding of self in terms of gender, race, culture, and abilities; of self in relation to family, peers, and community; and an increase in the capacity for empathy. These authors add that by ages 9 to 12 children begin to form an identification with causes, aspirations, and privileges of groups they belong to, which provides the motivation for them to think and act in certain ways. A key social ability in children is empathy, which involves understanding the feelings of others, being able to take others' perspective, and respecting differences in how people feel about things. This empathy includes being able to understand distress beyond an immediate situation and to feel for the plight of an entire group such as those who are oppressed or live in poverty (Goleman, 2006).

According to Erikson (1963), the major struggle of middle childhood is between **industry and inferiority**. The central task of this period is to achieve a sense of industry; failure to do so results in a sense of inadequacy and inferiority. Development of a sense of industry includes focusing on creating and producing and on attaining goals. Starting school is a critical event of this time. The first 4 years of school are vital to successful completion of a healthy outcome of this stage. The child's self-concept is especially fragile before the fourth grade; if teachers are critical of a child's performance, this could have a lasting impact. Children who encounter failure during the early grades may experience severe handicaps later on. A child with early learning problems, such as dyslexia, may begin to feel worthless as a person. Such a feeling may, in turn, drastically affect his or her relationships with peers, which are also vital at this time. Helen's story illustrates some of the common conflicts of the elementary school years.

HELEN'S STORY

I started kindergarten a bit too early and was smaller than most of the other children. I had looked forward to beginning school, but I soon felt overwhelmed. I began to fail at many of the tasks other children were enjoying and mastering. Gradually, I began to avoid even simple tasks and to find excuses for my failures. I became increasingly afraid of making mistakes, and I thought that everything I did had to be perfect.

My teachers thought I was sensitive and needed a lot of encouragement and direction, but I continued to quit too soon because I didn't think my work was "good enough." When I was in the third grade, I was at least a grade level behind in reading, despite having repeated kindergarten. I began to feel stupid and embarrassed because I couldn't read as well as the other children, and I did not want to read aloud. Eventually, I received instruction in remedial reading. I liked this attention, but then they gave me some reading tests and I didn't do well. I hate taking tests, and I always think I will fail.

I might have given up on school a long time ago, but many people helped me continue in spite of my fears. I am in college now, and I am still anxious about taking tests. I am learning to control my feelings of inadequacy and self-doubt, and I am arguing back to those old voices that say I am basically inadequate.

Helen's case indicates that the first few years of school can have a powerful impact on a child's life and future adjustment to school. Her school experiences colored her view of her self-worth and affected her relationships with other children.

At this point ask yourself these questions:

▶ Can I identify in any ways with Helen's feelings?

▶ What struggles did I experience in forming my self-concept?

▶ Does Helen remind me of anyone I know?

Forming a self-concept is a major task of middle childhood. Let's take a closer look at what this entails.

Developing a Self-Concept

The term self-concept refers to your awareness about yourself. It is your picture of yourself that includes your perceptions about the kind of person you are; your view of your worth, value, and possibilities; the way you see yourself in relation to others; the way you ideally would like to be; and the degree to which you accept yourself as you are. From ages 6 to 12 the view you have of yourself is influenced greatly by the quality of your school experiences, by contact with your peer group and with teachers, by your cultural context, and by your interactions with your family. To a large extent, your self-concept is formed by what others tell you about yourself, especially during the formative years of childhood. Whether you develop a positive or negative outlook on yourself has a good deal to do with what people close to you have expected of you. One's self-concept also may be negatively affected by the presence of disabilities or illnesses such as cerebral palsy (Nadeau & Tessier, 2011), deafness (van Gent, Goedhart, & Treffers, 2011), or dyslexia (Burden, 2008), to name just a few.

This view of yourself influences how you present yourself to others and how you act and feel when you are with them. For example, you may feel inadequate around authority figures. Perhaps you tell yourself that you have nothing to say or that whatever you might say would be stupid. More often than not, others will see and respond to you in the way you "tell" them you are, both verbally and nonverbally. Monitor the messages you are sending to others about yourself, and become aware of the patterns you might be perpetuating. It is difficult for those who are close to you to treat you in a positive way when you consistently discount yourself. Others cannot give you what you will not give to yourself. In contrast, people with a positive self-concept are likely to behave confidently, which causes others to react to them positively.

Once we have established our self-concept, a variety of strategies are available to help us maintain and protect it from outside threats. Next we discuss how these various ego-defenses are aimed at coping with anxiety.

Protecting the Self: Ego-Defense Mechanisms

Ego-defense mechanisms are psychological strategies we use to protect our self-concept from unpleasant emotions. We use these protective devices at various stages of life to soften the blows of harsh reality. Ego defenses typically originate during the early and middle childhood years, and later experiences during adolescence and adulthood reinforce some of these self-defense styles. At times external reality can threaten our perception of being capable of dealing with stress, which creates anxiety. To reduce the anxiety temporarily, we develop ego-defense mechanisms that distort either the sense of self or the realities of the world. We often carry these habitual responses into adulthood as a way to cope with anxiety. These distortions ultimately inhibit our capacity to develop and grow.

We will use Helen's story to illustrate the nature and functioning of some of these ego defenses. For the most part Helen made poor adjustments to her school and social life during her childhood years. Other children stayed away from her because of her aggressive and unfriendly behavior. She did not like her elementary school experience, and her teachers were not helpful to her. Helen's behavioral style in coping with the pressures of school included blaming the outside world for her difficulties. In the face of these failures in life, she might have made use of any one or a combination of the following ego-defense mechanisms.

Repression The mechanism of repression is one of the most important processes in psychoanalytic theory, and it is the basis of many other ego defenses. By pushing threatening or painful thoughts and feelings from awareness, we sometimes manage the anxiety that grows out of situations involving guilt and conflict. Repression may block out stressful experiences that could be met by realistically facing and working through a situation. Helen was unaware of her dependence/independence struggles with her parents; she was also unaware of how her painful experiences of failure were contributing to her feelings of inferiority and insecurity. Helen had unconsciously excluded most of her failures and had not allowed them to come to the surface of awareness.

Denial Denial plays a defensive role similar to that of repression, but it generally operates at a preconscious or conscious level. In denial there is a conscious effort to suppress unpleasant reality. It is a way of distorting what the individual thinks, feels, or perceives to be a stressful situation. Helen simply "closed her eyes" to her failures in school. Even though she had evidence that she was not performing well academically, she refused to acknowledge this reality.

Displacement Displacement involves redirecting emotional impulses (usually hostility) from the real object to a substitute person or object. In essence, anxiety is coped with by discharging impulses onto a "safer target." For example, Helen's sister Joan was baffled by the hostility she received from Helen. Joan did not understand why Helen was so critical of her every action. Helen used Joan as the target of her aggression because Joan did exceptionally well at school and was very popular with her peers.

Projection Another mechanism of self-deception is projection, which consists of attributing to others our own unacceptable desires and impulses. We are able to clearly see in others the very traits that we disown in ourselves, which serves the purpose of keeping a certain view of ourselves intact. Typically, projection involves seeing clearly in others actions that would lead to guilt feelings in ourselves. Helen tended to blame everyone but herself for her difficulties in school and in social relationships. She complained that her teachers were unfairly picking on her, that she could never do anything right for them, and that other children were mean to her.

Reaction Formation One defense against a threatening impulse is to actively express the opposite impulse. This involves behaving in a manner that is contrary to one's real feelings. A characteristic of this defense is the excessive quality of a particular attitude or behavior. For example, Helen bristled when her teachers or parents offered to give her help. She was convinced that she did not need anyone's help. Accepting their offers would have indicated that she really was stupid.

Rationalization Rationalization involves manufacturing a false but "good" excuse to justify unacceptable behavior and explain away failures or losses. Such excuses help restore a bruised ego. Helen was quick to find many reasons for the difficulties she encountered, a few of which included sickness, which caused her to fall behind in her classes; teachers who went over the lessons too fast; other children who did not let her play with them; and siblings who kept her awake at night.

Compensation Another defense reaction is compensation, which consists of masking perceived weaknesses or developing certain positive traits to make up for limitations. The adjustive value in this mechanism lies in keeping one's self-esteem intact by excelling in one area to distract attention from an area in which the person is inferior. The more Helen experienced difficulties at school and with her peers, the more she withdrew from others and became absorbed in artwork that she did by herself at home.

Regression Faced with stress, some people revert to a form of immature behavior that they have outgrown. In regression, they attempt to cope with their anxiety by clinging to such inappropriate behaviors. Faced with failure in both her social and school life, Helen had a tendency to engage in emotional tirades, crying a lot, storming into her room, and refusing to come out for hours.

Fantasy Fantasy involves gratifying frustrated desires by imaginary achievements. When achievement in the real world seems remote, some people resort to screening out unpleasant aspects of reality and living in their world of dreams. During her childhood, Helen developed a rich fantasy in which she imagined herself to be an actress. She played with her dolls for hours and talked to herself. In her daydreams she saw herself in the movies, surrounded by famous people.

Although ego-defense mechanisms have some adaptive value, their overuse can be problematic. Self-deception can soften harsh reality, but the fact is that reality does not change through the process of distorting those aspects of it that produce anxiety. When these defensive strategies do not work, the long-term result is an even greater degree of anxiety. Overreliance on these defenses leads to a vicious circle—as the defenses lose their value in holding anxiety in check, people step up the use of other defenses.

All defenses are not self-defeating, however, and there is a proper place for them, especially when stresses are great. In the face of certain crises, for example, defenses can enable people to cope at least temporarily until they can build up other resources, both from their environment and from within themselves. For instance, people of all ages can be encouraged to adopt positive coping strategies such as relaxation, reflection/journaling, positive self-talk, and mindfulness.

Spend some time reflecting on the defense mechanisms you used during your childhood years.

1. Do you see any similarities between the defenses you employed as a child and those you sometimes use at this time in your life? _____

_____

_____

2. List some of the defenses you use, and examine how they protect you and hinder you.

_____

_____

3. How would your life be different if you had no ego defenses? _My life__

might not be in existence if I did not gather my

ego defenses.

4. What are some positive coping skills you might use instead of ego defenses to help strengthen your self-concept? _____

_____

_____

PUBESCENCE

The years from about 11 to 14 constitute a stage of transition between childhood and adolescence. For girls, **pubescence** generally occurs between the ages of 11 and 13; for boys it is between the ages of 12 and 14. This stage is sometimes called the "tween" period—not quite a child, not quite a teenager. During this phase, boys and girls experience major physical, psychological, and sexual changes. Most people find the pubescent period particularly difficult. It is a paradoxical time. Preadolescents are not treated as mature adults, yet they are often expected to act as though they had reached maturity. Fashion marketing, music advertising, and social networking promote a pseudomaturity. Continually testing the limits, young people have a strong urge to break away from dependent ties that restrict their freedom. It is not uncommon for preadolescents to be frightened and lonely, but they may mask their fears with rebellion and cover up their need to be dependent by exaggerating their independence. They typically find that they have a voice, and they are willing to use it.

Much of preadolescent rebellion is an attempt to declare their uniqueness and to establish a separate identity. This is the time when individuals assert who and what they want to be. With the proliferation of social networking sites, preadolescents are increasingly using technology to express their individuality. Among youths 12 and 13 years old, 55% have a social networking profile page (Lenhart, Purcell, Smith, & Zickuhr, 2010). The benefits associated with social networking include opportunities for sociability and self-expression, but concerns about the frequent use of this technology are also expressed. Some young people spend so much time on the sites that time available for other activities such as schoolwork and face-to-face social pursuits is diminished (Baker & White, 2010). With the constant information flow on Facebook, Twitter, and other platforms, could preadolescents be destined to experience socially induced attention problems?

As infants we must learn to trust ourselves and others; as preadolescents we need to find a meaning in life and adult role models in whom we believe. As toddlers we begin to assert our rights as independent people by struggling for autonomy; as preadolescents we make choices that will shape our future. As preschoolers we try to achieve a sense of competence; as preadolescents and as adolescents we explore choices about what we want from life, what we can succeed in, what kind of education we want, and what career may suit us. Preadolescents are increasingly focused on the important tasks of learning how to select friends and on developing the social and interpersonal skills necessary to form healthy friendships. The foundation for building good relationships throughout our life span is laid during this life stage.

ADOLESCENCE

Adolescence spans the period from about age 13 for girls and age 14 or 15 for boys until the late teens or to about age 20. Adolescence is a critical period in the development of personal identity. It is a time marked by the interplay of biological, social, and psychological factors. Armstrong (2007) describes the unique "gift" of this stage of life as *passion*. A powerful set of changes in the adolescent body is reflected in sexual, emotional, cultural, and spiritual passion and a deep inner zeal for life.

The adolescent period is a time of searching for an identity and clarifying a personal system of values. One of the most important needs of this period is to experience successes that will lead to a sense of individuality and connectedness, which in turn lead to self-confidence and self-respect. Adolescents need opportunities to explore and understand the wide range of their experiences and to learn how to communicate with significant others in such a way that they can make their wants, feelings, thoughts, and beliefs known. Young people often look beyond their own needs and may identify with causes as a way to establish their identity. They want to address injustices, and their increasing sense of empathy is revealed in a dedication to helping others (Goleman, 2006).

Adolescence is a time when young people evolve their sexual and gender identities, learn to form intimate relationships, and learn to function in an increasingly independent manner. Adolescents renegotiate their identity and relationship with their parents, acquire a range of new attitudes and skills, develop an ethical and spiritual sense, and continue the process of defining their gender-role identity. Adolescence is marked by intrapersonal discovery and **self-authorship**, which starts in adolescence and continues well into the 20s. A sense of **self-efficacy** develops from learning to take control of one's life when one often feels out of control. A related theme is a sense of **self-sufficiency**, which is expressed by making decisions, assuming personal responsibility for one's choices, and achieving a degree of financial independence (Newman & Newman, 2012). This move toward autonomy is an important developmental milestone for many young adults.

For Erikson (1963), the major developmental conflicts of adolescence center on clarification of who they are, where they are going, and how they are going to get there. He sees the core struggle of adolescence as **identity versus role confusion**. Failure to achieve a sense of identity results in role confusion. Young people are moving from a relatively egocentric orientation to a perspective that includes acknowledging the thoughts, feelings, and values of others. As adolescents struggle with feeling unfairly treated, unduly judged, harshly punished, and misunderstood, their capacity to begin to think outside of themselves fosters individual growth and development.

Young people may feel pressured to make an occupational choice, to compete in the job market or in college, to become financially independent, or to commit themselves to physically and emotionally intimate relationships. In Western cultures it is ideal for the adolescent to have opportunities to make these decisions with the faith and support of caring adults. Teens with immigrant parents in the United States see their peers having the right to exercise freedom to make their own decisions and are exposed to academic and media messages reinforcing these freedoms. Their parents, who have values and traditions from their own culture, may see parents' wishes for their children as more important than the wishes of teens. The differences in assimilation to the dominant American culture can create conflict for parents and teens in immigrant families. Consider the dilemma that Jin-Sang is facing.

JIN-SANG'S STORY

We immigrated to Boston when I was around 10. My parents said that my sister and I would have better educational opportunities in the United States, and they made a lot of sacrifices so we could attend prestigious private schools. As the oldest child in my family, there is a lot of pressure on me to succeed academically and one day earn an MD from a prestigious medical school such as Harvard or Johns Hopkins.

I have discovered that many of my American peers have a lot more leeway to decide what they want to do with their lives, and if I am honest, it makes me resentful of my own parents. It is hard to be surrounded by people who have the freedom to pursue what *they* want instead of what their parents want for them. My classmates tease me because they think I am too childlike for not standing up to my parents and breaking free from their control. So I feel caught between these two cultures much of the time. I feel pressure from my parents, and I feel pressure from my friends at school.

My real desire is to become a science fiction writer, but I could never tell my parents this. They would feel disrespected and would be ashamed of me. In fact, my whole extended family back in Korea would be disappointed and would consider me ungrateful because my parents moved to Boston for my sake. I would bring shame to my family. That's kind of a heavy burden. At this time, I haven't decided how I am going to handle this dilemma. Am I going to disappoint my family by following my dream, or am I going to disappoint myself by following their dream for me?

The question of options is made even more urgent by the myth that the choices we make during adolescence bind us for the rest of our lives. Adolescents who believe this myth will be hesitant to experiment and test out many options. Too many young people yield to pressures to decide too early what they will be and what serious commitments they will make. Thus they may never realize the range of possibilities open to them. To deal with this problem, Erikson (1963) suggested a **psychological moratorium**—a period during which society would give permission to adolescents to experiment with different roles and values so they could sample life before making major commitments.

In their struggle to separate themselves from their parents and establish their own identity, peer groups become increasingly important. In today's world, many adolescents connect with their peer groups via their cell phones and the Internet. An extremely high percentage (82%) of youths between the ages of 14 and 17 have embraced social networking sites such as Facebook and MySpace (Lenhart et al., 2010). The peer group can be the most influential and positive force in a teenager's life, outweighing parents' wishes and other social forces, but it also can be a very negative force. Some adolescents bend to peer pressure and conform to the expectations of their friends, losing a sense of themselves. If the need to be accepted and liked is stronger than the need to be true to their own values, adolescents will most likely find themselves behaving in inauthentic ways and increasingly looking to others to tell them what and who they should be. One potential danger associated with exercising poor judgment in the age of social networking is that prospective employers, teachers, administrators, counselors, law enforcement, and college admissions officers may use the Internet as a tool to learn more about an individual's character (Patchin & Hinduja, 2010). Significant real-world consequences, such as sabotaging future academic and professional activities, can result from posting distasteful or incriminating content online.

For the typical adolescent, social relationships assume primary importance. Adolescents utilize these relationships to learn about self, the world, and others. When there are problems in this domain, the adolescent years can be extremely lonely ones; it is not unusual for adolescents to feel that they are alone in their conflicts and self-doubt. It is a period of life when young people feel a need for universal approval, yet they must learn to distinguish between living for others' approval and earning their own. This orientation toward the social world enhances their need for independence.

A crucial part of the identity-formation process is **individuation**, separating from our family system and establishing our own identity based on our experiences. This process of psychological separation from parental ties is the most agonizing part of the adolescent struggle and lays the foundation for future development. Although achieving psychological

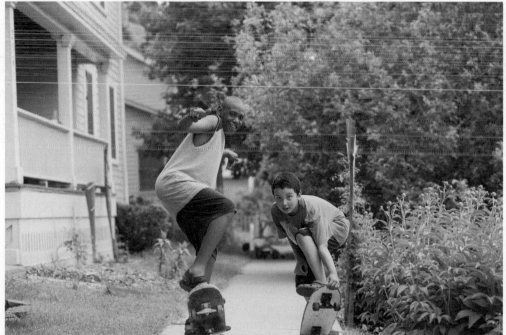

>> Adolescents have a need for self-expression and establishing a separate identity.

separation from one's family is a common theme in Western cultures, the wishes of parents continue to have a major influence on the behavior of adult children in some cultures. Adolescent development cannot be understood without taking into consideration the cultural context. Adolescents often delve deeper into exploring their unique sense of what their cultural identity means to them during this time period. Some collectivistic cultures foster dependence as a means of building bonds and community, keeping children dependent well beyond when mainstream Americans do. Children reared in collectivistic cultures often feel nurtured, not ashamed.

Feminist therapists view the early adolescent period as a time for expanding relationships with parents—not "getting rid" of parents (Miller & Stiver, 1997). More than needing "separation" from their parents, both preadolescents and adolescents need to *change* their relationship with their parents. If adolescents are able to maintain trustworthy connections with parents, they will be better able to undertake other changes they need to make. The most resilient adolescents have strong social skills and open, healthy relationships with their parents. This connection to their family is crucial for long-term success.

Adolescents confront dilemmas similar to those faced by older people in our society. Both age groups need to find a meaning in life and must cope with feelings of uselessness. Older people may be forced to retire and may encounter difficulty replacing work activities; young people have not completed their education or acquired the skills necessary for many occupations. Instead, they are in a constant process of preparation for the future. Even in their families, adolescents may feel unneeded.

Forming a philosophy of life is a central task of adolescence, as young people are defining who they want to be as adults. Sexual, religious, spiritual, moral, and racial issues take on a new perspective and are subject to new understanding and revision (McGoldrick et al., 2011b). Systems in the young person's ecological context (school, neighborhood, and socioeconomic status) have an influence on this search for identity and the development of beliefs, goals, and attitudes. Young people are also developing critical thinking skills and making choices that will affect the rest of their lives. Many adolescents are faced with an array of complex choices such as peer pressure for using drugs and biological drives (sexual urges) before they have developed the cognitive capacity to make fully considered choices. Adolescents are faced with choosing the beliefs and values that will guide their actions as adults. In meeting this challenge, young people need adequate models because a sense of moral living is largely learned by example. Adolescents are especially sensitive to duplicity and are quick to spot insincere people who tell them how they ought to live while themselves living in very different ways. They learn values by observing and interacting with adults who are positive examples rather than by being preached to. Of course, not all role models are positive. In some cases adolescents adopt drug dealers or other criminals as role models, and they may acquire a negative identity by seeking affiliation with a gang.

Today's adolescents also have to cope with violence at school and violence in the world. It is not uncommon for adolescents, and even children, to bring guns or knives to school. News reports of an adolescent injuring fellow classmates or a teacher are all too common. Not only do today's teens have to contend with peer pressure, parental pressure, and the confusion and pain that accompanies finding their identities, they also have to worry about being shot by a schoolmate or being the victim of some other form of violence or intimidation. This fear of the unpredictability of daily life often generates a good deal of realistic anxiety.

Cyberbullying is "the use of electronic communication technologies to intentionally engage in repeated or widely disseminated cruel acts towards another that results in emotional harm" (Willard, 2011, p. 75). A formidable threat among teens, this kind of electronic aggression is a contributing factor in altercations that occur on school campuses, and it can lead to a number of physical, social, and emotional problems. These include somatic symptoms such as headaches, stomache aches, and sleeping difficulties as well as low self-esteem and depression, and avoidance of school, resulting in academic failure. And the unthinkable can occur too—suicide or homicide. Perpetrators of school-based homicides are twice as likely to have been victims of bullying (Anderson et al., 2001). Equally as alarming, Hinduja and Patchin (2010) found that adolescents who experienced either traditional bullying or cyberbullying, as an offender or a victim, were more inclined to have suicidal thoughts and were more likely to attempt suicide than those who had not experienced such forms of peer aggression. Willard (2011) adds that **sexting**, a more recent trend that entails sending nude images via cell phone texting, is an increasingly challenging concern. Willard views cyberbullying and sexting as related matters.

Adolescents who belong to certain racial or cultural groups are the targets of racism, and they often encounter discrimination and oppression both at school and in society at large. Beverly Daniel Tatum (1999) writes about racial identity development in adolescence and raises the question, "Why are all the Black kids sitting together in the cafeteria?" When a group of Black teens sit together in the cafeteria, school administrators want to understand why this is so and how this can be prevented. Tatum's (1999) response is that such a racial grouping is a developmental process in response to the environmental stressor of racism. She adds:

> Joining with one's peers for support in the face of stress is a positive coping strategy. What is problematic is that the young people are operating with a very limited definition of what it means to be Black, based largely on cultural stereotypes. (p. 62)

Tatum's racial identity development concept can be applied to young people from other racial and ethnic groups as well. During adolescence, race becomes personally salient for people of color as they search for answers to questions such as "What does it mean to be a young person in my racial and cultural group?" "How should I act?" "What should I do?" These teens absorb many of the beliefs and values of the dominant society and may come to value the role models and lifestyles that are portrayed by the dominant group more highly than those of their own cultural or racial group. As a result of their heightened awareness of the significance of race, young people of color often grapple with what it means to be targeted by racism. In response to their growing awareness of the systematic exclusion of people from their racial and cultural group from full participation in the dominant society, many of these youths experience anger and resentment. This may lead to the development of an oppositional social identity, which protects young people of color from the psychological assault of racism and keeps the dominant group at bay.

Our childhood experiences have a direct influence on how we approach the adolescent years, and how well we master the tasks of adolescence has a bearing on our ability to cope with the critical turning points of adulthood. If we do not develop a clear sense of identity during adolescence, finding meaning in adult life becomes extremely difficult. As we progress from one stage of life to the next, we at times meet with roadblocks and detours and may experience anxiety, depression, or alienation. These barriers are often the result of having failed to master basic psychological competencies at an earlier period. When we encounter such obstacles, we can accept them as signposts and continue down the same path or use them as opportunities for growth. Miller and Stiver (1997) contend that these roadblocks can be turned to pathways of connection between people, which leads to the development of healthy individuals.

In sum, for most people adolescence is a difficult period, characterized by paradoxes: they strive for closeness, yet they also fear intimacy and often avoid it; they rebel against control, yet they want direction and structure; although they push and test limits imposed on them, they see some limits as a sign of caring; they are not given complete autonomy, yet they are often expected to act as though they were mature adults; they are typically highly self-centered, self-conscious, and preoccupied with their own world, yet they are expected to cope with societal demands to go outside themselves by expanding their horizons; they are asked to face and accept reality, and at the same time they are tempted by many avenues of escape; and they are exhorted to think of the future, yet they have strong urges to live for the moment and to enjoy life.

Adolescence is typically a turbulent and fast-moving period of life, often marked by feelings of powerlessness, confusion, and loneliness. It is a time for making critical choices, even the ultimate choice of living fully or bringing about one's own death. Decisions are being made in almost every area of life, and these decisions to a large extent define our identity. Adolescence is a time of tremendous growth and development, and teens are keenly interested in understanding how their early experiences have shaped their current feelings and behaviors. The following Take Time to Reflect provides an opportunity for you to identify some of the choices you made during your adolescent years and to clarify the impact these experiences continue to exert on you today.

TAKE TIME TO REFLECT

Review the choices open to adolescents, and especially think of the choices you remember having made at this time in your life. How do you think those choices have influenced the person you are today?

1. What major choices did you struggle with during your adolescent years? _____
_____
_____

2. How do you think your adolescence affected the person you are today? _____
_____
_____

3. What positive skills or strengths did you gain from your adolescence that influence the way you solve problems and approach the world as an adult? _____
_____
_____

4. What factors in your environment influenced development of your identity as an adolescent? _____
_____
_____

SUMMARY

A road map of the developmental tasks of the life span reveals that each stage presents certain challenges and offers particular opportunities. Crises can be seen as challenges to be met rather than as catastrophic events that happen to us. In normal development, critical turning points and choices appear at each developmental stage. Our early experiences influence the choices we make at later stages in our development, and each stage helps lay the foundation on which we build our adult personality. Developmental stages are not discrete but blend into one another. We all experience each period of life in our own unique ways.

The struggle toward autonomy, or psychological independence, begins in early childhood, takes on major proportions during adolescence and young adulthood, and extends into later adulthood. The process of individuation and the values attached to it are greatly influenced by culture. Actualizing our full potential as a person and learning to stand alone in life, as well as to stand beside others, is a task that is never really finished. Although major life events during childhood and adolescence have an impact on the way that we think, feel, and behave in adult life, we are not hopelessly determined by such events. Instead, we can choose to change our attitude toward these events, which in turn will affect how we behave today.

Critical turning points in our lives are influenced by a variety of biological, psychological, and social factors. Although we may not have direct control of some key elements of our development, such as early experiences and genetics, we have choices about how we interpret these experiences and use them to further our growth. At key turning points in our life we can either successfully resolve the basic conflict or get stuck on the road to development. Understanding your childhood is a key component in developing self-awareness and an appreciation for the growth and discovery you have made. Learning from your childhood experiences and applying these lessons to adult life will help you become the author of your life. As you will see in the next chapter, mastery of these earlier challenges is essential if we are to cope with the problems of adult living.

Where Can I Go From Here?

1. Write an account in your journal of the first 6 years of your life in the journal pages provided at the end of the chapter. Although you may think that you cannot remember much about this time, you can learn more by following these guidelines:

   a. Write down a few key questions that you would like answered about your early years.

   b. Seek out your relatives, and ask them some questions about your early years.

   c. Collect any reminders of your early years, particularly pictures.

   d. If feasible, visit the place or places where you lived and went to school.

2. When you reflect on your childhood and adolescent years, how did your ability to cope with experiences influence the way you cope with present life situations? What healthy coping mechanisms did you adopt? What maladaptive coping mechanisms did you adopt?

3. From among the many exercises in this chapter, choose those that you are willing to integrate into a self-help program during your time in this course. What things are you willing to do to bring about some of the changes you want in your life?

4. Pictures often say more about you than words. What do your pictures reveal about you? Look through any pictures of yourself as a child and adolescent, and see if there are any striking themes. What do most of your pictures suggest about the way you felt about yourself? Bring some of these pictures to class. Have other members look at them and tell you what they think you were like then. Pictures can also be used to tap forgotten memories, which can elicit powerful emotions. Be sure to honor your boundaries and assess your comfort level when you decide what to share with your classmates.

5. Identify individuals who, despite the odds, have proven to be resilient as well as those who have not been so resilient. Think of people you know personally, celebrities and others in the media, and people who are the focus of biographies or autobiographies for this exercise. What are some commonalities among those who are resilient? What do those who fail to thrive have in common?

6. The lives of children and adolescents growing up today are inarguably affected in both positive and negative ways by technology. With your classmates, hold a debate exploring the pros and cons of social media and technology and the central role they play in the lives of youth today.

7. Suggested Readings. The full bibliographic entry for each of these sources can be found in the References and Suggested Readings at the back of the book. For a discussion of the unique "gifts" of each of the stages of life, see Armstrong (2007). A useful book that deals with a psychosocial perspective of the developmental stages of life is Newman and Newman (2012). For a treatment of emotional competence, see Goleman (2006), and for social competence, see Goleman (2007).

WEBSITE RESOURCES

Included here are some valuable websites. For access to these websites, video activities, and other supporting materials, visit Cengage Learning's Counseling CourseMate website for *I Never Knew I Had a Choice*, 10th Edition, at **www.cengagebrain.com.**

ADOLESCENT DIRECTORY ONLINE
http://education.indiana.edu/aboutus/AdolescenceDirectoryonLineADOL/tabid/4785/Default.aspx

Recommended Search Words: "adolescent directory online"

The Center for Adolescent and Family Studies at Indiana University, Bloomington offers resources about adolescents that cover a range of health, mental health, and parenting issues.

AMERICAN ACADEMY OF CHILD AND ADOLESCENT PSYCHIATRY (AACAP): FACTS FOR FAMILIES
www.aacap.org

Recommended Search Words: "American academy of child and adolescent psychiatry"

The materials available from this site deal with a range of psychological concerns of children and adolescents.

AMERICAN ACADEMY OF PEDIATRICS
http://www.aap.org/

Recommended Search Words: "American academy of pediatrics"

This website offers a great deal of information about advocacy and community-based initiatives for the health and well-being of children and adolescents. The site contains links to research and professional resources.

NATIONAL CRIME PREVENTION COUNCIL
http://www.ncpc.org/topics

Recommended Search Words: "National crime prevention council"

Visit this website for information about bullying and cyberbullying, Internet safety, gang violence prevention, school safety, and other issues about safety in the lives of children and adolescents.

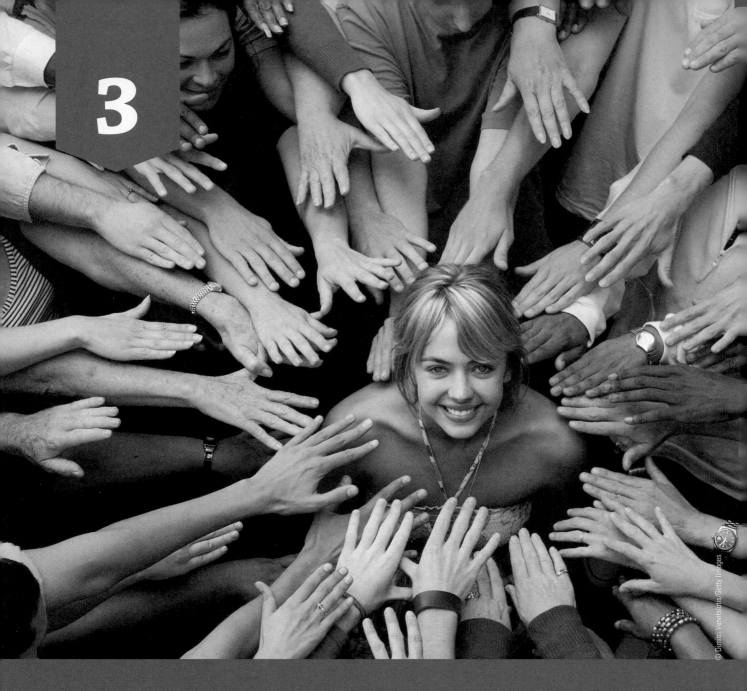
© Dimitri Vervitsiotis/Getty IImages

ADULTHOOD AND AUTONOMY

> Where Am I Now?

> The Path Toward Autonomy and
  Interdependence

> Stages of Adulthood

> Early Adulthood

> Middle Adulthood

> Late Middle Age

> Late Adulthood

> Summary

> Where Can I Go From Here?

> Website Resources

> *Independence means not being lonely even when you are alone.*
>
> —Bernie Siegel

WHERE AM I NOW?

Use this scale to respond to these statements:

4 = I *strongly agree* with this statement.
3 = I *agree* with this statement.
2 = I *disagree* with this statement.
1 = I *strongly disagree* with this statement.

1. My family of origin has greatly influenced my values and beliefs.

2. I'm an independent person more than I am a dependent person.

3. I think about early messages I received from my parents.

4. I am psychologically separated from my parents and have become my own parent.

5. As I get older, I feel an urgency about living.

6. Much of my life is spent doing things that I do not enjoy.

7. I look forward with optimism and enthusiasm to the challenges that lie ahead of me.

8. I expect to experience a meaningful and rich life when I reach old age.

9. There are many things I cannot do now that I expect to do when I retire.

10. I have fears of aging.

In this chapter we continue our discussion of the life-span perspective by focusing on the transitions and turning points in adulthood. Our childhood and adolescent experiences provide the foundation for our ability to meet the developmental challenges of the various phases of adulthood. But throughout adulthood many choices remain open to us. Before taking up early, middle, and late adulthood, we examine how you can become more independent and interdependent. One facet of the struggle toward autonomy involves recognizing the early life decisions you made and realizing that you can change them if they are no longer appropriate or useful. This change entails questioning some of the messages you received and accepted during your early childhood. You can also learn to engage in a dialogue with your self-defeating thoughts and beliefs and acquire a more positive and constructive set of beliefs.

We describe some typical developmental patterns, but we are not trying to lock you into categories of what is "normal" at each of the stages of development. Everyone goes through these stages in different ways, at different times. It is up to you to assess how you have dealt with the tasks of the various stages of life and to determine what meaning your earlier experiences have for you today.

Your family and your culture influence the manner in which you deal with developmental tasks. It is important to understand the ways your culture and family-of-origin experiences have contributed to influencing the person you are today. Your passage through adulthood is characterized by the choices you make in response to the demands made on you. You may find that you are primarily adapting yourself to others, or you may discover a pattern of choosing the path of security rather than risking new adventures. You may be pleased with many of the decisions you have made, or you may wish you had decided differently. As you think about these choices at critical turning points in your adulthood, look for a unifying theme beginning in childhood. Once you become aware of patterns of choices in your life, you can work to change these patterns if you decide that some of them are not serving you well. When you understand how earlier experiences have influenced you, it is possible to revise these decisions and create a different life.

If you are a young adult, you may wonder why you should be concerned about middle age and later life. You can expand the range of your choices by looking at the choices you are making now that will have a direct influence on the quality of your later adulthood. As you read this chapter, reflect on what you hope to be able to say about your life when you reach later adulthood.

THE PATH TOWARD AUTONOMY AND INTERDEPENDENCE

Our cultural background plays a role in how we interpret the central tasks of adulthood and in how we weigh our needs for increased responsibility and independence. Although we may have physically moved away from our parents, our extended family, and often our community, not all of us have done so psychologically. To a greater or lesser degree, the people who have been significant in your early years will have a continuing influence on your life. For this reason it is essential that you gain awareness of how you are presently influenced and determine whether these forces are enhancing your life or restricting your development as a mature adult. Many people may have significantly influenced you during your childhood and adolescent years, but the focus of this chapter is on the role parents (or caretakers) continue to have in your development. In later chapters we more fully discuss other significant relationships.

Autonomy, or **psychological maturity**, entails accepting responsibility for the consequences of your choices rather than holding others accountable for your choices. Finding your own identity is not something you do at a given time once and for all. The path toward maturity begins in early childhood and continues throughout life.

In writing about genuine maturity from the self-in-context perspective, McGoldrick and colleagues (2011b) remind us that the ultimate goal is to develop a mature, interdependent self. To do this requires that we recognize our dependence on each other and on nature. We must establish a solid sense of our unique self in the context of our connection to others. This systemic perspective is based on the assumption that maturity requires the ability to empathize, communicate, collaborate, connect, trust, and respect others. The degree to which we are able to form meaningful connections with a diverse range of people "is strongly influenced by how our families of origin, cultures of origin, and our society as a whole have dealt with difference" (p. 21).

The feminist approach to psychological development stresses connections and disconnections in relationships. In *The Healing Connection: How Women Form Relationships in Therapy and in Life,* Jean Baker Miller and Irene Pierce Stiver (1997) explain how we create connections with others and how disconnections derail us throughout our lives. Miller and Stiver use the word **connection** to mean "an interaction between two or more people that is mutually empathic and mutually empowering" and contrast that with **disconnection**, which represents "an encounter that works against mutual empathy and mutual empowerment" (p. 26). Miller and Stiver believe the source of psychological problems is disconnection, or the "psychological experience of rupture that occurs whenever a child or adult is prevented from participating in a mutually empathic and mutually empowering interaction" (p. 65). The goal is to learn to be an authentic individual who finds meaningful connections or relationships with others. Optimum mental health involves creating relationships based on caring for others, or a sense of mutual empathy. Mutually empowering relationships are characterized by both parties in the relationship fulfilling their needs and feeling good about each other. In contrast, a relationship in which one person gains power at the expense of the other is characterized as a disconnection.

Cultural factors play a significant role in determining the kinds of relationships that govern our lives (see Chapter 2). Some cultures value cooperation and a spirit of interdependence over independence and autonomy. In some cultures, parents, extended family, and the community continue to have a significant influence on individuals throughout the life cycle. In many Asian and Black families, respect and honor for parents and extended family members are values that may be extolled above individual freedom by these adult children.

Regardless of your cultural background, your parents had some influence on your decisions and behavior throughout your childhood and adolescent years. In your move toward autonomy and connection with others, it is probably wise to evaluate your past decisions to determine how well these decisions are working for you today. You very well may share many of your parents' values, but striving for maturity implies a degree of self-direction and self-determination. The self-in-relation theory stresses the interdependence of people rather than independence, and Jordan and her colleagues (1991) state:

> Thus, the self develops in the context of relationships, rather than as an isolated or separate autonomous individual. We are emphasizing the importance of a two-way interaction model, where it becomes as important to understand as to be understood, to empower as well as to be empowered. (p. 59)

Making decisions about the quality of life you want for yourself and affirming these choices is partly what psychological maturity is about. Another part of autonomy is the quality

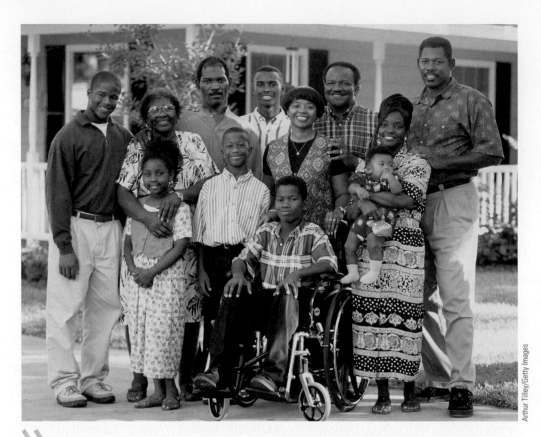

Arthur Tilley/Getty Images

》 It is important that you understand the ways your culture and your family-of-origin experiences have contributed to influencing the person you are.

of relationships with people who are significant in your life. To be able to relate to others in a meaningful way—to form connections—you first need self-knowledge and a mature sense of yourself. Autonomy includes far more than being a separate self; our conception of autonomy includes *self-in-relation* and *self-in-context*.

It is clear that becoming your own person is not "doing your own thing" irrespective of your impact on those with whom you come in contact. Instead, being a mature person implies that you have questioned the values you live by and made them your own; part of this process includes concern for the welfare of others. At this point, consider how you would answer these questions:

▶ To what degree do you think you can live your own life and still be sensitive to the needs and wants of others?

▶ In what areas of your life are you functioning independently? How does being independent affect your emotions and self-perceptions?

▶ To what degree do you want to become more autonomous, even if it involves some risk?

Recognizing Early Learning and Decisions

Transactional analysis (TA) offers a useful framework for understanding how our learning during childhood extends into adulthood. TA is a theory of personality and a method of counseling that was originally developed by Eric Berne (1975) and later extended by practitioners such as Claude Steiner (1975) and Mary and Robert Goulding (1978, 1979). The theory is built on the assumption that adults make decisions based on past premises—premises that were at one time appropriate to their survival needs but may no longer be valid. It stresses the capacity of the person to change early decisions and is oriented toward increasing awareness, with the goal of enabling people to alter the course of their lives. Through TA people learn how their current behavior is affected by the rules and regulations they received and incorporated as children and how they can identify the "life script," and also the family script, that determines their actions. These scripts are almost like plots that unfold. Individuals are able to realize that they can now change what is not working while retaining that which serves them well.

The Life Script The concept of the life script is an important contribution of TA. A **life script** is made up of both parental teachings and the early decisions we make as children. Often, we continue to follow our scripts as adults.

Scripting begins in infancy with subtle, nonverbal messages from our parents. During our earliest years, we learn much about our worth as a person and our place in life. Later, scripting occurs in both subtle and direct ways. Here are some negative messages we might "hear": "Always listen to authority." "Don't act like a child." "We know you can perform well, and we expect the best from you, so be sure you don't let us down." "Never trust people; rely on yourself." "You're really stupid, and we're convinced that you'll never amount to much." These messages are often sent in disguised ways. For example, our parents may never have told us directly that sexual feelings are bad or that touching is inappropriate. However, their behavior with each other and with us may have taught us to think in this way. Moreover, what parents do not say or do is just as important as what they say directly. If no mention is ever made of sexuality, for instance, that very fact communicates significant attitudes. Not all scripting is negative; our parents also give us positive scripts that build us up. Here are some positive messages we might "hear": "Follow your dreams." "Trust in yourself." "You are capable." "You have talent." "You make us proud."

On a broader level than the messages we receive from our parents are the life scripts that are a part of our cultural context. Cultural values are transmitted in many ways in the family circle. Here are a few examples of cultural messages pertaining to the family:

▸ Older people are to be honored and respected.

▸ Don't bring shame to the family.

▸ Don't talk about family matters outside the family circle.

▸ Don't show affection in public.

▸ Always obey your parents and grandparents.

▸ The mother is the heart of the family.

▸ The father is the head of the family.

▸ Avoid conflict and strive for harmony within the family.

▸ Work hard for the good of the entire family.

Our life script, including the messages from both our family of origin and our culture, forms the core of our personal identity. Our experiences may lead us to conclusions such as these: "I can only be loved if I'm productive and successful." "I'd better not trust my feelings because they'll only get me in trouble." These basic themes running through our lives tend to determine our behavior, and very often they are difficult to unlearn. In many subtle ways these early decisions about ourselves can come back to haunt us in later life. Our beliefs about ourselves can even influence how long and how well we live.

Our experiences and the environment help us to put these scripts in context. For example, Lynn's father used to tell her, "You're dyslexic, you're an embarrassment, and you will never be successful." However, Lynn's school experiences and moments of success (such as graduations, obtaining degrees, good grades on papers) helped her to interpret the script in context and to distinguish her father's voice from her own inner voice. In essence, our experiences and environment can either reinforce or dispute the scripting. Although your life scripts were largely formed by your family and cultural experiences, you do have choices over the environments and experiences that you seek out as adults.

A personal example may help clarify how early messages and the decisions we make about them influence us in day-to-day living. In my (Jerry's) own case, even though I now experience myself as successful, for many years I felt unsuccessful and inadequate. I have not erased my old script completely, and I still experience insecurities at times. I do not think I can change such long-lasting feelings by simply telling myself "OK, now that I'm meeting with success, I'm the person I was meant to be." I continue to reflect on the meaning of my life and explore how what I am doing relates to my life's purpose. To some extent, my striving for success is one way of coping with feelings of inadequacy.

I am convinced that part of my motivational force toward success is linked to the acceptance I wanted from my parents, especially from my father. In many important ways my father did not feel successful, and I believe on some level that my own strivings to prove my worth are entangled with a desire to make up for some of the successes that could have been his. Even though my father died many years ago, on a psychological level I sometimes find I am still attempting to win his acceptance and make him proud of my accomplishments. Also, I feel some responsibility to make more of my talents in my life than he did in his life. Although my external reality has certainly changed from the time I was a child to now, I realize that my connection with my father is revealed in underlying patterns associated with my work. For me this does not mean that I need to put an end to my projects, but it is important that I remain aware of the driving force in my life.

Although I believe I can change some of my basic attitudes about myself, I cannot get rid of all vestiges of the effects of my early learning and decisions. I can use my experiences to put these vestiges in context and develop an identity that is more accurate and reflective of the person who I really am. In short, we need not be determined by our early decisions, but it is wise to be aware of manifestations of our old ways that interfere with our attempts to develop new ways of thinking and being.

Injunctions Let's look more closely at the nature of the early messages, or **injunctions**, that we incorporate in our lives. By making decisions in response to real or imagined injunctions, we are partly responsible for keeping some of these decisions alive. If we hope to free ourselves from the impact of early messages, we must become aware of what these "oughts" and "shoulds" are and of how we allow them to operate in our lives. Here are some common injunctions and some possible decisions that could be made in response to them (Goulding & Goulding, 1978, 1979).

1. *"Don't make mistakes."* Children who hear and accept this message often fear taking risks to avoid looking stupid. They tend to equate making mistakes with being a failure.

   ▶ *Possible decisions:* "I'm scared of making the wrong decision, so I simply won't decide." "Because I made dumb choices, I won't decide on anything important again!" "I have to be perfect if I hope to be accepted."

2. *"Don't be."* This lethal message is often given nonverbally by the way parents hold (or do not hold) the child. The basic message is "I wish you hadn't been born."

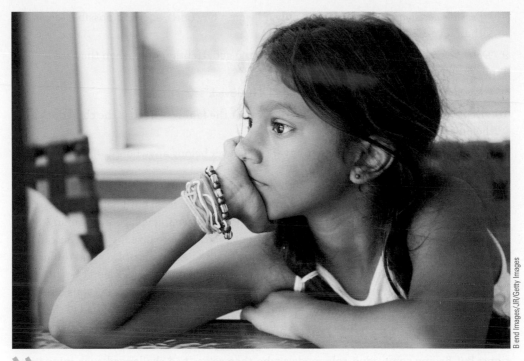

Childhood injunctions can affect our entire lives. This girl may have received the family message "don't belong" and could be a loner as an adult.

> *Possible decisions:* "I'll keep trying until I get you to love me."

3. *"Don't be close."* Related to this injunction are the messages "Don't trust" and "Don't love."

   > *Possible decisions:* "I let myself love once, and it backfired. Never again!" "Because it's scary to get close, I'll keep myself distant."

4. *"Don't be important."* If you are constantly discounted when you speak, you are likely to believe you are unimportant.

   > *Possible decisions:* "If, by chance, I ever do become important, I'll play down my accomplishments."

5. *"Don't be a child."* This message says: "Always act adult!" "Don't be childish." "Keep control of yourself."

   > *Possible decisions:* "I'll take care of others and won't ask for much myself." "I won't let myself have fun."

6. *"Don't grow."* This message is given by the frightened parent who discourages the child from growing up in many ways.

   > *Possible decision:* "I'll stay a child, and that way I'll get my parents to approve of me."

7. *"Don't succeed."* If children are positively reinforced for failing, they may accept the message not to seek success.

   > *Possible decisions:* "I'll never do anything perfect enough, so why try?" "I'll succeed, no matter what it takes." "If I don't succeed, then I'll not have to live up to the high expectations others have of me."

8. *"Don't be you."* This involves suggesting to children that they are the wrong sex, shape, size, color, or have ideas or feelings that are unacceptable to parental figures.

    ▸ *Possible decisions:* "They'd love me only if I were a boy (girl), so it's impossible to get their love." "I'll pretend I'm a boy (girl)."

9. *"Don't be sane"* and *"Don't be well."* Some children get attention only when they are physically sick or acting out.

    ▸ *Possible decision:* "I'll get sick, and then I'll be loved."

10. *"Don't belong."* This injunction may indicate that the family feels that the child does not belong anywhere.

    ▸ *Possible decisions:* "I'll be a loner forever." "I'll never belong anywhere."

Overcoming Injunctions I (Marianne) want to share some messages I heard growing up as a personal example of a struggle with listening to injunctions from both parents and society. I was born and spent my childhood and adolescence in a farming village in Germany. Some of the messages I received, though they were not typically verbalized, were "You can't do anything about it." "Things could be worse, so don't talk so much about how bad things are." "Accept what you have, and don't complain about what you don't have." "Don't be different. Fit in with the community. Do what everybody else does." "Be satisfied with your life."

Although my childhood was very good in many respects and I was satisfied with part of my life, I still wanted more than I felt I could get by remaining in the village and becoming what was expected of me. It was a continuing struggle not to surrender to these expectations, but having some adult role models who themselves had challenged such injunctions inspired me to resist these messages. As early as age 8 I felt a sense of daring to be different and hoping someday to go to the United States. Although I doubted myself at times, I still began saving every penny I could lay my hands on. Finally, at the age of 19 I asked my father for permission to take a ship to the United States and surprised him when I told him that I had saved enough money to buy a ticket.

Even though there were many obstacles, I seemed to be driven to follow a dream and a decision that I made when I was only 8 years old. When I did come to the United States, I eventually fulfilled another dream, and consequently challenged another injunction, by furthering my education. The theme of my struggles during my earlier years is that I was not willing to surrender to obstacles. I argued with myself about simply accepting what seemed like limited choices for a life's design, and in doing so I began writing a new life script for myself. It was important to me not to feel like a victim of circumstances. I was willing to do what was necessary to challenge barriers to what I wanted and to pursue my dreams and goals. Although I fought against these injunctions at an early age, they have not gone away forever. I continue to have to be aware of them and not allow them to control me as an adult.

It certainly can be challenging to identify and critically evaluate self-defeating assumptions and to learn new and constructive beliefs in their place. The following questions can assist you in evaluating childhood decisions you may have made about yourself and about life:

▸ What implicit and explicit messages have I listened to and accepted?

▸ How valid are the sources of these messages?

▸ What are some of the self-defeating sentences I say to myself?

▸ How do my core beliefs affect me?

▸ How can I challenge some of the decisions I made about myself and make new ones that will lead to a positive orientation?

▸ How would my life be different if I were successful in replacing some outdated beliefs with more realistic beliefs?

Once you have identified and become aware of these internalized "do's and don'ts," you are in a better position to critically examine these messages and determine whether you are willing to continue living by them. You can begin this process by learning to become a mindful observer of the injunctions you are repeating to yourself, by evaluating them, and then by making choices about how you will react or respond to these messages. At times it may seem that these injunctions control you and that you are powerless. However, by becoming mindful of these past messages, you can decide to put them into context and prevent them from unduly influencing your life today. You can make rational choices about how you want to be and how you want your scripting to affect your emotions, thinking, and behavior. Let's look at some ways to dispute these early messages.

Learning to Dispute Self-Defeating Thinking

As children and adolescents, we uncritically incorporate certain assumptions about life and about our worth as a person. **Rational emotive behavior therapy** and other cognitive behavioral therapies are based on the premise that emotional and behavioral problems are originally learned from significant others during childhood. Others gave us inaccurate beliefs, which we accepted automatically. We actively keep dysfunctional or inaccurate beliefs alive by the processes of self-suggestion and self-repetition (Ellis, 2001). Self-defeating beliefs are supported and maintained by negative and dysfunctional statements that we make to ourselves over and over again: "If I don't win universal love and approval, then I have no chance of being happy." "If I make a mistake, that would prove I am a failure."

Albert Ellis (2001), who developed rational emotive behavior therapy (REBT), describes some of the common ways people make themselves miserable by remaining wedded to their irrational beliefs. He holds that it is our faulty thinking, not actual life events, that creates emotional upsets and leads to our misery. He contends that we have the power to control our emotional destiny and suggests that when we are upset it is a good idea to critically examine our hidden dogmatic "musts," "oughts," and absolutist "shoulds."

Ellis's **A-B-C theory of personality** explains how people develop negative evaluations of themselves. For example, Sally experiences pain because her parents abandoned her when she was a child (A, the activating event). Sally's emotional reaction may be feelings of depression, worthlessness, rejection, and unlovability (C, the emotional consequence). However, Ellis asserts it is not A (her parents' abandonment of her) that caused her feelings of rejection and unlovability; rather, it is her belief system (B) that is causing her low self-esteem. She made her mistake when she told herself that there must have been something terrible about her for her parents not to want her. Her faulty beliefs are reflected through self-talk such as this: "I am to blame for what my parents did." "If I were more lovable, they would have wanted to keep me." This kind of thinking is what gets Sally into psychological trouble.

REBT is designed to teach people how to dispute faulty beliefs that get in the way of effective living. Let's apply REBT to our example. Sally does not need to continue believing she is basically unlovable. Instead of clinging to the belief that something must have been wrong with her for her parents to have rejected her, Sally can begin to dispute this self-defeating statement and think along different lines: "It hurts that my parents didn't want me, but perhaps they had problems that kept them from being good parents." "Maybe my parents didn't love me, but that doesn't mean that nobody could love me." "It's unfortunate that I didn't have parents in growing up, but it's not devastating, and I do not need to be controlled by this."

Donald Meichenbaum's (2007, 2008) **self-instructional training** also helps clients become aware of their negative self-talk and the stories they tell about themselves. Many people who are dissatisfied with their lives benefit from becoming more cognizant of their internal dialogue and can acquire positive coping skills. By changing our maladaptive internal dialogue, we become open to learning new skills and behaviors that will enhance our lives.

One member of a therapeutic group of ours had major struggles believing that he could have a long-term relationship without sabotaging it in some way. Through his group work, Samuel learned how to pay attention to his internal dialogue and realized how his thoughts influenced what he did and how he felt about himself. In this story, Samuel reports how his self-talk got in his way.

SAMUEL'S STORY

My parents divorced when I was 9, and my earliest memories are of them fighting. My mother remarried soon after the divorce, and within months she began arguing with my stepfather. That marriage lasted a couple of years at most. Before she filed for divorce, she started dating the man who would become her third husband. You guessed it—more fighting. More of the same. I could go on for days giving examples of how dysfunctional my mother's relationships with men were, but the main point is that it really resulted in distorting my view of adult relationships. I remember thinking as a kid, "I'm never getting married! It seems like a big hassle and it never works out."

For many years I sabotaged every relationship I had. I would tell myself that women were manipulative and deceitful and that I was weak if I caved in to their demands. It doesn't take a rocket scientist to figure out that my way of interacting with women was a recipe for disaster. Now that I am older and a bit wiser (hopefully), I recognize some of the errors in my thinking. I think I am finally ready for a committed relationship, and for things to work out, I need to replace my negative thoughts about women and about myself with more realistic ones. For instance, lately I have been reminding myself that some women are honest and stable and that choosing to compromise in relationships doesn't make me weak. I tell myself that I do not have to model my relationships after my mother's failed relationships. I can be happy in a committed relationship. My internal dialogue is starting to change, but it is something I have to consciously work on every day.

Samuel is a good example of a person who is changing his life by recognizing and exploring his self-destructive beliefs. Ellis stresses that your feelings about yourself are largely the result of the way you think. Thus, if you hope to change a negative self-image, it is essential to learn how to dispute the illogical sentences you now continue to feed yourself and to challenge faulty premises that you have accepted uncritically. Further, you also need to work and practice replacing these self-sabotaging beliefs with constructive ones.

Common Cognitive Distortions

In contrast to Ellis, who emphasizes irrational thinking processes, Aaron Beck, the founder of **cognitive therapy**, regards self-defeating beliefs as being more *inaccurate* than *irrational*. He asks his clients to conduct behavioral experiments to test the accuracy of their beliefs (Hollon & DiGiuseppe, 2011). One premise of this theory is that people with emotional difficulties commit "logical errors" that distort objective reality. The systematic errors in reasoning that lead to misconceptions and faulty assumptions are called **cognitive distortions** (J. Beck, 2011; Beck & Weishaar, 2011). As you continue reading this section, think about times when you have committed these cognitive errors:

- *Dichotomous thinking* occurs when you categorize experiences in either-or extremes. By labeling events in opposing terms, you might give yourself little room for error as a student. If you are not the top student, then you regard yourself as the worst student and a miserable failure.

- *Selective abstraction* entails forming conclusions based on an isolated detail of an event. You ignore other information and miss the total context. By assuming that the events that matter are those dealing with failure and weaknesses, you might measure your worth and value by your errors and shortcomings rather than by your successes. If you are an actor and mess up one line in a play, you might regard your performance as a total flop even though you receive many compliments and a standing ovation afterward.

- *Arbitrary inferences* refer to making conclusions without supporting evidence. Catastrophizing—thinking of the worst case scenario and the most horrendous outcome that could happen—is a common arbitrary inference. Even though you seem to get along well with others, you might not initiate new friendships because you are certain people will dislike you and see all of your flaws.

- *Overgeneralization* occurs when you form extreme beliefs based on a single incident and apply them inappropriately to events or settings that are dissimilar. Suppose you do poorly on an exam because you feel ill on the day of the test. You would be overgeneralizing if you assumed that you will do poorly on exams in all subject areas, even when you feel well.

- *Personalization occurs* when individuals relate external events to themselves, even when there is no basis for drawing this conclusion. If one of your coworkers announces she is leaving the company and starting a new job, you might convince yourself that your behavior led to her decision to quit. In reality, your behavior may not have influenced your coworker's decision at all.

- *Magnification and minimization* consist of perceiving a situation in a greater or lesser light than it deserves. If your significant other comes home from work late on rare occasions, you might be magnifying matters by accusing him or her of being totally unreliable and undependable. Conversely, if your significant other is chronically late and unreliable, yet you regard that behavior as acceptable, you might be minimizing the situation.

- *Labeling and mislabeling* involve portraying one's identity on the basis of past mistakes or imperfections and allowing them to define one's true identity. If you experienced a painful breakup or divorce in the past and felt like you failed in some way, you might fall into the trap of believing that you will always be a failure in intimate relationships.

Identify any cognitive distortions that are interfering with your life satisfaction, and test these automatic thoughts against reality by examining and weighing the evidence for and against them. We provide an opportunity for you to do this in the next Take Time to Reflect exercise.

Learning to Challenge Your Inner Critic

We would like to expand a bit on the general concepts of transactional analysis and rational emotive behavior therapy and discuss some related ideas about challenging early messages and working toward autonomy. The term **inner parent** refers to the attitudes and beliefs we have about ourselves and others that are a direct result of things we learned from our parents or parental substitutes. As we move through life, we tend to internalize messages we received from parents and authority figures. Our willingness to question and challenge the critical voices we have internalized is one of the hallmarks of maturity. Being bombarded with harsh messages from parents can leave an indelible impression on us, making it difficult to develop healthy self-esteem. Rachel's story illustrates this struggle.

Many of the qualities we incorporated from our parents may be healthy standards for guiding our behavior. No doubt our past has contributed in many respects to the good qualities we possess, and many of the things we like about ourselves may be largely due to the influence of the people who were important to us in our early years. However, part of maturity entails looking for the subtle ways we have acquired our values, perhaps without making a conscious choice about certain values.

How do we learn to recognize the continuing influence of early messages? One way to begin is by thinking about where we acquired our values and beliefs about ourselves. Notice things you do and avoid doing, and ask yourself why. For instance, suppose you avoid enrolling in a college course because you long ago categorized yourself as "not smart enough." You may tell yourself that you would never be able to pass the class, so why even try? In this case an early decision you made about your intellectual capabilities prevents you from branching out to new endeavors. Rather than stopping at this first obstacle, however, you could challenge yourself by asking, "Who says I'm too stupid? Even if my teachers have told me that I'm slow, is it really true? Why have I accepted this view of myself uncritically? Let me check it out and see for myself." By engaging in this new dialogue, you can begin to change your self-perceptions.

Hal and Sidra Stone (1993) developed a therapeutic process aimed at transforming this "inner critic" from a crippling adversary to a productive ally. The Stones claim that the **inner critic** is our inner voice that criticizes us and makes constant judgments about our worth. This aspect of our personality develops early in life and absorbs the judgments of people in our environment. The inner critic checks our thoughts, controls our behavior, kills our spontaneity and creativity, and leads to feelings of shame, anxiety, depression, exhaustion, and low self-esteem. Developed as a way to protect us from the pain and shame of being discovered as being less than we should be, this inner voice reflects the concerns of our parents, church, and significant others from our early years. Here are some of the characteristics of this inner critic:

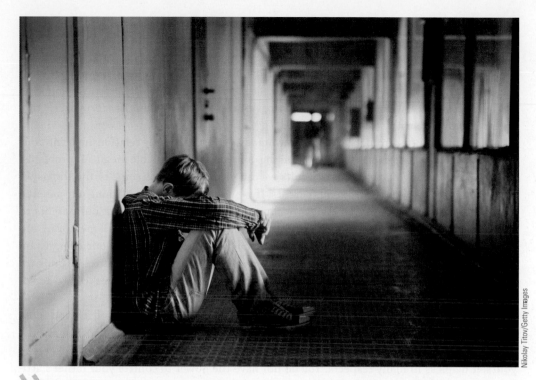

Nikolay Titov/Getty Images

>> When you become aware of negative self-talk, it is useful to challenge your critical voices.

▶ It constricts your ability to be creative.

▶ It prevents you from taking risks.

▶ It makes you particularly vulnerable to fearing mistakes and failure.

▶ It warns you never to look foolish.

▶ It takes the fun out of life.

▶ It makes you susceptible to the judgments of others.

The content of the inner critic may vary from culture to culture, according to the value system of each particular culture, but this critical voice is universal and seems to have the power to immobilize people and render them less effective than they might be. The Stones explain how to minimize the negative impact of this self-destructive internal dialogue and how to transform this negative force by developing an internal source of support very much like an internal parent who protects you and your creative process. You do not conquer your inner critic by attempting to destroy it; paradoxically, you lessen its negative impact by embracing it.

Another way of challenging your inner critic is found in a process known as **mindfulness**, which involves becoming increasingly observant and aware of external and internal stimuli in the present moment and adopting an open attitude of accepting *what* is rather than judging the present situation (Kabat-Zinn, 1994; Segal, Williams, & Teasdale, 2002). Mindfulness is a way to access our resources for growing, healing, and self-compassion (Kabat-Zinn, 1995). When we practice living mindfully, we enhance our capacity to be more fully in the present moment. "Mindfulness is vast, because it is fundamentally about wakefulness, about paying attention in one's life—all of it" (p. 110). Kabat-Zinn emphasizes that we are only alive in the present moment. When people discover the ways they are not living in the present, they become aware that they have been functioning on automatic pilot and are more asleep than awake. "When you have that realization, you begin to see differently and then act differently" (p. 112). **Acceptance** involves a process of connecting with your present experience without judgment or self-criticism, but with curiosity and kindness, and becoming aware of your mental activity from moment to moment (Germer, Siegel, & Fulton, 2005). By practicing mindfulness and acceptance, we increase the joy of living. We discuss mindfulness as a form of self-care and as way to cope with stress in Chapter 5.

Many of us suffer from psychological wounds as a result of early relationships with our parents. We often keep the past alive by holding our parents responsible for all our problems. Instead of criticizing our parents, as adults we can give to ourselves some of the things we may still expect or hope for from our parents. If we do not get beyond blaming our parents, we end up resenting them. As long as we cling to our resentments, expect our parents to be different than they are, or wait for their approval, we are keeping painful memories and experiences alive. If we harbor grudges against our parents and focus all our energies on changing them, we have little constructive energy left over to assume control of our own lives. Forgiveness and letting go of resentments and regrets are essential steps toward acceptance, which enable us to live fully in the present.

If you want a closer relationship with your father and insist that he talk to you more and approve of you, for example, you are likely to be disappointed. He may not behave the way you want him to, and if you make changing him your central goal, you are keeping yourself helpless in many respects. You do not have the power to control your father's attitudes or behavior, yet you do have choices with respect to how you will relate to your father. As long as you are stuck in a blaming mode, you will not be able to recognize the power you have within you to change the influence that you allow your father to have in your life. You can learn to ask yourself before you act, "Will doing or saying what I am about to do or say bring us closer together? If it won't, then I won't do or say it." If you make some significant changes in the way you talk to your father and in the way you treat him, you may be greatly surprised at how he might change. You will increase your chances of success if you do what you want him to do.

To be at peace with yourself, it is important to let go of resentments, to work through unresolved anger, and to stop blaming others. These factors not only poison relationships but also take a toll on the way you feel about yourself. It is only when you find a sense of inner peace that you can hope to make peace with the significant people in your life. You do have a choice! Even though your family situation may have been far from ideal, you now can choose the attitude you take toward your past circumstances and determine how some aspects of your past continue to affect you. If you choose to assume responsibility for the person you are now, you are moving in the direction of becoming your own parent.

There are many ways to engage in self-exploration, and no one way is the best method. To achieve emotional maturity, you need to decide what you can do about the experiences that have shaped your life. One choice is deciding how you will allow your early perceptions of yourself to influence your adult life.

TAKE TIME TO REFLECT

The first part of this self-inventory is designed to increase your awareness of the injunctions you have incorporated and to help you challenge the validity of messages you may not have critically examined. You are then asked to reflect on any cognitive distortions that you have held.

1. Place a check (✓) in the space provided for each of these "don't" injunctions that you think applies to you.

_____ Don't be you.

_____ Don't think.

_____ Don't feel.

✓ Don't be close.

✓ Don't trust.

_____ Don't be sexy.

✓ Don't fail.

_____ Don't be foolish.

_____ Don't be important.

_____ Don't brag.

_____ Don't let us down.

✓ Don't change.

List any other injunctions you can think of that apply to you: _____Don't be annoying ✓_____

_____

_____

2. Check the ways you sometimes badger yourself with "do" messages.

_____ Be perfect.

_____ Say only nice things.

_____ Be more than you are.

_____ Be obedient.

_____ Work up to your potential.

_____ Be practical at all times.

_____ Listen to authority figures.

_____ Always put your best foot forward.

_____ Put others before yourself.

_____ Be seen but not heard.

List any other injunctions you can think of that apply to you: _____

_____

_____

3. What messages have you received concerning

your self-worth? _____

your ability to succeed?_____

your gender role? _____

your intelligence? _____

your trust in yourself? _____

trusting others? _____

making yourself vulnerable? _____

your security? _____

your aliveness as a person? _____

your creativity? _____

your ability to be loved? _____

your capacity to give love? _____

4. Because your view of yourself has a great influence on the quality of your interpersonal relationships, we invite you to look carefully at some of the views you have of yourself and also to consider how you arrived at these views. To do this, reflect on these questions:

a. How do you see yourself now? Use as many adjectives as you can think of to describe yourself. _____

_____

_____

b. Do others generally see you as you see yourself? What are some ways others view you differently from how you view yourself? _____

_____

_____

c. Who in your life has been most influential in shaping your self-concept? How did this person do this? _____

_____

_____

5. List examples of the cognitive distortions that you have held. What strategies did you use to cope with these cognitive errors? How well did the strategies work? _____

_____

_____

_____

6. For each cognitive distortion you have identified, devise a way to test it to see whether the evidence supports your thoughts. _____

_____

_____

_____

7. Review your responses to these exercises and identify areas where you would like to change. In the journal pages at the end of the chapter list some of your ideas about how you can begin the process of detecting the messages you now give yourself. How can you dispute some of the messages that are self-sabotaging or unhelpful?

STAGES OF ADULTHOOD

Some developmental theorists reject the notion of well-defined stages of adulthood, contending that adult development is highly individualized. Other researchers conceptualize the life cycle in general periods of development. We will continue to discuss the developmental process from the point of view of Erikson's psychosocial stages and the self-in-context perspective, concentrating on the core struggles and choices from early adulthood through late adulthood (see Table 3.1). Levinson (1996) conducted in-depth interviews with 45 women and found that women go through the same sequence of seasons as men, and at the same ages, making a case for the underlying order in the course of human development. However,

	TABLE 3.1	**Overview of Developmental Stages From Early Adulthood to Late Adulthood**		
Life Stage	**Self-in-Context View**	**Erikson's Psychosocial View**	**Potential Problems**	
Early adulthood (ages 21–34)	The major goals of this period of life are being able to engage in intimate relationships and find satisfying work. Some developmental issues include caring for self and others, focusing on long-range goals, nurturing others physically and emotionally, finding meaning in life, and developing a tolerance for delayed gratification to meet long-range goals.	*Young adulthood.* Sense of identity is again tested by the challenge of achieving intimacy. Ability to form close relationships depends on having a clear sense of self. Core struggle: *intimacy* versus *isolation*. Theme: love.	The challenge of this period is to maintain one's separateness while becoming attached to others. Failing to strike a balance leads to self-centeredness or to an exclusive focus on the needs of others. Failure to achieve intimacy can lead to alienation and isolation.	
Middle adulthood (ages 35–55)	A time for "going outside oneself." This period sees the reassessment of one's work satisfactions, of involvement in the community, and of accepting choices made in life. A time for solidifying one's philosophy of life. Tasks include nurturing and supporting one's children, partner, and older family members. One challenge is to recognize accomplishments and accept limitations.	*Middle age.* Individuals become more aware of their eventual death and begin to question whether they are living well. The crossroads of life; a time for reevaluation. Core struggle: *generativity* versus *stagnation*. Theme: care.	Failure to achieve a sense of productivity can lead to stagnation. Pain can result when individuals recognize the gap between their dreams and what they have achieved.	
Late middle age (56–69)	This is the beginning of the wisdom years, in which key themes are helping others, serving the community, and passing along one's values and experiences. A few critical tasks of this period include dealing with declining physical and intellectual abilities, coming to terms with the choices one has made in life, planning for work transitions and retirement, defining one's senior roles in work and community, and dealing with the death of parents.			
Late adulthood (age 70 onward)	Themes of this final stage of life are grief, loss, resiliency, retrospection, and growth. This is a time to find new levels of meaning in life and to appreciate what one has accomplished. Some tasks of this period are responding to loss and change, remaining connected to others, coming to terms with death, focusing on what else one can do for others and oneself, engaging in a life review, accepting increased dependence on others, accepting death of a spouse or loved ones, and dealing with diminished control of one's life.	*Later life.* Ego integrity is achieved by those who have few regrets, who see themselves as living a productive life, and who have coped with both successes and failures. Key tasks are to adjust to losses, death of others, maintaining outside interests, and adjusting to retirement. Core struggle: *integrity* versus *despair*. Theme: wisdom.	Failure to achieve ego integrity often leads to feelings of hopelessness, guilt, resentment, and self-rejection. Unfinished business from earlier years can lead to fears of death stemming from a sense that life has been wasted.	

Levinson emphasizes that although there is a single human life cycle there are myriad variations related to gender, class, race, culture, historical epoch, specific circumstances, and genetics. In short, there are wide variations between and within genders as well as in the specific ways individuals traverse each season of life. It is best to keep this variation in mind as we examine the stages of adulthood.

In *New Passages*, Gail Sheehy (1995) describes a new map for the stages of adult life. Contending that we need new markers for life transitions, she states that "the old demarcation points we may still carry around—an adulthood that begins at 21 and ends at 65—are hopelessly out of date" (p. 7). People who are today in their 20s, 30s, and early 40s are confronted with a different set of conditions than was the case 20 years ago. Today, people at 50 are dealing with transitions that were characteristic of people at 40 just a couple of decades ago. Sheehy's research, based on a collection of life histories of people facing the challenges of "second adulthood" (age 45 and beyond), results in this conclusion: "There is no longer a standard life cycle. People are increasingly able to customize their life cycles" (p. 16).

EARLY ADULTHOOD

Early adulthood encompasses ages 21 through 34. There are many changes during this stage of adulthood, and the decisions made here will have far-reaching effects. Armstrong (2007) identifies the principle of *enterprise* as a key characteristic of this stage of life. For young adults to accomplish the tasks facing them (such as finding a home and a partner, establish a career), enterprise is required. This characteristic serves us well at any stage of life when we must go into the world to make our mark. According to Erikson (1963, 1968), we enter adulthood after we master the adolescent conflicts over identity versus role confusion. Our sense of identity is tested anew in adulthood, however, by the challenge of **intimacy versus isolation**.

One characteristic of the psychologically mature person is the ability to form intimate relationships. Before we can form such relationships, we must have a clear sense of our own identity. Intimacy involves sharing, giving of ourselves, and relating to another out of strength and a desire to grow with the other person. Failure to achieve intimacy can result in isolation from others and a sense of alienation. If we attempt to escape isolation by clinging to another person, however, we rarely find success in the relationship. As you will see in Chapter 7, there are many types of intimate relationships, a few of which include a parent, a partner, or a best friend. As long as you have established some form of intimate relationship, you are not failing, even if you are not involved in a committed life partnership.

The self-in-context theory of McGoldrick and colleagues (2011b) places the early adulthood period from about 21 to 34. At this stage the major aim is development of the ability to engage in intense relationships committed to mutual growth and in satisfying work. They acknowledge the differences in the pathways at this phase, depending on the person's culture, race, gender, class, and sexual orientation. In general, they view this phase as one of generativity in terms of partnering, working, and rearing children, but barriers to healthy development (such as discrimination due to race, gender, class, or sexual orientation) can derail potentially productive people. For example, gay and lesbian young adults may have difficulties at this stage because of the social stigma attached to their partnering and parenting or to the necessity of keeping their identity a secret. Haldeman (2001) indicates that social stigma affects people powerfully, especially when it is part of their early life experiences. Gay, lesbian, and bisexual parents frequently encounter the misconception that same-sex parents influence a child's gender-role identity, conformity, and sexual identity. However, research indicates no grounds for concerns as to a child's gender-role identity being associated with having same-sex parents (Haldeman, 2001).

Emerging Adulthood

The late teens and early 20s are characterized by change and exploration of possible life directions. Arnett (2000) proposes a theory of human development focusing on the period from roughly ages 18 to 25 that he calls the period of **emerging adulthood**. The term *emerging* captures the dynamic, rich, complex, changeable, and fluid quality of this period of life:

> Emerging adulthood is a time of life when many different directions remain possible, when little about the future has been decided for certain, when the scope of independent exploration of life's possibilities is greater for most people than it will be at any other period of the life course. (p. 469)

What matters most to emerging adults are three individualistic qualities: accepting responsibility for one's self, making independent decisions, and becoming financially independent. This notion of becoming a self-sufficient person is similar to the concept of autonomy described earlier in this chapter.

Arnett (2000, 2011) characterizes emerging adulthood as a time of change and exploration for most young people in industrialized societies—a time when they examine life's choices regarding love, work, and worldview:

▶ *Love.* Explorations in love during emerging adulthood generally involve a deeper level of intimacy than in adolescence. The emerging adult considers the kind of person he or she is and questions what kind of person he or she wishes to have as a partner through life.

▶ *Work.* Emerging adults consider how their work experiences are apt to set the foundation for the jobs they may have throughout adulthood. Identity issues are closely related to the exploration of work possibilities. Questions typically raised include: "What kind of work will best fit the person that I am?" "What kind of work will be satisfying in the long term?" "What are the chances of securing a job in the field that seems to best suit me?"

▶ *Worldview.* Emerging adults often find themselves questioning the worldview they were exposed to during childhood and adolescence. Many young people go through a process of reexamining the religious beliefs and values they learned as children. This explanation sometimes results in forming a different value system, but oftentimes it leads to rejecting an earlier belief system without constructing a new set of values.

Emerging adulthood must be understood within a cultural context, for this period exists only in cultures that allow young people a prolonged period of independent exploration during their late teens and 20s (Arnett, 2011). This is a time when personal freedom and exploration are higher for most people than at any other time in life.

Entering the Twenties

During their 20s, young adults are faced with a variety of profound choices. They move away from the safe shelter of the family and confront insecurity about the future as they attempt to establish independence. This time is often characterized by considerable agitation, excitement, and change.

If you are in this age group, you are no doubt facing decisions about how you will live. Your choices probably include questions such as these: "Will I choose the security of staying at home, or am I willing to endure financial and psychological challenges in order to live on my own?" "Will I stay single, or will I get involved in a committed relationship with a part-ner?" "Will I stay in college full time, or will I begin a career?" "What are some of my dreams, and how might I make them become reality?" "What do I most want to do with my life at this time, and how might I find meaning?" Add your own questions to this list.

Choices pertaining to work, education, marriage, family life, and lifestyle are complex and very personal, and it is common to struggle over what it is we really want. Although emerging adults may begin to find their own direction, smooth sailing is not guaranteed. A faltering economy and a divisive political climate are likely to curtail some options and opportunities for emerging adults today. Even those who are more psychologically independent may need to remain financially dependent on their parents for a longer period than they desire. Mastery of some life tasks typically associated with young adulthood may be delayed, as Jason's story illustrates.

JASON'S STORY

I always thought I would be living on my own by the time I was 24. I figured I would be done with college, I'd have an awesome job, and I would be supporting myself. That's not how things have worked out. I'm still in college and won't be finished for at least another year if all goes well. Because the economy is so bad right now, I can't count on finding a decent job after I graduate. In fact, I may have to move back in with my parents after I graduate so I can pay off some of my college debt. I think my parents are pretty cool, but I'd rather not live with them. I should be moving forward with my life, not backward. It's frustrating.

Although some young adults may choose to continue living with their parents into their 20s, and others find it is expected of them for cultural reasons, Jason's expectations were quite different. Each person's situation must be viewed within his or her cultural context. Jason and others experiencing similar circumstances are faced with the challenge of not succumbing to feelings of hopelessness and powerlessness. Although it may be tempting to become less moti-vated during tough times, it is important to the well-being of emerging adults that they contin-ue their efforts to attain their existing goals or to establish new ones (Shulman & Nurmi, 2010).

Transition From the Twenties to the Thirties

The transition from the late 20s to the early 30s is a time of changing values and beliefs for most people. Inner turmoil often increases during this period, and commitments to relationships and careers are often made. Others may defer these responsibilities for various reasons, and couples may delay having children until their late 30s.

During this transition, people often take another look at their long-term dreams, and they may reevaluate their life plans and make significant shifts. Some become aware that their dreams may not materialize. This recognition often brings anxiety, but it can be the catalyst for making new plans and working hard to attain them. Consider Pam's evolution in her process of striving to make her dreams become reality.

PAM'S STORY

When I was growing up, a college education was not considered essential for a female. The belief in my family was that as a female I would grow up, get married, have children, and be financially supported by my husband.

When I turned 17 I attended college for a couple of years, but I did not take my studies seriously. I got married and very soon my husband and I had marital problems, and we eventually divorced. Reality turned out to be very different from the dreams I had while growing up.

In my late 20s I began taking inventory of my life. I realized that I wanted a meaningful career. I wanted financial security and a nice home in which to raise my children. Although I had remarried by this time, I did not want to make the same mistake again of depending on someone else to fulfill my goals and secure my future. For me, education seemed to be the key to achieve these goals. At 30, I returned to college and completed my last 2 years with a 4.0 grade point average.

What I learned is that dreams become reality by working hard. I did not understand the value of an education earlier in my life and how having a college education could change my life and help me achieve my goals. I see things very differently now. I see how life is not about luck. Life is about excitement about what I'm doing, choices, personal responsibility, and hard work.

TAKE TIME TO REFLECT

1. Think about a few of the major turning points in your young adulthood. Write down two significant turning points, and then state how you think they were important in your life. What difference did your decisions at these critical times make in your life?

Turning point: _____

Impact of the decision on my life: _____

_____

Turning point: _____

Impact of the decision on my life: _____

_____

2. Complete the following sentences by giving the first response that comes to mind:

a. To me, being an independent person means_____

b. If I could change one thing about my past, it would be _____

c. My fears of being independent are _____

d. One thing I most want for my children is _____

e. I find it difficult to be my own person when _____

f. I feel the most free when_____

g. The thing I find most empowering about being independent is _being me_____

3. Identify any discrepancies between what you were taught about adulthood and your actual experiences as an adult. _____

_____

_____

_____

MIDDLE ADULTHOOD

The period of life between the ages of 35 and 55 is characterized by a "going outside of ourselves." **Middle adulthood** is a time when people are likely to engage in a philosophical reexamination of their lives and, based on this evaluation, may reinvent themselves in their work and their involvement in the community to fit changing circumstances (McGoldrick et al., 2011b). Armstrong (2007) refers to *contemplation* as the "gift" of middle adulthood. People in midlife reflect upon the deeper meaning of their lives, which is an important resource that can be drawn upon to enrich life at any age. At this time, individuals reexamine life decisions they made earlier and make choices about what changes they want to make. The developmental tasks of middle adulthood are complex and demand persistence. At this time in life, people assess their self-worth mainly in relation to their contributions to family, work, and community (Newman & Newman, 2012). This period involves a time for learning how to live creatively with ourselves and with others, and it can be the time of greatest productivity in our lives. In middle age we reach the top of the mountain yet at the same time realize that we eventually will begin the downhill journey. In addition, we may painfully experience the discrepancy between the dreams of our 20s and 30s and the hard reality of what we have achieved.

The Late Thirties

People in their 30s often experience doubts and reevaluate significant aspects of their lives, and it is not uncommon for them to experience a crisis. These crises center on doubts about their earlier commitments and on concerns over getting locked into choices that make it difficult for them to move in new directions. During this period of unrest, disillusionment, and questioning, people often modify the rules and standards that govern their lives. They also realize that their dreams do not materialize if they simply wish for things to happen, but that they need to actively work at attaining their goals.

At this stage of life, even if our life choices have served us well to date, we often find that we are ready for some changes. This is a time for making new choices and perhaps for modifying or deepening old commitments. We are likely to review our commitments to career, marriage, children, friends, and life's priorities. With many opportunities to review and revise our commitments and goals, transitions in our work and family roles are typical, and we encounter a widening circle of relationships and new responsibilities (Newman & Newman, 2012). Because we realize that time is passing, we often make a major reappraisal of how we are spending our time and energy. We are awakened to the reality that we do not have forever to reach our goals. This can be a very positive force, filling us with excitement as we pursue different possibilities and directions in life.

We may find ourselves asking questions such as these: "Is this all there is to life?" "What do I want for the rest of my life?" "What is missing from my life now?" "Am I excited about how I am living?" A woman who has primarily been engaged in a career may now want to spend more time at home and with the children. A woman who has devoted most of her life to being a homemaker may want to begin a new career outside the home. As you will see, Maria's desires are even more complex and difficult to fulfill. Men may do a lot of questioning about their work and wonder how they can make it more meaningful. It is likely that they will struggle with defining the meaning of success. They may be exteriorly focused in measuring success, which puts the source of the meaning of life in jeopardy. They are likely to begin to question the price of success, and they may give more thought to what success means to them.

MARIA'S STORY

Up to this point in my life, I have been pretty satisfied. My mother never had the means or the emotional support from her parents to attend college, but my situation was completely different. My mother and stepfather supported my decision to pursue higher education 100%, including my decision to attend law school. I am now 37 and have a thriving law practice. The one thing weighing on me is that I am still single, and I wish desperately to have a child. My biological clock is ticking, and I feel the constant pressure to figure this out. I could adopt a child on my own; I have the financial resources to do so. However, I never imagined being a single parent, and it is difficult to keep up with the demands of my career and make time to date to meet a prospective husband. I feel like I am at a crossroads in my life.

Life During the Forties

For Erikson (1963), the stimulus for continued growth in middle age is the core struggle between **generativity and stagnation. Generativity** includes being productive in a broad sense—for example, through creative pursuits in a career, in leisure-time activities, in teaching or caring for others, or in some meaningful volunteer work. Two basic qualities of the productive adult are the ability to love well and the ability to work well. Adults who fail to achieve a sense of productivity begin to experience a form of psychological death.

When we reach middle age, we come to a crossroads. During our late 30s and into our mid-40s, we are likely to question what we want to do with the rest of our lives. We face both dangers and opportunities—the danger of slipping into predictable routines and the opportunity to choose to rework the narrow identity of the first half of our life.

During middle age we realize the uncertainty of life, and we discover more clearly that we are alone. We may also go through a grieving process because many parts of our old self are dying, and we may reevaluate and reintegrate an emerging identity that is not the sum of others' expectations. During this evolution we may uncover talents that lead to rich periods of self-exploration and positive change. Here are a few seemingly negative events that may contribute to a midlife transformation:

▶ We may come to realize that some of our youthful dreams will never materialize.

▶ We begin to experience the pressure of time, realizing that now is the time to accomplish our goals.

▶ We recognize our accomplishments and accept our limitations.

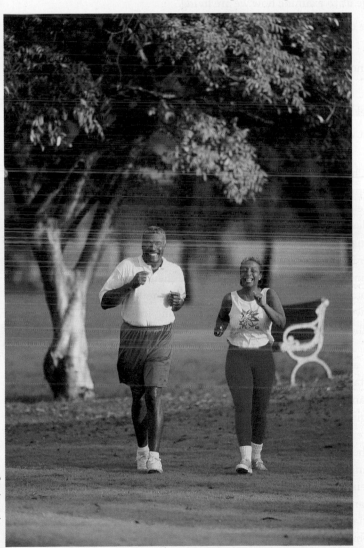

© Stockbyte/Getty Images

The second half of life enlarges the boundaries of vital living.

▶ We may realize that life is not necessarily just and fair and that we often do not get what we had expected, yet we can also make choices about how to make the most of what we have in our lives.

▶ There might be marital crises and challenges to old patterns. A spouse may have an affair or seek a divorce. These crises may also lead to a deepening of the partnered relationship, which can open up a new dimension of intimacy.

▶ Coping with getting older is difficult for many; the loss of some of our youthful physical qualities can be hard to face.

▶ Our children grow up and leave home at this time. People who have lived largely for their children now may face emptiness. However, many experience a period of rejuvenation and self-discovery as they embrace having time to themselves.

▶ We may be confronted with taking care of our elderly parents while we are still taking care of our children or as our children are leaving home.

▶ The death of our parents drives home a truth that is difficult for many to accept; it brings to awareness our own mortality and can challenge us to examine how we are living.

Along with these factors that can precipitate a crisis, new choices are available to us at this time:

▶ We may decide to go back for further schooling and prepare for a new career.

▶ We may deepen our friendships.

▶ We may develop new talents and embark on novel hobbies.

▶ We may look increasingly inward to find out what we most want to do with the rest of our life and begin doing what we say we want to do.

Carl Jung, to whom you were introduced in Chapter 1, was the first modern voice to address the possibility of adult personality development (see Schultz & Schultz, 2013, for an in-depth look at Jung's influence). He took the position that personality development simply cannot progress very far by the end of adolescence and young adulthood. According to Jung, we are confronted with major changes and possibilities for transformation when we begin the second half of life between 35 and 40. For many, this is a time to make choices about solidifying our philosophy of life and deepening our spirituality. Jung's therapy clients consistently revealed signs of experiencing a pivotal middle-age life crisis. Although they may have achieved worldly success, they typically were challenged with finding meaning in projects that had lost meaning. Many of Jung's clients struggled to overcome feelings of emptiness and flatness in life.

Jung believed major life transformations are an inevitable and universal part of the human condition at this juncture in life. He maintained that when the zest for living sags it can be a catalyst for necessary and beneficial changes. To undergo such a transformation requires the death of some aspect of our psychological being, so new growth can occur that will open us to far deeper and richer ranges of existence. To strive for what Jung called **individuation**—integration of the unconscious with the conscious and psychological balance—people during their middle-age years must be willing to let go of preconceived notions and patterns that have dominated the first part of their lives. Their task now is to be open to the unconscious forces that have influenced them and to deepen the meaning of their lives.

For Jung, people can bring unconscious material into awareness by paying attention to their dreams and fantasies and by expressing themselves through poetry, writing, music, and art. Individuals need to recognize that the rational thought patterns that drove them during the first half of life represent merely one way of being. At this time in life, you must be willing to be guided by the spontaneous flow of the unconscious if you hope to achieve an integration of all facets of your being, which is part of psychological health (Schultz & Schultz, 2013).

You may be some distance away from middle age right now, but you can reflect on the way your life is shaping up and think about the person you would like to be when you reach middle age. To help you in making this projection, consider the lives of people you know who are over 40. Do you have any models available in determining what direction you will pursue? Are there some ways you would not want to live? Some of the issues facing middle-aged people are illustrated in Linda's story.

LINDA'S STORY

As a young woman I tried too hard to be superwife, mother, daughter, and friend. I had the role of peacemaker, was very quiet, stayed in the background, and desired to help a star to shine. I had always been there for others, sometimes to the neglect of my own needs and wants. I put too much effort into doing and little into just being. As a result of my personal therapy and other learning, I knew I wanted to change. I started to embrace being genuine and took more risks. I became more verbal and enjoyed participating in class. I began to notice where I could shine. I let go of the self-talk that kept me feeling stupid. I saw hope.

LATE MIDDLE AGE

The time between approximately the early 50s and the early 70s can be considered **late middle age** blending into early aging. This is also a time when many adults are beginning to consider retirement, pursue new interests, and think more about what they want to do with the rest of their lives. This time in the life cycle is often characterized by the beginning of wisdom or the reclaiming of the wisdom of interdependence. This tends to be a time when serving others and passing along experiences become manifest. If a society is to thrive, it is essential that adults direct their resources to preserving the quality of life for future generations. For individuals to grow and thrive, a society must provide adults with opportunities to express and fulfill their generative strivings. During this period of life both individual and societal development are interwoven (Newman & Newman, 2012).

The Fifties

People often begin the process of preparing for older age in their 50s. Many are at their peak in terms of status and personal power, and this can be a satisfying time of life. They do not have to work as hard as they did in the past, nor do they have to meet others' expectations. They can enjoy the benefits of their long struggle and dedication rather than striving to continually prove themselves. It is likely that rearing children and work are moving toward a culmination. Adults at this stage often do a lot of reflecting, contemplating, refocusing, and evaluating, so they can continue to discover new directions.

Rather than focusing on the 50s as a time of decline, we can enhance our lives by looking for what is going right for us. Although many women may experience this as an exciting time, they are often challenged to cope with both the physical and psychological adjustments surrounding menopause. Some women, fearing that menopause means losing their youthful looks, sink into depression.

For men, the 50s can be a time to awaken their creative side. Instead of being consumed with achievement strivings, many men reveal human facets of themselves beyond rational thinking that can result in a richer existence. But men, too, are challenged to find new meaning in their lives. Projects that once were highly satisfying may now lack luster. Some men, like Brent, become depressed when they realize that they have been pursuing empty dreams. They may have met goals they set for themselves only to find that they are still longing for a different kind of life. For both women and men in their 50s, examining priorities often leads to new decisions about how they want to spend their time.

BRENT'S STORY

I have worked as an accountant for many years. My job has paid the bills, so I can't complain. It has enabled me to support my family and even pay for my son's college tuition, which in today's economy means a lot. I feel good about that, but the thought that my job no longer excites me and that it is too late to start a different path has crossed my mind more than once. It actually has sent me into a panic. I want to be able to look back on my life and say that my work made a difference in people's lives.

The Sixties

As we approach advanced age, many physical and psychological changes take place. How we adapt to these changes is influenced by our past experiences, coping skills, beliefs about changing, and personality traits. Many people in their 60s are very able, both physically and mentally, to function independently. A challenge during this phase of the life cycle is coming to terms with the reality that not all the goals that people set for themselves earlier in life will be completed. People must let go of some of their dreams, accept their limitations and unmet goals, stop dwelling on what they cannot do, and focus on what they *can* do (McGoldrick et al., 2011b). As Eugene's story shows, there is much to look forward to during this life transition. Those who have reached mature adulthood have typically raised families, established themselves in their careers, and contributed to the betterment of society in various ways. For Armstrong (2007), the "gift" of this period is *benevolence*. Through their example, others are able to learn ways of striving to make the world a better place.

EUGENE'S STORY

I am looking forward to my retirement from the postal service next year. When I started as a postal carrier, I only intended to do it for a few years. I had bigger dreams, but as the saying goes "life happened" and my plans changed. It doesn't matter now. Everything worked out well. Working a government job gave me a decent living and good benefits. I have no regrets. I have met a lot of amazing people during my career. I used to deliver mail to a nonprofit organization that feeds homeless people. When I retire next year, I am eager to start some volunteer work there. It will give my life meaning.

If you have reached middle age, use the journal pages at the end of this chapter to write down your reactions to a few of these questions that have the most meaning for you. If you have not reached middle age, think about how you would like to be able to answer these questions when you reach that stage in your life. What do you need to do now to meet your expectations? Do you know a middle-aged person who serves as a role model for you?

▶ Is this a time of "generativity" or of "stagnation" for you? Think about some of the things you have done during this time of life that you feel the best about.

▶ Do you feel productive? If so, in what ways?

▶ Are there some things that you would definitely like to change in your life right now? What prevents you from making these changes?

▶ Have you experienced a midlife crisis? If so, how has it affected you? How has it affected others who are important in your life?

▶ What losses have you experienced?

▶ What are some of the most important decisions you have made during this time of your life?

▶ What do you look forward to in your remaining years?

▶ If you were to review the major successes of your life to this point, what would they be?

LATE ADULTHOOD

Late adulthood spans the period from age 70 onward, yet it is imprecise to define late adulthood strictly in terms of chronological age. Newman and Newman (2012) write of a longevity revolution and describe a new psychosocial stage called **very old age**, from age 75 until death. There is a great deal of individual variation at this final stage of life, and many more older people are in good health today as they age. In the United States and other industrialized countries, people in their 70s are the fastest growing portion of the population, and many 75-year-olds have the energy of middle-aged people. How people look and feel during late adulthood is more than a matter of physical age; it is largely a matter of attitude. To a great degree, vitality is influenced by state of mind as much as by the actual years lived.

As I (Jerry) read about this new psychosocial stage (very old age of 75 years onward), I was taken aback, realizing that I fall into this category. But I do not experience myself as a "very old person," and I do not recognize many of the characteristics associated with old age as applying to me. From a personal perspective, I realize that the typical characteristics of the various stages of life are simply rough markers rather than accurate signs of development. Perhaps I am in denial, but I believe I can still to do everything I was able to do in my 50s, although it may take me a bit longer. My family makes it easy for me to stay in denial by referring to me as a "perpetual adolescent."

Themes During Late Adulthood

The death of parents and the loss of friends and relatives confront us with the reality of preparing ourselves for our own death. A basic task of late adulthood is to complete a life review in which we put our life in perspective and come to accept who we are and what we have done. Late adulthood is a time in life when spirituality may take on a new meaning and provide us with a sense of purpose, even as we face an increasing dependence on others (McGoldrick et al., 2011b).

Prevalent themes for people during late adulthood include loss; loneliness and social isolation; feelings of rejection; finding meaning in life; dependency; feelings of uselessness, hopelessness, and despair; fears of death and dying; grief over others' deaths; sadness over physical and mental deterioration; and regrets over past events. Today, many of these themes characterize people in their mid-80s more than people in their 60s and even 70s. Those individuals who are very old have an opportunity to travel uncharted territory. Indeed some would say "life begins at 80" because there are so few norms for behavior for people who reach very old age that they are free to do whatever they want to do (Newman & Newman, 2012).

According to Erikson (1963), the central issue of this age period is **integrity versus despair**. Those who succeed in achieving **ego integrity** feel that their lives have been productive and worthwhile and that they have managed to cope with failures as well as successes. They can accept the course of their lives and are not obsessed with thoughts of what might have been and what they could or should have done. They can look back without resentment and regret and can see their lives in a perspective of completeness and satisfaction. They accept themselves for who and what they are, and they also accept others as they are. They believe that who they are and what they have become are to a great extent the result of their choices. They approach the final stage of life with a sense of integration, balance, and wholeness. They can view death as natural, even while living rich and meaningful lives until the day they die. One reason it is so important for older people to demonstrate integrity is that it gives hope to younger people that life is worth living.

Some older people fail to achieve ego integration. Typically, such people fear death. They may develop a sense of hopelessness and feelings of self-disgust. They approach the final stage of their lives with a sense of personal fragmentation. They often feel that they have little control over what happens to them. They cannot accept their life's cycle, for they see whatever they have done as "not enough" and feel that they have a lot of unfinished business. They yearn for another chance, even though they realize that they cannot have it. They feel inadequate and have a hard time accepting themselves, for they think that they have wasted much of their lives and let valuable time slip by. For other older people, this may be a time of forming a new community. As they move into assisted living or participate in senior center services, they may form new relationships that are quite positive and engaging. The field of geriatrics is developing, and seniors now have many more options than previous generations had.

From Armstrong's (2007) perspective, people in late adulthood give the "gift" of *wisdom*. Older adults represent the source of wisdom that exists in each of us, which helps us avoid the mistakes of the past and reap the benefits of life's lessons. In many traditional societies, the oldest members are looked to for their wisdom and guidance in solving problems of society. A new international group of independent global leaders working together for peace and humanity, known as The Elders,* has the aim of bringing about social change. An Elder is a changemaker in the sense that he or she leads by example and creates positive social change and inspires others to do the same. The Elders, who were brought together by Nelson Mandela, offer their collective wisdom and experience to help alleviate the causes of human

*For more information on The Elders, go to their website at www.theelders.org.

suffering. Here are a few of The Elders whose names you may be familiar with who have led by example:

Nelson Mandela: Former President of South Africa and Nobel Peace Laureate; a leader who has dedicated his life to the anti-apartheid struggle, democracy and equality; founder of The Elders.

Graca Machel: International advocate for women's and children's rights; former freedom fighter, and first Education Minister of Mozambique.

Gro Brundtland: First woman Prime Minister of Norway; a medical doctor who champions health as a human right; put sustainable development on the international agenda.

Ela Bhatt: The "gentle revolutionary"; a pioneer in women's empowerment and grassroots development, founder of the more than 1-million-strong Self-Employed Women's Association in India.

Desmond Tutu: Archbishop Emeritus of Cape Town, Nobel Peace Laureate and Chair of The Elders; a veteran anti-apartheid activist and peace campaigner widely regarded as "South Africa's moral conscience."

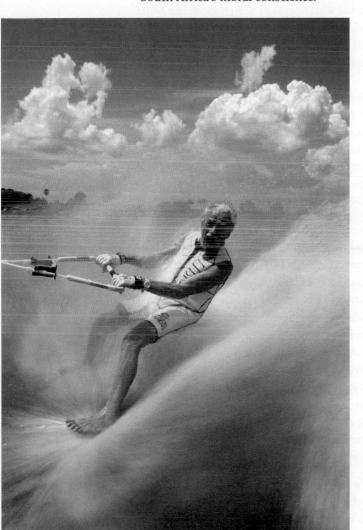

» Stereotypes of older people need to be challenged.

Older people do not have to belong to The Elders to share their life experiences and wisdom. The group believes that everybody can make a difference and bring about change in his or her own way.

Stereotypes of Late Adulthood

It is a challenge for us to change the image of late adulthood, which is based on myths and stereotypes. What gets in the way of understanding older people as individuals with this capacity for great variation are the common stereotypes many people hold about older adults.

Ageism refers to prejudice toward or stereotyping of people simply because they are perceived as being "old" (American Psychological Association [APA], 2004). Ageism predisposes us to discriminate against old people by avoiding them or in some way victimizing them primarily because of their age. Here are some of the stereotypes associated with older people that need to be challenged:

▶ All older individuals eventually become senile.

▶ It is disgraceful for an old person to remarry.

▶ Old people are not creative.

▶ Growing old always entails having a host of serious physical and emotional problems.

▶ Older people are set in their ways, stuck on following rigid patterns of thinking and behaving, and are not open to change.

▶ When people grow old, they are no longer capable of learning or contributing.

- An older person will die soon after his or her mate dies.

- Most older persons are socially isolated.

- Old people are no longer interested in sex or intimacy.

- Depression is a natural consequence of aging.

- Preoccupation with death and dying is typical of older adults.

These negative perceptions and stereotypes of older people are common in our society. The attitudes older people have about aging are extremely important. Like adolescents, older adults may feel a sense of uselessness because of how others view them. It is easy to accept the myths of others and turn them into self-fulfilling prophecies. Older people themselves can harbor ageist attitudes and stereotypes (APA, 2004), and they can be rendered helpless if they accept such erroneous beliefs. Older people can benefit from critically examining these stereotypes and challenging these negative messages.

Challenging the Stereotypes

Old age does not have to be something we look toward with horror or resignation; nor must it be associated with bitterness. However, many older adults in our society do feel resentment, and we have generally neglected this population, treating them as an undesirable minority that is merely tolerated. Their loss is doubly sad because older people can make definite contributions to society.

Older adults have a wealth of life experiences and coping skills, and they are likely to share this wisdom if they sense that others have a genuine interest in them. Many older adults are still very capable, yet the prejudice of younger adults often keeps us from acknowledging the value of the contributions older adults offer us.

Do you know some older people who are living testimony that growing old does not mean that life is over? Do you know anyone in late adulthood who refuses to be caught up in the stereotypes of aging? Here are some older people whose lives are evidence that aging is more than simply a chronological process.

Aunt Mary We often imagine that people in their 80s and 90s live in rest homes and convalescent hospitals. We forget that many people of advanced age live by themselves and take care of themselves quite well. For instance, I (Marianne) occasionally visited with one of Jerry's aunts who lived to be 101 years old. We always had good discussions about the past as well as the present. Aunt Mary had an incredible memory and showed interest in what was happening in the world. Until a few years before her death, she was active through gardening, sewing, and taking care of her household. At times she resisted fully accepting her limitations, but eventually she was willing to receive the help needed to make her life more comfortable. She had a deep religious faith, which gave her the strength to cope with many of the hardships she had to endure. Another source of vitality was her involvement with her children, grandchildren, and great grandchildren. I always walked away from my visits with Aunt Mary feeling uplifted, positive about aging, and saying to myself "I hope I will feel as positive about life should I be fortunate enough to reach beyond 100."

Art Art was widowed several years ago. No one would guess that he is 88 by looking at him. A few years ago he moved 200 miles from the home he and his wife resided in for 30 years to make a new home with some of his family. His occupation was carpentry, and although he has been retired for many years, he is actively engaged in a number of building projects for others and for himself. Just recently he began to teach at-risk youth and ex-gang members the art of carpentry. In addition to learning carpentry from Art, one youth acknowledged that he also benefits from Art's wisdom on life. Art is still spry, is able to laugh and cry with the young people he teaches, and just 2 years ago he remarried.

Bob and Betty A couple in their 90s who have been married for 70 years, Bob and Betty still enjoy each other's company. In addition to what they have as a couple, they are also blessed as individuals. They enjoy relatively good health, live independently in their own home, are involved with a large extended family, enjoy many grandchildren and great grandchildren, and assume leadership roles in their church. They take a walk together each day for at least a mile. They spend many hours doing volunteer work. Routinely, they make trips to Mexico where they serve as missionaries, providing assistance to an orphanage and a local church. Those who know them marvel at their ability to handle the strain connected with devoting countless hours to missionary work. What is most notable about them is their love for their family and their strong religious faith. Betty's quiet strength and gentleness blend nicely with Bob's incredible sharp wit and humor.

The Delany Sisters In their inspirational book, *Having Our Say* (Delany & Delany, 1993), Bessie and Sarah Delany show us, even at the ripe ages of 102 and 104, that it is possible to maintain an interest in the world about them. The two women illustrate a wonderful example of aging with integrity. Both of them, of African American descent, were professional women, one a teacher and the other a dentist. The two sisters reflect on their long life and give us some insight about what led to their longevity. Although surprised at their longevity, they continued to live a healthy lifestyle that included exercise and a good diet. The sisters depended on each other as well as on family to care for them, yet they were able to retain a degree of independence. They gave a flavor of the challenge of growing old in their own words:

> But it's hard being old, because you can't always do everything you want, exactly as *you* want it done. When you get as old as we are, you have to struggle to hang on to your freedom, your independence. We have a lot of family and friends keeping an eye on us, but we try not to be dependent on any one person. (p. 238)

Most people who have read their book or listened to their interviews are surprised by their incredible interest and definite opinions on a range of current affairs. The Delany sisters offer us a good illustration of remaining vital in spite of living more than 100 years.

Many octogenarians lead exemplary lives. Willard Scott, a national weatherman, often recognizes people on the morning news who have reached age 100 or above. Many of these individuals are described as living an active life, which shows us that aging is partially a state of mind. The Delany sisters, and others who have lived long and rich lives, frequently cite a host of elements that contributed to their advanced age:

▶ Being fortunate to have good genes

▶ Work that has provided meaning and fulfillment

▶ Involvement with family and friends

- An interest in doing good for others
- Staying involved in life and not retiring from life
- Having strong religious convictions
- A sense of humor
- The ability to grieve losses
- The willingness to forgive and not to be bitter
- Expressing rather than holding onto irritations
- A sense of pride in self
- Regular physical exercise
- Practicing good nutritional habits

The people briefly described here do not fit the stereotypes of older adults. They are living proof that one can age and at the same time live a full and rich life. There is no formula for growing old with grace and dignity. One of the ways to increase the chances of reaching an active old age is to make choices at earlier ages that will provide the foundation for these later years. Although you may not have reached old age, we hope you won't brush aside thinking about your eventual aging. Your observations of the old people you know can provide you with insights about what it is like to grow older. From these observations you can begin to formulate a picture of the life you would like to have as you get older.

TAKE TIME TO REFLECT

Imagine yourself being old. Think about your fears and about what you would like to be able to say about your life—your joys, your accomplishments, and your regrets. To facilitate this reflection, consider these questions:

- What do you most hope to accomplish by the time you reach old age?
- What are some of your greatest fears of getting old?
- What are you doing now that might have an effect on the kind of person you will be as you grow older?
- Do you know an older person who is a role model for you? If so, what is it about him or her that stands out the most?
- What are some things you hope to do during the later years of your life? How do you think you will adjust to retirement?
- How would you like to be able to respond to your body's aging? How do you think you will respond to failing health or to physical limitations on your lifestyle?
- What would you most want to be able to say about yourself and your life when you are an older adult?

In the journal pages at the end of this chapter write down some impressions of the kind of old age you hope for as well as the fears you have about aging.

SUMMARY

Adulthood involves the struggle for autonomy, which means that we know ourselves and that we are able to form meaningful connections with others. Our quest for autonomy and maturity is truly a lifelong endeavor. Each stage of adulthood presents us with different tasks. Meeting the developmental tasks of later life hinges on successfully working through earlier issues. One part of this quest is learning to evaluate our early decisions and how these decisions currently influence us.

Transactional analysis can help us recognize early learning and decisions. Our life script is made up of both parental messages and decisions we make in response to these injunctions. The events of childhood and, to some extent, adolescence contribute to the formation of our life script, which we tend to follow into adulthood. By becoming increasingly aware of our life script, we are in a position to revise it. Instead of being hopelessly "scripted" by childhood influences, we can use our past to change our future. In short, we can shape our destiny rather than being passively shaped by earlier events.

During early adulthood, it is important to learn how to form intimate relationships. To develop intimacy, we must move beyond the self-preoccupation that is characteristic of adolescence. This is also a time when we are at our peak in terms of physical and psychological powers and can direct these resources to establish ourselves in all dimensions of life. Choices that we make pertaining to education, work, and lifestyle will have a profound impact later in life.

As we approach middle age, we come to a crossroads. Midlife is filled with a potential for danger and for new opportunities. At this phase we can assume a stance that "it's too late to change," or we can make significant revisions. There are opportunities to change careers, to find new ways to spend leisure time, and to find other ways of making a new life.

Later life can be a time of real enjoyment, or it can be a time of looking back in regret to all that we have not accomplished and experienced. A key task of the last stage of life is the completion of a life review, in which we evaluate turning points and the significance of our life. It is important to recognize that the quality of life in later years often depends on the choices we made at earlier junctures in life.

The experiences and events that occur during each developmental stage are crucial in helping to determine our attitudes, beliefs, values, and actions regarding the important areas of our lives that will be discussed in the chapters to come: gender-role identity, work, the body, love, sexuality, intimate relationships, loneliness and solitude, death and loss, and meaning and values. For this reason we have devoted considerable attention to the foundations of life choices. We recognize that conditions in society such as widespread financial hardship may put a damper on the choices we make as adults and may affect how smoothly we transition through the developmental stages. Understanding how we got where we are now is a critical first step in deciding where we want to go from here.

Where Can I Go From Here?

1. Reflect on some critical turning points in your life. Draw a chart in your journal showing the age periods you have experienced so far and indicate your key successes, joys, failures, conflicts, and memories for each stage. In your journal write down some examples of new decisions or turning points that have made a significant difference in your life.

2. After you have described some of the significant events in your life, list some of the decisions you have made in response to these events. How were you affected by these milestones in your life? Think about what you have learned about yourself from doing these exercises. What does all of this tell you about the person you are today?

3. To broaden your perspective on human development in various cultural or ethnic groups, talk to someone you know who grew up in a very different environment from the one you knew as a child. Find out how his or her life experiences have differed from yours by sharing some aspects of your own life. Try to discover whether there are significant differences in values that seem to be related to the differences in your life experiences. This could help you reassess many of your own values.

4. Talk with some people who are significantly older than you. For instance, if you are in your 20s, interview a middle-aged person and an older adult. Try to get them to take the lead and tell you about their lives. What do they like about their lives? What have been some key turning points for them? What do they most remember about the past? You might even suggest that they read the section of the chapter that pertains to their present age group and react to the ideas presented there.

5. Now that you have studied each stage of life, reflect on the meaning of these stages to you. If you have not yet arrived at a particular stage, think about what you can do at this time to assure the quality of life you would like in a future phase.

6. **Suggested Readings.** The full bibliographic entry for each of these sources can be found in the References and Suggested Readings at the back of the book. Books you may find useful in learning how to dispute negative self-talk include Ellis (2001), Burns (1981), Beck (2011). For interesting reading on the path toward living mindfully, see Kabat-Zinn (1990, 1994). For a book describing key developmental tasks of the stages of adulthood, see Armstrong (2007). A useful book that deals with a psychosocial perspective of early adulthood, middle adulthood, and late adulthood is Newman and Newman (2012).

WEBSITE RESOURCES

Included here are some valuable websites. For access to these websites, video activities, and other supporting materials, visit Cengage Learning's Counseling CourseMate website for *I Never Knew I Had a Choice*, 10th Edition, at **www.cengagebrain.com.**

ERIKSON TUTORIAL HOME PAGE
http://web.cortland.edu/andersmd/ERIK/welcome.HTML
Recommended Search Words: "erikson tutorial homepage"

This site provides handy information about Erik Erikson's eight stages of psychosocial development, including a summary chart of key facts for each stage, an introduction to each stage, and other links to information on Erikson and psychosocial development.

SENIORNET
www.seniornet.org
Recommended Search Words: "seniornet"

SeniorNet seeks to provide access and education about computer technology and the Internet to those who are 50+ years old. The site offers links, information, and discussion groups on a wide variety of topics of interest to seniors. If you are interested in learning about computers and the Internet, you can look up their learning centers online here or call them at (571) 203-7100 for the location nearest you.

ADULT DEVELOPMENT AND AGING: APA DIVISION 20
http://apadiv20.phhp.ufl.edu/
Recommended Search Words: "APA division 20"

Division 20 of the American Psychological Association is devoted to the study of the psychology of adult development and aging. Here you will find information on instructional resources for teachers, resources for students, and links for publications, conferences, and other related websites.

THE ELDERS
http://www.theelders.org
Recommended Search Words: "the elders"

The Elders is an independent group of global leaders who work together for peace and human rights. These older adults are living examples of people who are bringing their wisdom to bear on some of the most pressing social problems of our time.

107

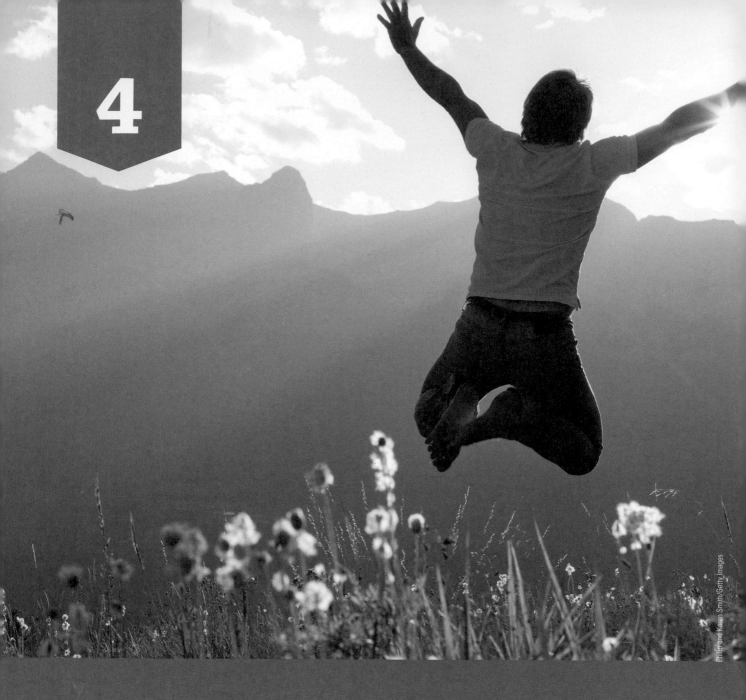

4

YOUR BODY AND WELLNESS

> Where Am I Now?

> Wellness and Life Choices

> Maintaining Sound Health Practices

> Your Bodily Identity

> Summary

> Where Can I Go From Here?

> Website Resources

Philip and Karen Smith/Getty Images

Wellness stresses positive health rather than merely the absence of disabling symptoms.

WHERE AM I NOW?

Use this scale to respond to the following statements:

4 = I *strongly agree* with this statement.
3 = I *agree* with this statement.
2 — I *disagree* with this statement.
1 = I *strongly disagree* with this statement.

1. Making changes in my lifestyle to improve my health is not something I often think about.

2. The way I treat my body expresses the way I feel about myself.

3. When I look in the mirror, I feel comfortable with my physical appearance.

4. When something ails me, I want a quick fix.

5. I like to give hugs and receive hugs.

6. My diet consists mainly of fast food.

7. Exercise is a priority in my life.

8. I am motivated to take better care of myself in all respects.

9. I set aside sufficient time for rest and sleep.

10. I take care of my physical and emotional needs.

In this chapter we begin by exploring the topic of our general state of wellness. We take a holistic approach to wellness, which involves considering all aspects of our being. We look at the ways self-image is influenced by people's perceptions of their body. We also address how bodily identity, which includes the way people experience themselves and express themselves through their body, affects their beliefs, decisions, and feelings about themselves.

Think about these questions: Do you take care of the physical you? How comfortable are you with your body? How do your feelings and attitudes about your body affect your self-worth, sexuality, and love? How aware are you of the impact your emotional state has on your physical state? How does the quality of your relationships affect your physical health?

We also explore the goal of wellness as a lifestyle choice that enhances body and mind, which includes making decisions about rest, exercise, and diet and learning to accept responsibility for our health. Although most of us would readily say that we desire the state of wellness as a personal goal, many of us have experienced frustrations and discouragement in attaining this goal. Wellness is not something that merely happens to us. It is the result of many choices we make every day about taking care of ourselves on all levels. Wellness is more than the absence of illness. In some ways the medical model ignores wellness and focuses on the removal of symptoms, which results in a limited view of health. Often physicians do not explore with their patients those aspects of their lifestyle that may contribute to their health problems.

An examination of the choices you are making about your body and your overall wellness reveals a great deal about how you feel about your life. We are in charge of our general health, and the way we lead our life affects our physical and psychological well-being. This includes accepting responsibility for what we eat and drink, how we exercise, and the stresses we experience. (Stress and approaches to managing stress are the subjects of Chapter 5.)

The body gives us critical information that we can choose to listen to, ignore, or deny. If you listen to your body, you can make life-enhancing choices. Think about these questions as you read this chapter: At this time in your life, what priority do you place on your own wellness? What resources do you require to begin modifying those parts of your lifestyle that affect your bodily well-being? If you are not taking care of yourself, what beliefs, thought patterns, and assumptions may be getting in the way? A main challenge many of us face is, "What can I do to discontinue any habitual, unhealthy choices and replace them with healthy patterns of living?" The purpose of this chapter is to assist you in reflecting on what you want for yourself in the long term and on the range of choices available to you for staying healthy.

WELLNESS AND LIFE CHOICES

Traditional medicine focuses on identifying symptoms of illness and curing disease. It aims at removing disease and the cause of disease whenever possible, although sometimes symptom relief is all that can be done. By contrast, **holistic health** focuses on all facets of human functioning, which involves our taking responsibility for maintaining all aspects of our well-being. **Wellness** entails a lifestyle choice and involves a lifelong process of taking care of our needs on all levels of functioning. Well people are committed to creating a lifestyle that contributes to taking care of their physical selves, challenging themselves intellectually, expressing the full range of their emotions, finding rewarding interpersonal relationships, and searching for meaning that will give direction to their lives. Hales (2013) captures the essence of wellness:

> Wellness can be defined as purposeful, enjoyable living or, more specifically, a deliberate lifestyle choice characterized by personal responsibility and optimal enhancement of physical, mental, and spiritual health. (p. 4)

Wellness encompasses more than the absence of illness and disabling symptoms; it is the result of a conscious commitment to our physical and psychological well-being. Wellness is a process of making choices that lead to zest, peace, vitality, and happiness in our whole being.

In *The Wellness Workbook*, Travis and Ryan (2004) describe wellness as a bridge supported by two piers: self-responsibility and love. They write that self-responsibility and love flow from the appreciation that we are not merely separate individuals, nor are we simply the sum of separate parts. The essence of wellness involves a way of life aimed at achieving our highest potential; it entails an integration of body, mind, and spirit.

The wellness process involves identifying personal goals, prioritizing your goals and values, identifying any barriers that might prevent you from reaching your goals, making an action plan, and then committing yourself to following through on your plans to reach your goals. This may seem a rather simple pathway, but simplicity is not to be confused with ease of doing. Many people who desire general wellness are reluctant to put what they know into a plan designed to bring about changes. We suggest you review the section on making an action plan in Chapter 1 and apply these principles to some health behavior you may target for change.

Wellness and Responsible Choices

Although many of us know *what* to do, we oftentimes do not put what we know into action. We may deny our part in our level of wellness and think of getting sick as something that is beyond our control. Although most of us have a great deal of knowledge about wellness, our challenge is to use the knowledge we have in a way that works for us, rather than against us.

A combination of factors contributes to a sense of well-being, and a holistic approach pays attention to specific aspects of our lifestyle: how we work and play, how we relax, how and what we eat, how we think and feel, how we keep physically fit, our relationships with others, our values and beliefs, and our spiritual needs and practices. When something is amiss in our lives, we are generally failing to take proper care of one or more of these basic human dimensions.

Bernie Siegel (1988), a psychologically and spiritually oriented physician, has investigated the quality of his patients' psychological and spiritual lives as the key to understanding the mystery of illness and how to foster health. As a physician, Siegel views his role not simply as finding the right treatments for a disease but also as helping his patients resolve emotional conflicts, find an inner reason for living, and release the healing resources within.

Siegel's works point to the power we have to keep ourselves well and to heal ourselves. Scores of self-help books and home videos address the subjects of stress management, exercise, meditation, diet, nutrition, weight control, control of smoking and drinking, and wellness medicine. As a society, we have begun to recognize the value of preventive medicine, and wellness clinics, nutrition centers, and exercise clubs have become popular in recent years. Because a direct relationship between students' general health and well-being and their academic success has been observed, "many universities are constructing or remodeling facilities to combine state-of-the-art student recreation and fitness centers with university health centers, thus creating a one-stop shop for their students' health, wellness, and fitness needs" (Fullerton, 2011, p. 63).

Despite the increased emphasis on holistic health practices and wellness in our society, the fight against unhealthy lifestyle choices is far from over. Childhood obesity is such a formidable threat to the well-being of an entire generation of young Americans that First Lady Michelle Obama introduced *Let's Move*, a comprehensive initiative aimed at combating childhood obesity. Although wellness encompasses more than diet and fitness, poor choices in these two areas alone can have far-reaching consequences later in life. Serious physical problems including diabetes, heart disease, asthma, high blood pressure, and cancer are linked to childhood obesity, not to mention the psychological and emotional repercussions that are likely to result. As alarming as these facts are, some U.S. secondary schools do not have physical education programs due to limited budgets and other constraints.

Take a few moments to reflect on the priority you are placing on your physical and psychological well-being.

One Man's Wellness Program

Kevin was in one of our therapeutic groups, and when we first met him, Kevin seemed closed off emotionally, rigid, stoic, and defensive. For many years he had thrown himself completely into his work as an attorney. Although his family life was marked by tension and bickering with his wife, he attempted to block out the stress at home by burying himself in his law cases and by excelling in his career. Kevin's story underscores the truth that many of us are not motivated to change until we have faced a serious health concern. Here is his own account of his life.

KEVIN'S STORY

When I reached middle age, I began to question how I wanted to live the rest of my life. My father suffered a series of heart attacks. I watched my father decline physically, and this jolted me into the realization that both my father's time and my own time were limited. I finally went for a long-overdue physical examination and discovered that I had high blood pressure, that my cholesterol level was abnormally high, and that I was at relatively high risk of having a heart attack. I also learned that several of my relatives had died of heart attacks. I decided that I wanted to reverse what I saw as a self-destructive path. I decided to change my patterns of living in several ways. I was overeating, my diet was not balanced, I was consuming a great deal of alcohol to relax, I didn't get enough sleep, and I didn't do any physical exercise. My new decision involved making contacts with friends. I learned to enjoy playing tennis and racquetball on a regular basis. I took up jogging. If I didn't run in the morning, I felt somewhat sluggish during the day. I radically changed my diet based on suggestions from my physician. As a result, I lowered both my cholesterol level and my blood pressure without the use of medication; I also lost 20 pounds and worked myself into excellent physical shape. Getting into personal counseling was extremely helpful, because my sessions with a counselor helped me make some basic changes in the way I approach life and also helped me put things into perspective.

Let's underscore a few key points in Kevin's case. First of all, he took the time to seriously reflect on the direction he was going in life. He did not engage in self-deception; rather, he admitted that the way he was living was not healthy. On finding out that heart disease was a part of his family history, he did not assume an indifferent attitude. Instead, he made a decision to take an active part in changing his life on many levels.

With the help of counseling, Kevin realized the price he was paying for bottling up emotions like hurt, sadness, anger, guilt, and joy. Although he did not give up his logical and analytical dimensions, he added to his range of emotional expression. He learned that unexpressed emotions would find expression in some form of physical illness or symptom. He continued to question the value of living exclusively by logic and calculation, in both his professional and personal life. As a consequence, he cultivated friendships and let others who were significant to him know that he wanted to be closer to them. Kevin was challenged to review his life to determine what steps he could take to get more from the time he had to live. He took a proactive stance in making basic changes in the way he was living. Perhaps his experience will inspire you to review your own life and the choices you are currently making.

Accepting Responsibility for Your Body

The American public is becoming increasingly informed about exercise, diet, and ways to manage stress. Many health insurance companies are paying for preventive medicine as well as remediation, and some are asking clients to complete lifestyle surveys to identify positive and negative habits that affect their overall health. Many communities provide a wide variety of programs aimed at helping people improve the quality of their lives by finding a form of exercise that suits them.

Physicians report that it is not uncommon for patients to be more interested in getting pills and in removing their symptoms than in changing a stressful lifestyle. In describing this trend, positive psychologist Tal Ben-Shahar (2011) commented: "Last semester one of my students was devastated after he received his first-ever B, and after thirty minutes in the doctor's office—the first time he had ever visited a psychiatrist—he was prescribed an antidepressant" (p. 188). Some people see themselves as victims of their ailments rather than as being responsible for them. However, with increased attention being paid to the possible side effects of drugs and medications, many people are taking steps to educate themselves about prescription drugs and to question their physicians about the medications they prescribe. Perhaps it will come as no surprise that "consumers' use of the Internet for acquiring important health care information is growing sharply" (Wymer, 2010, p. 187).

The perceived benefits and risks of medications often change as more is learned through experience. We may be advised to take cholesterol-lowering medications to reduce the chances of a heart attack or a stroke but later learn of serious side effects such as damage to our organs from those same medications. A particular drug may be praised as being life saving initially but taken off the market a few years later due to serious side effects, including death. Some people still prefer to give full authority for health care to their physicians, and many trust pharmaceutical companies to provide information to consumers that is credible, comprehensive, and accurate, without considering that there may be a conflict of interest (Wymer, 2010). Others take a more active role and assume more responsibility for their health care.

Psychologically oriented physicians emphasize the role of *choice* and *responsibility* as critical determinants of our physical and psychological well-being. They invite their patients to look at what they are doing to their bodies through lack of exercise, the substances they take in, and other damaging behavior. Although they may prescribe medication to lower a person's extremely high blood pressure or cholesterol, they inform the patient that medications can do only so much and that what is needed is a change in lifestyle. The patient is encouraged to share with the physician the responsibility for maintaining wellness.

We cannot control every aspect of our overall health however, and there are limits to our responsibility. Consider the medical problems Christa has battled for years. Despite the severity of her conditions, she has chosen to take control of those aspects of her health that are within her power.

CHRISTA'S STORY

I recently celebrated an accomplishment that I never dreamed I'd achieve. At the age of 22 I graduated from college. Now, that may not seem that out of the ordinary, but when you consider that I have battled one medical crisis after another since I was a child, it is nothing short of a miracle. I have had an ongoing problem with seizures for years, not to mention two brain tumors (one in childhood and the other in late adolescence), which were both successfully removed, and most recently, a diagnosis of kidney disease. My identity has been shaped to some extent by these problems, but I refuse to allow them to completely define who I am. This is very difficult at times. Some of the medication I have had to take has had the unfortunate side effect of weight gain. When I get down on myself about my body image, I remind myself that being several pounds overweight is better than having seizures constantly. In fact, being overweight is better than "not being" at all. I do the best I can in terms of watching my diet and exercising a few times a week, but I try not to be too hard on myself when I don't perfectly adhere to my diet or exercise routine. My body has gone through way too much for me to spend energy berating myself for something I have limited control over.

If you see yourself as an active agent in maintaining your health, this can make a world of difference. If you believe you simply catch colds or are ill-fated enough to get sick, and if you do not see what you can do to prevent bodily illnesses, your body is not getting your support. But if you recognize that the way you lead your life has a direct bearing on your physical and psychological well-being, you can be more in control of your health. Psychological factors play a key role in enhancing physical well-being and preventing illness. Likewise, our level of physical health affects us psychologically. The Take Time to Reflect exercise can help you answer the question, "Who is in charge of my health?"

TAKE TIME TO REFLECT

1. Here are some common rationalizations people use for not changing patterns of behavior that affect their bodies. Look over these statements and decide which ones, if any, fit you.

_____ I don't have time to exercise several times a week.

_____ No matter how I try to lose weight, nothing seems to work.

_____ I sabotage myself, and others sabotage me, in my attempts to lose weight.

_____ I'll stop smoking soon.

_____ When I have a vacation, I'll relax.

_____ I drink a lot (or use drugs), but it calms me down and has not interfered with my life.

_____ I need a drink or a smoke to relax.

_____ Food isn't important to me.

_____ I don't have time to eat three balanced meals a day.

_____ If I stop smoking, I'll surely gain weight.

_____ I simply cannot function without several cups of coffee.

_____ If I don't stop smoking, I might get lung cancer or die a little sooner, but we all have to go sometime.

What other statements could you add to this list? _____

_____

_____

2. Complete the following sentences with the first word or phrase that comes to mind:

a. One way I take care of my body is _____.

b. One way I neglect my body is _____.

c. When people notice my physical appearance, I think that _____.

d. When I look at my body in the mirror, I _____.

e. I could be healthier if _____.

f. One way to cut down the stress in my life is to _____.

g. If I could change one aspect of my body, it would be my _____.

h. One way that I relax is _____.

i. I'd describe my diet as _____.

j. For me, exercising is _____.

3. As you review your responses to this exercise, what changes, if any, do you want to make? What steps can you take at this time to bring about these changes? _____

_____

_____

MAINTAINING SOUND HEALTH PRACTICES

Maintaining a balanced life involves attending to our physical, emotional, social, mental, and spiritual needs. Developing sound habits pertaining to sleeping, eating, exercising, and cultivating our spirituality is basic to any wellness program. As you read the following sections, reflect on your own practices pertaining to rest and sleep, exercise and fitness, diet and nutrition, and spirituality and think about changes you may want to make.

Rest and Sleep

Sleep is a fundamental aspect of being healthy. Rest is restorative. During sleep our physical body is regenerated, we recover from the stresses we experience during the day, and we are provided with energy to cope effectively with challenges we will face tomorrow. If we sleep between 6 and 9 hours each night, we are in the normal range. Experts in sleep tell us that the quality of sleep matters more than the quantity. The amount of sleep that is normal for different individuals can vary. It is important to pay attention to your body and to adjust your sleeping habits based on what you need.

Sleep deprivation leads to increased vulnerability to emotional upset and leaves us susceptible to the negative consequences of stress. Weiten (2013) reports that researchers have investigated the notion that sleep deprivation could have serious health consequences. Sleep loss can affect physiological processes in ways that may undermine physical health. Individuals' attention, motor coordination, reaction time, and decision making may be

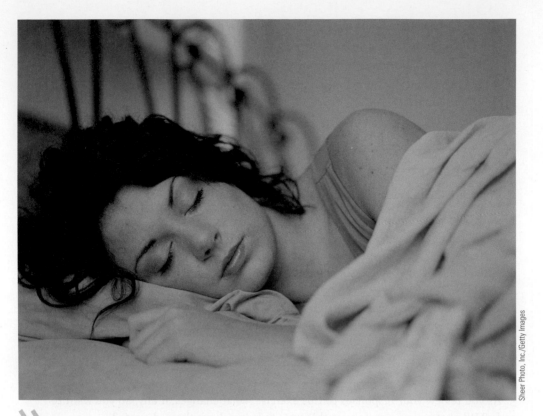

Sheer Photo, Inc./Getty Images

Getting proper sleep is a fundamental aspect of being healthy.

impaired. "If we deprive ourselves of sleep on a regular basis and rely instead on chemical stimulants to keep us awake, we pay a price in the form of decreased creativity and productivity, as well as an increased risk of depression and anxiety" (Ben-Shahar, 2011, p. 145).

There is variability among individuals in how sensitive they are to sleep deprivation, but researchers have found that people who consistently sleep less than 7 hours or those who sleep more than 8 hours show elevated mortality risk. Mortality rates are especially high for people who sleep more than 10 hours (Weiten, 2013). In a recent study, Brigham Young University researchers Eric Eide and Mark Showalter (2012) found that 16- to 18-year-olds need 7 hours of sleep, not the often cited recommendation of 8 or 9, to perform better on standardized tests. Among 12-year-olds, the optimal amount of sleep ranges between 8 and 8.5 hours, and among 10-year-olds, the optimal number of hours per night is 9 to 9.5. Their research, based on a representative sample of 1,724 primary and secondary school students across the United States, suggests that the ideal amount of sleep decreases with age.

Your needs tend to change as you grow older and variation among individuals is to be expected, so how can you tell whether you are getting the quantity and quality of sleep you need? Some of the signs that you may not be getting adequate sleep include moodiness, tiredness, difficulty concentrating, and falling asleep in class or when trying to study. Sleep disturbances or insufficient sleep tend to result in increased irritability, difficulty concentrating, memory loss, increased physical and emotional tension, and being overly sensitive to criticism. Insomnia can be caused by stress and is often the result of not being able to "turn off thinking" when you are trying to sleep. If you are interested in sleeping well, make efforts to take your mind off your problems. Ruminating about your difficulties is one of the key factors contributing to insomnia.

It is a good idea to monitor how well and how often you get the sleep and rest you require to function optimally. One of the most common sleep disorders is **insomnia,** which refers to chronic problems in getting adequate sleep. Most of us experience occasional insomnia and difficulty in falling or staying asleep. This kind of transient insomnia is often associated with an event that is disturbing to us or some series of stressful events. Sleep disorders have been linked to hypertension, increased stress hormone levels, irregular heartbeats, and increased inflammation (Hales, 2013). If sleeplessness becomes a chronic problem, consider taking steps to change these patterns. If you find that you have serious problems getting adequate sleep, you may want to consult your physician, your campus health center, or a sleep disorder specialist.

Exercise and Fitness

A sedentary lifestyle is more common than a physically active lifestyle in our present society. That wasn't always the case:

> Thirty years ago, most people led lives that kept them at a healthy weight. Kids walked to and from school every day, ran around at recess, participated in gym class, and played for hours after school before dinner....
>
> Today, children experience a very different lifestyle. Walks to and from school have been replaced by car and bus rides. Gym class and after-school sports have been cut....
>
> Eight to 18-year old adolescents spend an average of 7.5 hours a day using entertainment media, including TV, computers, video games, cell phones and movies, and only one-third of high school students get the recommended levels of physical activity. ("How Did We Get Here?" 2012, para. 1, 2, & 6)

Hales (2013) reports that a sedentary lifestyle is a hazard to health; it increases all causes of mortality and accounts for 10% of all deaths in the United States each year. As a risk factor for heart disease, physical inactivity ranks as high as smoking, high blood pressure, and elevated cholesterol. Sedentary living doubles the risk of cardiovascular diseases, diabetes, and obesity; it increases the risk of colon cancer, high blood pressure, osteoporosis, depression, and anxiety.

Regular exercise is a central component to achieving physical fitness and maintaining wellness. It helps prevent disease, and it can prolong and enhance our life. Regular exercise promotes health, improves psychological functioning, and reduces the risks of developing various diseases (Whitney, DeBruyne, Pinna, & Rolfes, 2011). Exercise is a natural means of reducing the negative effects of stress. One form of exercise that most people can do on a regular basis is walking. Brisk walking for just 30 minutes a day helps your heart, lungs, and circulatory system; walking also controls body weight, relieves stress, and invigorates your body and mind. The benefits of walking are similar to those for running, without the wear and tear on your joints. A consistent walking program can relieve stress and is an excellent way to prevent a host of illnesses. It is important to select a form of exercise that you enjoy, that you can realistically do on a regular basis, and that fits your interests. You might consider the social benefits of exercising with others. This can be intrinsically enjoyable, and exercising with others can serve as a motivational resource.

Being physically fit has a number of benefits, some of which are described by Whitney and colleagues (2011):

▶ More restful sleep

▶ Better nutritional health

▶ Improved bone density

- Resistance to colds and other infectious diseases
- Lower risk of some types of cancers
- Reduced risk of heart disease
- Stronger circulation and lung function
- Lower risk of Type 2 diabetes
- Lower incidence and severity of anxiety and depression
- Longer life and higher quality of life in the later years

Other benefits to regular physical activity and physical fitness include the following:

- Releases stress, anger, tension, and anxiety
- Increases feelings of well-being, self-esteem, and self-concept
- Prevents hypertension
- Improves work efficiency
- Decreases negative thinking
- Provides a source of enjoyment

Although there are many benefits to keeping physically fit, there are some risks involved with exercise. Overexercising can have a negative impact on us both physically and psychologically. Hazards associated with physical activity include exercise addiction, exercise-related injuries, becoming obsessed with body image, and sudden death while exercising (Brannon & Feist, 2004). Some people approach exercise in a driven manner, which may undo some of its potential benefits. We may get inspired to exercise only to discover that we are overly ambitious in our goals and become discouraged. It is good to keep in mind that the experts tell us that even moderate exercise is beneficial. There are some hazards to jogging,

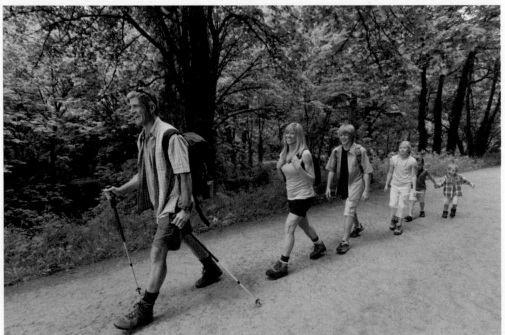

Jupiter Images/Getty Images

>> Brisk walking for 20 to 30 minutes several times a week is an easy way to get regular exercise and keep fit.

especially the risk of muscular and skeletal injuries. Moderation is a good course to follow. Before embarking on a rigorous physical fitness program, it is important to discuss your proposed exercise program with a physician.

An exercise program needs to be planned with care to minimize the risks and maximize the gains to your overall wellness. Having said this, we want to add that you are never too old to take up a form of exercise you might enjoy, which is illustrated by Buster Martin from England who decided he wanted to complete a marathon, so he began training for the event. While this may not seem unusual, what truly distinguished Buster was the fact that he finished his first marathon in 10 hours—at age 101 (reported on the NBC Nightly News, April 13, 2008). When a reporter running alongside Buster asked him why he waited so long to take up jogging, he replied that he never had time before because he was so busy working. Another centenarian, Fauja Singh, fulfilled a lifelong wish when he completed the Toronto marathon (26.2 miles) in 8 hours in September 2011. Singh, who began running in his 80s after the tragic loss of his wife and child, earned eight world records for this amazing feat (Casey, 2011). These stories are a good reminder that it pays to challenge our assumptions about the factors we think may limit us from engaging in healthy activities.

It was not until my (Jerry) mid-20s that I gave much thought to exercising. Although no crisis nudged me into beginning an exercise program, I eventually realized that I was somewhat lethargic and needed to move to increase my energy level. When I began my career in high school teaching, I decided to bicycle from our apartment to school each day. I enjoyed this and began to feel more invigorated, but I didn't realize then that bicycling would remain such a major source of enjoyment and exercise for me 50 years later. For many years I have been committed to making the time to exercise—walking, hiking, and bicycling every day, rain or shine! Maintaining fitness in all areas has become a priority for me. I (Marianne) have made exercising a consistent part of my life too, and I enjoy the forms of exercise I choose. Jerry and I started a competition several years ago, recording the time we devote daily to exercising. I must admit that he is ahead of me!

Designing an adequate and enjoyable program of physical activity is difficult for many people. If you are not physically fit, your initial attempts can be painful and discouraging. It is tempting to give up. If you are not satisfied with this aspect of your life, we encourage you to discover an exercise routine that you find enjoyable. Devise your own plan to keep yourself physically active and psychologically engaged. Doing something you detest may be of little benefit, and chances are you won't stick with it. You can increase your likelihood of success by choosing exercises suitable for your age, physical condition, and life circumstances—try something that you want to make a part of your life.

Create healthy and realistic goals for your exercise program. If you complete a goal that you set for yourself, reward yourself for sticking to your plan. Appreciate what you have done and avoid chastising yourself for what you cannot yet do. If you approach exercise compulsively, it might become another demand on you, which may increase your stress. Exercise, like rest, can be a break from the grind of work and can refresh you.

Diet and Nutrition

There is a lot of truth in the axiom "You are what you eat." Your daily diet affects your long-term health more than any other factor within your control. Brenner (2002) writes: "Diet, like health, is a state of mind. Diet is a relationship between yourself and the food you choose to eat. And perhaps most importantly, it's what you think and feel about the food you eat" (p. 113).

Within the limits set by genetics, the foods we choose to eat have a lot to do with our health. Nutrition experts advise us to eat a variety of foods that supply all the nutrients

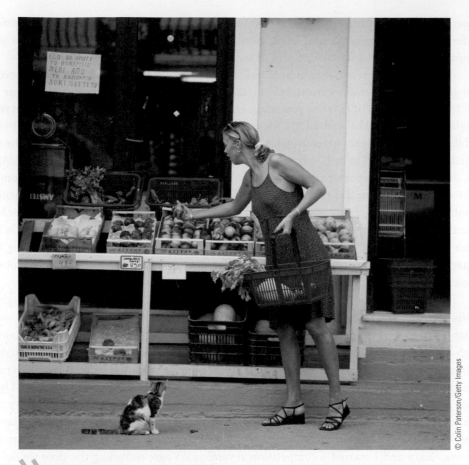

© Colin Paterson/Getty Images

Your diet is the relationship between yourself and the food you choose to eat.

our bodies need, and whole sections in bookstores are devoted to this topic (Whitney et al., 2011). But what is the best course to follow? One source might recommend certain foods that provide specific benefits, yet another source may suggest that we avoid these foods. Some sources recommend that we take vitamin supplements to maintain health, whereas other sources tell us to avoid them. We are often left wondering what an ideal nutritional program is and what supplements to take or to avoid.

If your primary diet is poor, you will not have the energy to meet the demands of everyday life. Irregular and inconsistent eating patterns are a key nutritional problem for many. We often hear students say they do not have time to eat. It is difficult to develop sound diet and nutrition practices when the consequences of not doing so may not be immediate. Healthy nutritional habits do not have to take an abundance of time, especially when new patterns are developed and a varied diet becomes part of your daily life.

By learning how to eat wisely and well, how to manage your weight, and how to become physically fit, you can begin a lifelong process toward wellness. Many of us consume too much sugar, salt, and fat, especially saturated fat. By being aware of this, we can make changes that will enhance our health. Making healthy choices about diet and nutrition entails having specific knowledge about what we eat, so it is well for us to become smart nutrition consumers. Besides eating to live, eating can bring increased satisfaction to living.

Eating for health and eating for pleasure are not incompatible. From Andrew Weil's (2000) perspective, *eating well* means using food to influence health and well-being and, at the same time, to satisfy your senses and to provide pleasure and comfort. It is possible to eat in ways that best serve our body while also getting the enjoyment we expect from food. Weil believes *what* and *how* we eat are critical determinants of how we feel and how we age. He also believes food can function as medicine to influence a variety of common ailments.

Weil teaches physicians and other health professionals lifestyle medicine, which is oriented toward prevention of diseases. He encourages people to change their lifestyle habits before disease appears. Eating well is one aspect of lifestyle, which is only one set of variables in the mix accounting for healthy living. Weil contends that there are multiple determinants of health, starting with genetics and including a great many environmental, psychosocial, and spiritual factors. But diet is one of the lifestyle factors over which we have a large degree of control. We cannot change our genes. We cannot always control the quality of air we breathe, and we cannot completely avoid the stresses of everyday life. But we can decide what to eat and what not to eat.

Spirituality and Purpose in Life

Spirituality is another key ingredient in a balanced life and an important facet of wellness and health. According to Hales (2012), spiritual practices can provide an inner source of strength and calmness and enhance your sense of well-being. Your spirituality can serve as a compass and a guide for the life choices you make. "Spiritually healthy individuals identify their own basic purpose in life; learn how to experience love, joy, peace, and fulfillment; and help themselves and others achieve their full potential" (p. 5).

Spirituality has many meanings and plays greater or lesser roles in different people's lives. For us, **spirituality** encompasses our relationship to the universe and is an avenue for finding meaning and purpose in living. It is an experience beyond the merely physical realm that helps us discover unity in the universe. One definition of spirituality is the practice of letting go of external noise and connecting with your inner self. Religion may be a vital aspect of your spirituality, but many people perceive themselves as being deeply spiritual, but not religious, beings. **Religion** refers to a set of beliefs that connect us to a higher power or a God. For many people, affiliation with a church is an organized means by which they express their religion. It encompasses three loves: love of God, love of neighbor, and love of self. In addition to formal prayer and religious practices, meditation, mindfulness, and living in the moment are some of the paths that can lead you to a greater sense of spirituality.

His Holiness the Dalai Lama is the spiritual leader of the Tibetan people. In *Ethics for the New Millennium* (1999), he makes what he considers to be an important distinction between religion and spirituality. He views religion as being concerned with some form of faith tradition that involves acceptance of a supernatural reality, including perhaps the belief in a heaven or nirvana. A part of religion includes dogma, ritual, and prayer. The Dalai Lama sees spirituality as being concerned with qualities of the human spirit, which include love and compassion, patience, tolerance, forgiveness, contentment, a sense of responsibility, and a sense of harmony. Spiritual acts presume concern for others' well-being.

Some people find it helpful to view spirituality as a developmental process. James Fowler's faith development theory (1981), for example, offers a model of spiritual development that emphasizes the adaptive qualities of faith as well as those qualities that have the potential to be maladaptive (Parker, 2011). Regardless of one's specific religious beliefs, Fowler (1981) suggests that people tend to progress through a series of faith stages and may encounter life crises during stable stage periods as well as stage transitions.

We like Walt Schafer's (2000) personal guiding philosophy, which balances self-care with social responsibility. Schafer writes that true wellness involves being concerned about the well-being of others and having a commitment to the common good, which certainly can be an expression of spirituality in practice. He invites his readers to reflect on his four-part philosophy:

1. Continually have visions and dreams, some of which have social significance—that will benefit others.

2. Work hard, at least partly with others, to bring these dreams and visions to reality.

3. Balance this hard work with play, care of body and spirit, intimacy, friendship, and healthy pleasures.

4. Enjoy the process. (pp. 482–483)

From our perspective, having a guiding personal philosophy is at the heart of wellness. Finding meaning and purpose in life is a never-ending spiritual process. Nourishing your soul may be as important as nourishing your body for overall health. There are many ways to nourish the spirit, some of which include spending some time in quiet reflection, appreciating natural beauty in silence, lying on the ground and watching the clouds go by, visiting a sick person, planting some seeds or flowers in a garden, engaging in volunteer work, attending a church service, kissing or hugging someone you love, writing a letter to someone you have not seen in a long time, reading something inspirational or spiritual, praying for yourself and others, writing in your journal, or watching an inspirational movie. Recall the last time you did something to nourish your spirit, or the spirit of someone else. What did you do? What was it like for you to participate in a spiritual experience? How important is spirituality for you? We return to the topic of spirituality and meaning in life in a later chapter.

Other components essential to wellness are discussed in subsequent chapters. They include our capacity to give and receive love (Chapter 6), the quality of our interpersonal relationships (Chapter 7), the way we approach our work and leisure activities (Chapter 10), and the meaning in life (Chapter 13). These factors also have a major impact on our overall well-being.

Reflect on the balance in your life. Are there some aspects of daily living that you want to modify? The Take Time to Reflect exercise will help you assess the degree of balance in your life.

> ## TAKE TIME TO REFLECT

1. Do you get adequate sleep? What changes, if any, might you want to make? _____
_____
_____

2. What physical activity do you enjoy most? Is there anything you are interested in changing?
_____
_____

3. How open are you to making changes in your diet, nutrition, and eating habits? _____
_____
_____

4. Reflect on the meaning of spirituality in your life. How do you define your spirituality? What gives you a purpose in life? _____
_____
_____

5. What are your thoughts about balancing self-care with a sense of social commitment? To what extent is personal wellness dependent upon having a concern for the welfare of others? _____

_____

_____

6. What other aspects do you consider essential in maintaining a balanced life? _____

_____

_____

YOUR BODILY IDENTITY

We are limited in how much we can actually change our bodies, but we can do a lot working with the material we have. First, pay attention to what you are expressing about yourself through your body, so you can determine whether you *want* to change your bodily identity. This involves increasing your awareness of how you experience your body through touch and movement.

In this section, reflect on how well you know your body and how comfortable you are with it. Then you can decide about changing your body image, if you so desire.

Experiencing and Expressing Yourself Through Your Body

For some of us the body is simply a vehicle that carries us around. If someone asks us what we are thinking, we are likely to come up with a quick answer. If asked what we are experiencing and sensing in our body, however, we may be at a loss for words. Yet our body can be eloquent in its expression of who we are. Much of our life history is revealed through our bodies. We can see evidence of stress and strain in people's faces. Some people speak with a tightened jaw. Others walk with a slouch and shuffle their feet, as if expressing their hesitation in presenting themselves to the world. Their bodies may be communicating more than their speech. What story does your body tell about you? Here are some ways that your body can express your inner self:

▶ Your eyes can express excitement or emptiness.

▶ Your mouth can be tight or at ease.

▶ Your neck can hold back your anger or tears and can also hold your tensions.

▶ Your chest can develop armor that inhibits your ability to freely express your crying, laughing, or breathing.

▶ Your diaphragm can block the expression of anger and pain.

▶ Your abdomen can develop armor that is related to fear of attack.

Unexpressed emotions do not simply disappear. The chronic practice of "swallowing" emotions can take a physical toll on the body and manifest itself in physical symptoms such as severe headaches, ulcers, digestive problems, and a range of other bodily dysfunctions. If people seal off certain emotions, such as grief and anger, they also keep themselves from experiencing intense joy. Golda Meir once said, "Those who don't know how to weep with their whole heart don't know how to laugh either." Ben-Shahar (2011) urges us to give ourselves permission to be human and to accept our emotions:

> While it's at times necessary to keep certain emotions out of sight (when we are with others), it may be harmful to try to keep them out of mind (when we

are alone). We are taught that it is improper to display our anxiety or to cry in public, so we hold our emotions back in private as well. Anger does not win us friends, and over time we lose our ability to express and experience anger altogether. We extinguish our anxiety, fear, and rage for the sake of being pleasant and easy to get along with—and in the process of getting others to accept us, we reject ourselves. (p. 42)

By allowing painful emotions to flow through us naturally and freely, pressure is alleviated and our emotions eventually subside. It may be helpful to think of suppressed emotions as blocks to our energy.

Let's take a closer look at what it means to experience yourself through your body.

Experiencing Your Body One way of experiencing your own body is by paying attention to your senses of touch, taste, smell, seeing, and hearing. Simply pausing and taking a few moments to be aware of how your body is interacting with the environment is a helpful way of learning to make better contact. For example, how often do you allow yourself to really taste and smell your food? How often are you aware of the tension in your body? How many times do you pause to smell and touch a flower? How often do you listen to the chirping of birds or the other sounds of nature?

We often fail to enjoy our physical selves. Treating ourselves to a massage, for example, not only can be exhilarating but can give us clues as to how alive we are physically. Singing and dancing are yet other avenues through which we enjoy our physical selves and express ourselves. Dance is a popular way to teach people to "own" all parts of their bodies and to express themselves more harmoniously. Engaging in sports and other forms of physical exercise can be approached with the same playful attitude as dancing and singing. These are a few ways to become more of a friend and less of a stranger to your body.

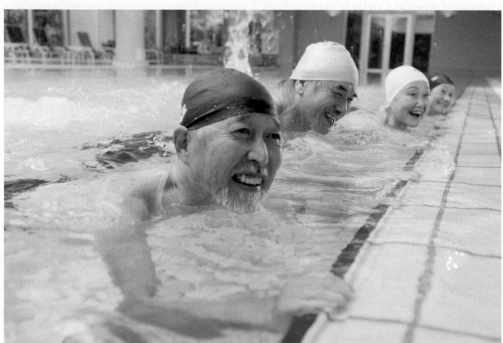

Indeed/Getty Images

》》Our body can be an eloquent expression of who we are.

The Importance of Touch Some people are very comfortable with touching and with being touched by others. They require a degree of touching to maintain a sense of physical and emotional connection. Other people show a great deal of discomfort in touching themselves or allowing others to be physical with them. They may stiffen and quickly move away if they are touched accidentally. If such a person is embraced by another, he or she is likely to become rigid and unresponsive. For instance, in Jerry's family of origin there was very little touching. He had to recondition himself to feel comfortable being touched by others and touching others. In contrast, Marianne grew up in a German family characterized by much more spontaneous touching.

There are critical periods in development when physical stimulation is essential for normal development. In most cultures, touching is important for developing in healthy ways physically, psychologically, socially, and intellectually. "[T]ouch is a universal aspect of human interaction ...but there are vast differences in the amount of touching that people do"; touching varies by culture, gender, and even age (Dibiase & Gunnoe, 2004, p. 49). In many cultures touching is a natural mode of expression; in others, touching is minimal and is regulated to clearly defined situations. Some cultures have taboos against touching strangers, against touching people of the same sex, against touching people of the opposite sex, or against touching in social situations. In spite of these differences, studies have demonstrated that physical contact contributes to the healthy development of body and mind.

Body Image

Body image involves more than size. A healthy body and a positive image of your body gives you pleasure and helps you do what you want to physically. You might ask yourself if your body keeps you from doing what you would like to do. If so, then you might explore what you are willing to do to change it. Judging yourself and blaming yourself do not bring about change. Accepting the body you have and deciding what you can and will do to enhance it is the beginning of change.

Many people are dissatisfied with their physical appearance, and some cannot tolerate any imperfections in the way they look. Many people have body image concerns over the size and proportion of body parts, skin blemishes and scars, and the straightness and whiteness of teeth. As a nation, we spend an astronomical amount each year to keep us looking younger or to change our physical appearance. Many undergo expensive operations, with some pain and side effects, to change their shape, to remove wrinkles, or to change some physical features. Piercings and tattoos are two body modification practices that are increasingly common choices in contemporary society (Tiggemann & Hopkins, 2011). Certainly, many people are obsessed with how they look to themselves and how they appear to others.

The task of understanding body image is not simple. There is a significant difference between the model who says "I don't like the way my body looks" and the man who continually struggles to keep his weight under control. Judging yourself and being impatient with your rate of progress are not helpful means of understanding your body. Once you reach these kinds of judgments, you limit the kind of feedback you will accept. Any feedback that does not support that self-perception is enjoyed for a few moments but will not endure. The most important component in effecting change in your bodily image is your own perception. This is where your program of change begins.

Your view of your body and the decisions you have made about it can have much to do with the choices you will make in other areas of your life. Some people see themselves as unattractive, unappealing, or physically inferior, and these self-perceptions are likely to affect other areas of their lives. They may say:

▶ If I had a better body, then I'd be happy.

▶ If I were physically more attractive, people would like me.

▸ I never look good enough.

▸ It's too much work to change the things I dislike about my body.

If you feel unattractive, you may tell yourself that others will see your defects and will not want to approach you. In this way you contribute to the reactions others may have toward you by your own internal messages. You may be perceived by others as aloof, distant, or judgmental. Even though you may want to get close to people, you may also be frightened of the possibility of meeting them.

You may answer that there is little you can do to change certain aspects of your physical being such as your height or basic build. Yet you *can* look at the attitudes you have formed about these physical characteristics. How important are they to who you are? How has your culture influenced your beliefs about what constitutes the ideal body? We can also develop feelings of shame if we unquestioningly accept certain cultural messages about our bodies. Sometimes the sense of shame remains with people into adulthood. The following brief descriptions represent some typical difficulties:

▸ Donna painfully recalls that during her preadolescence she was much taller and more physically developed than her peers. She was often the butt of jokes by both boys and girls in her class. Although she is no longer taller than most people around her, she still walks stoop-shouldered, for she still feels self-conscious and embarrassed over her body.

▸ Herbert, a physically attractive young man, is highly self-conscious about his body, much to the surprise of those who know him. He seems to be in good physical condition, yet he gets very anxious when he gains even a pound. As a child he was overweight, and he developed a self-concept of being the "fat kid." Even though he changed his physique years ago, the fear of being considered fat still remains.

Consider whether you, too, made some decisions about your body early in life or during adolescence that still affect you. Did you feel embarrassed about certain of your physical characteristics? Even though others may think of you as an attractive person, you may react with disbelief. If you continue to tell yourself that you are in some way inferior, your struggle to change your self-concept may be similar to that of Donna or Herbert.

Weight and Your Body Image

From years of experience reading student journals and counseling clients, we have concluded that many people are preoccupied with maintaining their "ideal weight." Some people view themselves as too skinny and strive to gain weight, but many more are looking for effective ways to lose weight. Young people are bombarded by unrealistic models of what constitutes an ideal body. In a television report, young college women were objecting to the unrealistic portrayal of ideal bodies by the use of models who did not look like them. These women took issue with the unrealistic standard of what it means to be physically fit and attractive. They refused to accept the image presented. They wanted models in advertisements to be more inclusive of the general population.

You may be one of those people who struggle with societal standards as to what makes a body attractive. You may find that your weight significantly affects the way you feel about your body. Do these statements sound familiar to you?

▸ I've tried every diet program there is, and I just can't seem to stick to one.

▸ I'm too occupied with school to think about losing weight.

▸ I love to eat, and I hate to exercise.

In our travels to Germany and Norway we have noticed how the ideal weight differs from culture to culture. The same thin person who is viewed as attractive in the United States might well be seen as undernourished in Germany. A person with a certain amount of weight is generally considered attractive and healthy looking in Germany. One young American woman who struggled with her weight and body image told us that when she spent some time in Norway she did not think of herself as being physically unattractive. There many people commented about her vitality. However, when she returned to her home in the United States, she was much more conscious of her appearance.

It may also help to examine how unrealistic societal standards regarding the ideal body can lead to the perpetual feeling that you are never physically adequate. For example, our society places tremendous pressure on women to be thin. Messages from the media reveal that thinness and beauty are often equated. For the many women who accept these cultural norms, the price they often pay is depression and loss of self-esteem and health. Men also obsess about having a perfect body. Andrew believed he had had a weight problem for most of his life. He began to diet and engaged in rigorous exercise, often pushing himself to the point of exhaustion. His physician was concerned that Andrew's drastic weight loss was affecting his health. He often had nightmares about gaining weight, and his obsession with creating the perfect body affected his personal relationships. With the help of his physician, Andrew developed a more realistic program of eating and exercising. However, for Andrew, keeping physically fit continues to be a daily concern.

The topic of body image applies to both men and women. However, in this society women are subject to greater pressures to live up to the ideal size, which results in their pre-occupation with weight and body image. In some ways, keeping women focused on achieving a "perfect" body is a form of oppression. Many eating problems that women face have to do with their internalized hatred of not being thin. Consider the case of Kate, who writes about her personal experience with weight problems and her body image.

KATE'S STORY

Although I have overcome a large degree of my body hatred, I continue to struggle with accepting and living with my body as it is. My last relationship ended with my partner justifying his disinterest with a critique of my body size. His words will probably sting me as long as I live.

Although part of me agrees with the negative comments people have made about my size, another part of me knows that their words are a form of oppression taught to them by our society. This does not excuse their behavior, but it helps me to understand that all of us are victims of our sexist standards. As a woman, I have worn my bad body image like a suit of armor. In many ways it protects me from having to examine other parts of my life.

The challenge in overcoming eating problems is multifold. Those of us who struggle with these issues need to continue to be brave and to ask ourselves if we can stand the thought of accepting ourselves for who we are. In recent months I have come to realize that my bad body image is not only a result of sociocultural factors but is also a form of self-preservation. I am used to being dismissed and rejected because of my body size. In an ironic way it has become a safe way to feel my pain. The challenge has been and continues to be for me to face those feelings within myself that have nothing to do with the size or shape of my legs, thighs, and stomach.

Kate's story illustrates a woman's struggle to accept her body, but other people are driven to meet societal standards of an attractive and "perfect" body. In its extreme form, this striving can lead to eating disorders. Although eating disorders tend to be associated with females, there is a growing body of literature on eating disorders among males (see Bayes & Madden, 2011; Darcy et al., 2012; Reyes-Rodriguez et al., 2011), and some evidence links social comparisons with celebrities to disordered eating (Shorter, Brown, Quinton, & Hinton, 2008). Anorexia and bulimia are frequently linked to the internalization of unrealistic standards that lead to negative self-perceptions and negative body images. Naomi's description of her struggle with anorexia illustrates how self-destructive striving for psychological and physical perfection can be.

NAOMI'S STORY

During my high school years, I attended a private boarding school on a scholarship. The high school in my home town was really bad, so my parents thought it was in my best interest to go to a boarding school. The vast majority of my new classmates were from wealthy families and had expensive tastes, but I came from a middle-class family on a tight budget. I wore hand-me-down clothes from my older sister while the girls at school shopped for clothes only at the finest stores. Image was everything to them. If you didn't own a Coach purse, you were considered a loser! Needless to say, I didn't fit in very well and became depressed. I had no respect for these girls, who were quite mean. They started to spread vicious rumors about me on Facebook and referred to me as fat and ugly. I desperately wanted to leave the school and return home, but I could not disappoint my parents. They were so proud of me for attending this school. Plus, I didn't want them to worry about me, so I pretended everything was wonderful when I talked to them.

During my sophomore year, my self-esteem took a nosedive, and I became increasingly withdrawn. I lost my appetite but didn't mind because I was hoping to lose a few pounds. After dropping 10 pounds, I became almost obsessed with losing more weight. It was as if something took me over. I started to exercise compulsively; I even missed class sometimes so I could work out. I became so preoccupied with food (because I was so starved) that no one could stand to be around me anymore. I couldn't even stand myself! By the time I was a high school junior, I had lost so much weight that my parents pulled me out of school and had me hospitalized. In my attempt to take control of my life, I had completely lost control.

It is easy to get trapped in self-destructive patterns of critical self-judgment. Being and feeling healthy—and choosing what that entails for you—are the real challenges to wellness.

Although weight is a significant health factor, nutritional and exercise habits are also crucial to your overall well-being. Rather than too quickly deciding that you need to either gain or lose weight or to change your nutritional habits, it is a good idea to consult your physician or one of the nutrition centers in your area. If you decide you want to change your weight, there are many excellent support groups and self-help programs designed for this purpose. If you are interested in learning how cognitive therapy techniques can aid in weight loss, Judith Beck (2008) has written a few books on this topic, including *The Complete Beck Diet for Life*. In addition, the counseling centers at many colleges offer groups for weight control and for people with eating disorders.

A basic change in attitude and lifestyle is important in successfully dealing with a weight problem. People with weight problems do not eat simply because they are hungry. They are typically more responsive to external cues in their environment. If you do not like what your body is saying, it is up to you to decide what, if anything, you want to change. Should you decide that you do not want to change, you need not be defensive about it. There is no injunction that you *must* change.

If you have not liked your physical being for some time but have not been able to change it, some genetic or physical factors may be making it extremely difficult for you to manage your weight. Some people's medical history prevents them from having a great deal of choice regarding their weight, in spite of exercise and healthy nutrition. In addition, some people may have a greater predisposition to develop eating disorders due to neurobiological factors (Kaye, Wagner, Fudge, & Paulus, 2011). Many aspects need to be considered in managing your weight; there are no simple solutions for this complex matter. You can begin with an awareness of your situation and learn the steps you can take in bringing about the changes you want. Before you embark on any fitness or weight-loss program, consider your own situation and talk with your physician about alternatives.

Many of us get stuck because we focus on what society dictates as being the ideal weight and body image. We hope you are able to raise your awareness about the societal messages under which you have operated, and we encourage you to challenge these cultural messages. The Take Time to Reflect exercise is designed to assist you in clarifying your attitudes about your perception of your body. Ask yourself these questions: "How satisfied am I with the body I have? How can I move toward increased self-acceptance?"

TAKE TIME TO REFLECT

1. What are your attitudes toward your body? Take some time to study your body and become aware of how you look to yourself and what your body feels like to you. Try standing in front of a good sized mirror, and reflect on these questions:

- ▶ Look at your face. What is it telling you?
- ▶ What are your eyes conveying to you?
- ▶ Can you see yourself smiling?
- ▶ Is your body generally tight or relaxed? Where do you feel your tension?
- ▶ Which parts, if any, of your body do you feel ashamed of or try to hide?
- ▶ What about your body would you most like to change? What do you like the most?

Each time you complete the exercise just described, record your impressions or keep an extended account of your reactions in your journal.

2. If you have modified a part of your body through piercings, tattoos, or surgical procedures, how has it changed the way you perceive yourself? When you see others who have modified their bodies in some way, what thoughts and impressions come to mind?

3. Imagine yourself looking more the way you would like to look. Let yourself think about how you might be different, as well as how your life would be different.

4. As a result of reading this chapter and doing these exercises, what actions are you willing to take to become more invested in taking care of yourself? _____

_____

_____

SUMMARY

The purpose of this chapter has been to invite you to think about how you are treating your body and

how you can take control of your physical and psychological well-being. Even if you are not presently concerned with health problems, you may have discovered that you hold some self-defeating attitudes about your body. A theme of this chapter has been to examine what might be keeping you from really caring about your body or from taking appropriate actions to ensure your wellness. It is not simply a matter of smoking or not smoking, of exercising or not exercising; the basic choice concerns how you feel about yourself and about your life. When you accept responsibility for the feelings and attitudes you have developed about your body and your life, you begin to free yourself from feeling victimized by your body.

We can enhance our experience of the world around us by seeing, hearing, smelling, tasting, and touching. We can become less of a stranger to our body through relaxation, dance, and movement. Touch is particularly important. For healthy physical and emotional development, we need both physical and psychological contact.

Remember that you are a whole being, composed of physical, emotional, social, intellectual, and spiritual dimensions. If you neglect any one of these aspects of yourself, you will feel the impact on the other dimensions of your being. Take a moment to think again about how well you are taking care of yourself in all areas of your life. How committed are you to a wellness perspective? Consider the value you place on taking good care of yourself through practices such as meditation, relaxation exercises, paying attention to your spiritual or religious life, maintaining good nutritional habits, getting adequate sleep and rest, and participating in a regular exercise program.

Making a change in your lifestyle is a process, not a single event. If you determine that you are not as healthy as you want to be, you do have a choice. You can choose to maintain unhealthy habits and risk health problems, possibly resulting in a shorter life, or you can choose to alter your lifestyle and live a healthier and potentially longer life.

Where Can I Go From Here?

1. Wellness means different things to different people. When you think of wellness, what aspects of your life do you most think of? Look at what you are doing to maintain a general state of wellness. How much of a priority do you place on wellness?

2. Assess how exercise (or the lack of exercise) is affecting how you feel physically and psychologically and how it influences your ability to deal with stress. If you are interested in engaging in some form of regular physical activity, decide on some exercise that you would enjoy doing. Start small so you don't get overwhelmed, but stick with your physical activity for at least 2 to 4 weeks to see if you begin to feel a difference.

3. In your journal record for a week all of your activities that are healthy for your body as well as those that are unhealthy. You may want to list what you eat, how much you smoke or drink

(if applicable), your sleep patterns, and what you do for exercise and relaxation. Then look over your list and choose one or more areas that you would be willing to work on during the next few months. Develop a specific plan of action to achieve your wellness goals and implement it. Make use of the journal pages at the end of this chapter to write about wellness as it applies to you.

4. Suggested Readings. The full bibliographic entry for each of these sources can be found in the References and Suggested Readings at the back of the book. For a comprehensive textbook on health and wellness, see Hales (2012). For an interesting book on health, illness, and healing, see Brenner (2002). For two comprehensive textbooks on the topic of nutrition and health, see Sizer and Whitney (2011) and Whitney, DeBruyne, Pinna, and Rolfes (2011).

WEBSITE RESOURCES

Included here are some valuable websites. For access to these websites, video activities, and other supporting materials, visit Cengage Learning's Counseling CourseMate website for *I Never Knew I Had a Choice*, 10th Edition, at **www.cengagebrain.com.**

GO ASK ALICE!

http://goaskalice.columbia.edu/

Recommended Search Words: "go ask alice"

Columbia University's Health Education Program has created a widely used website designed for undergraduate students. Alice! answers questions about relationships, sexuality, sexual health, emotional health, fitness and nutrition, alcohol, nicotine and other drugs, and general health. If you cannot find an answer to what you are looking for, you can "Ask Alice!" yourself.

CENTERS FOR DISEASE CONTROL AND PREVENTION

www.cdc.gov

Recommended Search Words: "centers for disease control"

The Centers for Disease Control and Prevention (CDC) offers news, fact sheets on disease information and health information, articles, statistics, and links regarding health and illness in the United States (also offered in Spanish).

NATIONAL WELLNESS INSTITUTE

www.nationalwellness.org

Recommended Search Words: "national wellness institute"

This site offers information and resources pertaining to optimal health and wellness.

JOHNS HOPKINS MEDICINE

www.hopkinsmedicine.org

Recommended Search Words: "johns hopkins medicine"

This site offers an extensive health library and a wealth of information about medical conditions.

MAYO CLINIC

www. mayoclinic.com

Recommended Search Words: "mayo clinic"

This site offers "reliable information for a healthier life" and provides news items, highlights, and specific health category centers for information and resources on various diseases, medications, and general health.

NATIONAL EATING DISORDERS ASSOCIATION

www.nationaleatingdisorders.org

Recommended Search Words: "national eating disorders association"

The website of this national organization provides access to information and news about eating disorders, resources and programs, research, and links to other relevant organizations dealing with eating disorders.

NATIONAL ASSOCIATION FOR HEALTH AND FITNESS

www.physicalfitness.org

Recommended Search Words: "national association for health and fitness"

This is a network of state and governors' councils that promotes physical fitness for persons of all ages and abilities.

FOOD PLATE

www.choosemyplate.gov

Recommended Search Words: "myplate"

This website stresses that optimal diets differ for different people and recommends personalized eating plans.

NATIONAL CENTER ON PHYSICAL ACTIVITY AND DISABLILITY

www.ncpad.org

Recommended Search Words: "national center on physical activity and disability"

This site promotes the "substantial health benefits that can be gained from participating in regular physical activity" and "provides information and resources that can enable people with disabilities to become as physically active as they choose to be."

SHAPE UP AMERICA!

www.shapeup.org

Recommended Search Words: "shape up America"

Shape Up America is a nonprofit organization dedicated to helping you achieve a healthy weight for life.

LET'S MOVE

www.letsmove.gov

Recommended Search Words: "let's move"

Program launched by First Lady Michelle Obama in 2010 to fight childhood obesity and to promote the physical and emotional health of today's youth. The program emphasizes that the economic health and security of our nation are at stake.

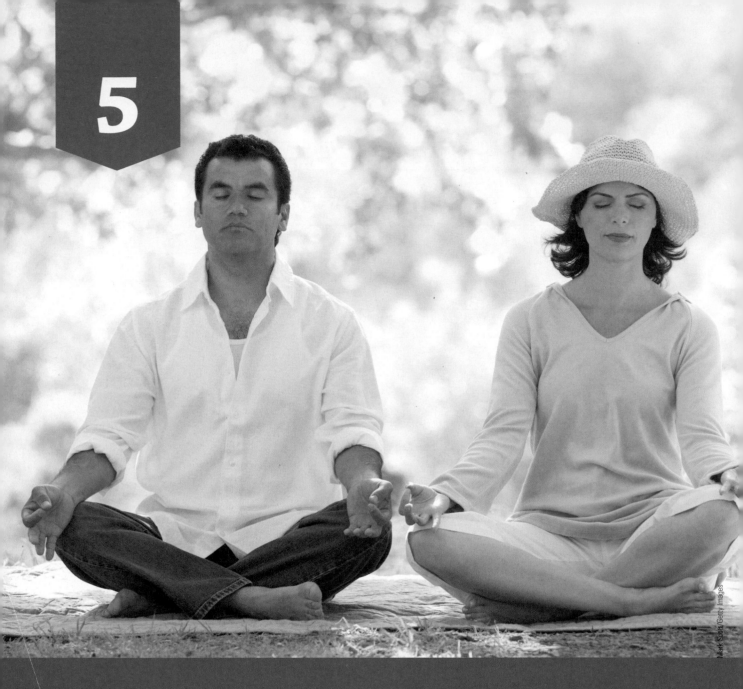

Mark Scott/Getty Images

MANAGING STRESS

> Where Am I Now?

> Sources of Stress

> Effects of Stress

> Ineffective Reactions to Stress

> Posttraumatic Stress Disorders

> Sexual Exploitation

> Vicarious Traumatization

> Constructive Responses to Stress

> Time Management

> Meditation

> Mindfulness

> Deep Relaxation

> Yoga

> Therapeutic Massage

> Summary

> Where Can I Go From Here?

> Website Resources

> *Either you control your stress, or stress controls you.*

WHERE AM I NOW?

Use this scale to respond to these statements:

4 = I *strongly agree* with this statement.
3 = I *agree* with this statement.
2 = I *disagree* with this statement.
1 = I *strongly disagree* with this statement.

1. My lifestyle is generally stressful.

2. I have relied on drugs or alcohol to help me through difficult times, but I do not abuse these substances.

3. It is relatively easy for me to fully relax.

4. Due to the way I live, I sometimes worry about having a heart attack.

5. I am able to recognize how my thoughts contribute to my stress.

6. Stress has sometimes made me physically ill.

7. If I do not control stress, I believe it will control me.

8. I meditate to reduce my stress.

9. Burnout is a real concern of mine.

10. I feel a need to learn more stress management techniques.

Stress is an event or series of events that leads to strain, which often results in physical and psychological health problems. Stress can involve external factors that threaten our well-being, internal factors, and physical responses to both external and internal demands. Everyday living involves coping with frustrations, conflicts, pressures, and change, and over our lifetime we will confront some severely stressful situations: the death of a family member or a close friend, a national crisis, a natural disaster, the loss of a job, a personal failure, or an injury. Even positive changes, such as being promoted, moving to a new location, or getting married, can be stressful and often require a period of adjustment.

Hans Selye (1974), a pioneer in stress research, believes stress has both positive and negative effects. Selye differentiates between *eustress* (pronounced "you-stress") and *distress*. **Eustress**, or good stress, challenges us to find creative solutions to the problems of everyday living. When we meet these challenges, we are rewarded with a sense of accomplishment, meaning, and balance. **Distress** refers to the negative effects of stress that can deplete, fragment, and harm us, leading to a sense of helplessness and exhaustion. Distress leads to negative physical and psychological states.

Stress is an inevitable part of life. We cannot totally eliminate stress, but we can learn to monitor and manage the physical and psychological impact of our stress. Our body or state of mind may be telling us that something in our life needs to change. Some of these signs include loneliness, insecurity, loss of concentration and memory, fatigue and sleeping difficulties, mood swings, impatience, restlessness, obsessive working, loss of appetite, and fear of silence. These signs often serve as an invitation to examine what we are doing and to create better ways of dealing with life's demands. Recognizing ineffective or harmful reactions to stress is a first step in dealing with it. Developing stress management skills and making them a basic part of our lifestyle is essential if we hope to maintain a sense of wellness (see Chapter 4).

Although many sources of stress are external, how we perceive and react to stress is subjective and internal. Therefore, our central task is learning how to recognize and respond constructively to the sources of stress rather than trying to eliminate them. Some constructive paths to stress management addressed in this chapter include learning time management, challenging self-defeating thinking and negative self-talk, developing a sense of humor, acquiring mindfulness, practicing meditation and other centering activities, and learning how to relax.

SOURCES OF STRESS

Stress of one kind or another is present in each of the stages in the life cycle (see Chapters 2 and 3). As you recall from Chapter 4, wellness is a central buffer against stress. Some of the stress we experience is self-imposed. For example, we may repeatedly choose to take on too many demands and feel overwhelmed. In such instances, we probably have more control over our feelings of stress than we realize. Other stressors, over which we have less or no control, can affect our lives in profound ways, leaving us with the arduous task of learning to cope with our stress reactions in a constructive manner. A prime example of this is the ongoing threat of terrorism, which unfortunately is a fact of life in today's world. Before we can exert control, however, we must identify the source of our stress. Two major sources of stress are environmental and psychological factors.

Environmental Sources of Stress

Many of the stresses of daily life come from environmental sources such as living in crowded conditions, noise, traffic congestion, and pollution. Stress also may be a by-product of the constant bombardment of news and information around the clock. Before cell phones became popular, people were not available to others 24 hours a day, seven days a week, 365 days a year. With the advent of trends such as tweeting and texting, however, that has changed. As Maggie Jackson, author of "*Distracted: The New News World and the Fate of Attention*" (2008b), asks, "In our rapid-fire, split-focus era, are we able to process, filter, and reflect well on the tsunamis of information barraging us daily?" (p. 27).

As a student, you are likely to confront many external stressors, especially at the beginning of a new semester. You may encounter problems finding a parking place on campus. You may stand in long lines and have to cope with many other delays and frustrations. Some of the courses you need may be closed; simply putting together a decent schedule of classes may be next to impossible. You may have difficulty arranging your work schedule to fit your school schedule, and this can be compounded by the external demands of friends and family and other social commitments. Financial problems and the pressure to work to support yourself (and perhaps your family too) make being a student a demanding task. Guo, Wang, Johnson, and Diaz (2011) have demonstrated that college students perceive immediate stressors such as future employment opportunities and current financial burden as high-stress triggers. The pressures associated with academic success—deadlines and competition—are external stressors that you need to address. Attempting to fit too many things into one day can add extra stress to the many new pressures you are facing. During your undergraduate education and beyond, you are faced with many critical choices that will influence your career path, and making these choices is often demanding.

Our minds and bodies are also profoundly affected by more direct physiological sources of stress. Illness, exposure to environmental pollutants, improper diet, lack of exercise, poor sleeping habits, and abusing our bodies in any number of other ways all take a toll on us.

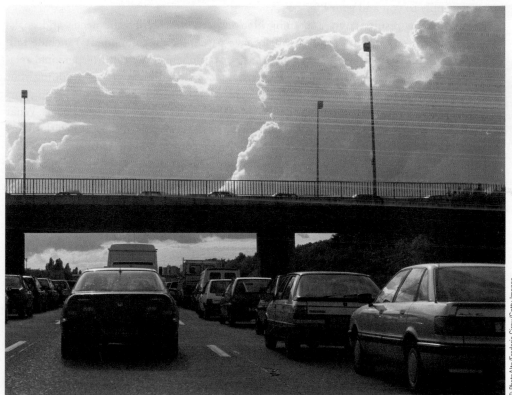

>> Many of the stressors of daily life come from external sources.

We must not forget societal stressors. Few would argue that we are currently living in a divisive political, economic, and social climate. Despite efforts to increase awareness, discrimination on the basis of race, nationality, age, gender, socioeconomic status, or sexual orientation creates stress in the lives of many people today. Immigrants, who may face discrimination, also have the stressful task of adapting to a new culture.

The national economic crisis, which has resulted in a dramatic increase in unemployment, home foreclosures, and bankruptcies, has shattered the American dream for many families. Disillusioned and in debt, people are under enormous stress and are worried about the future. Listening to news reports of the ravages of war and violence and watching politicians and other public figures act in their own self-interest rather than in the interests of their constituents affect us psychologically and physically. The tragic events of 9/11 activated a level of fear new for most Americans as we realized how vulnerable we are. Over the past decade, we have all witnessed the aftermath of 9/11 and are confronted daily with the reality that we can no longer assume that we are safe, which we once took for granted. This uncertainty is a source of stress that has profoundly affected the psyche of Americans and has had a global impact.

Psychological Sources of Stress

Any set of circumstances that we perceive as being threatening to our well-being puts a strain on our coping abilities. Stress is in the mind of the beholder, and our appraisals of stressful events are highly subjective. How we label, interpret, think about, and react to events in our lives has a lot to do with determining whether those events are stressful. Weiten and colleagues (2012) describe frustration, conflict, change, and pressure as four key elements of psychological stress. As we consider each of these sources of stress, think about how they apply to you and your life.

Frustration results from something blocking attainment of your needs and goals. External sources of frustration (all of which have psychological components) include failures, losses, job discrimination, accidents, delays, traffic jams, hurtful interpersonal relationships, loneliness, and isolation. Some internal factors can hinder you in attaining your goals as well. These include a lack of basic skills, physical handicaps, a lack of belief in yourself, and any self-imposed barriers you may create that block the pursuit of your goals. What are some of the major frustrations you experience, and how do you typically deal with them?

Conflict, another source of stress, occurs when two or more incompatible motivations or behavioral impulses compete for expression. Conflicts can be classified as approach-approach, avoidance-avoidance, and approach-avoidance.

▶ **Approach-approach conflicts** occur when a choice must be made between two or more attractive or desirable alternatives. Such conflicts are inevitable because we have a limited amount of time to do all the things we would like to do and be all the places we would like to be. An example of this type of conflict is being forced to choose between two job offers, both of which have attractive features.

▶ **Avoidance-avoidance conflicts** arise when a choice must be made between two or more unattractive or undesirable outcomes. These conflicts are the most unpleasant and the most stressful. You may have to choose between being unemployed and accepting a job you do not like, neither of which appeals to you.

▶ **Approach-avoidance conflicts** are produced when a choice must be made involving two or more linked outcomes, each of which has attractive and unattractive elements. For example, you may be offered a challenging job that appeals to you but that entails much traveling, which you consider a real drawback.

How many times have you been faced with two or more desirable choices and forced to choose one path? And how many times have you had to choose between unpleasant realities? Perhaps your major conflicts involve your choice of a lifestyle. For example, have you wrestled with the issue of being independent or letting others make choices for you? What about living a self-directed life or living by what others expect of you? Consider for a few minutes some of the major conflicts you have recently faced. How have these conflicts affected you? How do you typically deal with the stress you experience over value conflicts?

Change can exacerbate stress, especially life changes that involve readjustment in our living circumstances. Holmes and Rahe's (1967) classic study on the relationship between stressful life events and physical illness found that changes in personal relationships, career changes, and financial changes are often stressful, even if these changes are positive. Thus, within a relatively short period of time, you may get married, move into a new house, and begin a family. Any one of these changes can be stressful, but the combined effect of these changes often increases the intensity of stress you experience. However, the demands for adjustment to these life changes, along with your perceptions of these demands, are more important than the type of life changes alone.

Pressure, which involves expectations and demands for behaving in certain ways, is part of the "hurry sickness" of modern living. Also, we continually place internally created pressures on ourselves. Many of us are extremely demanding of ourselves, and we never quite feel satisfied that we have done all we could or should have done. Striving to live up to the expectations of others, coupled with self-imposed perfectionist demands, is a certain route to stress. If you find yourself in this situation, consider some of the faulty and unrealistic beliefs you hold. Are you overloading your circuits and heading for certain burnout? In what ways do you push yourself to perform, and for whom? How do you experience and deal with pressure in your daily life?

EFFECTS OF STRESS

Stress produces adverse physical effects. In our attempt to cope with everyday living, our bodies experience what is known as the **fight-or-flight response**. Our bodies go on constant alert status, ready for aggressive action to combat the many "enemies" we face. If we subject ourselves to too many stresses, the biochemical changes that occur during the fight-or-flight response may lead to chronic stress and anxiety. This causes bodily wear and tear, which can lead to a variety of what are known as psychosomatic or psychophysiological disorders. These are not a product of one's imagination. **Psychosomatic illnesses** are genuine physical maladies such as ulcers, hypertension, and asthma that are caused in part and exacerbated by emotional factors and the prolonged effects of stress. They are real bodily disorders and symptoms that range from minor discomfort to life-threatening conditions.

Hales (2012, 2013) reports that stress contributes to a range of major physical illnesses, including cardiovascular disease, cancer, endocrine and metabolic disease, skin rashes, ulcers, migraine and tension headaches, emotional disorders, musculoskeletal disease, infectious illnesses, breast cysts, and premenstrual syndrome. Explore how your physical symptoms may actually be a manifestation of stress. Ask yourself how your life might be different if you were symptom free.

Allan Abbott (a family-practice doctor) and Colony Abbott (a nurse) are two friends of ours who spent some time treating indigenous people in Peru. This experience stimulated their interest in the ways in which stress affects the body. The Abbotts became especially interested in coronary-prone behavior, which is so characteristic of the North American way of life. The leading causes of death in North America are cardiovascular diseases and cancer (diseases the Abbotts relate to stress), but these diseases rarely cause the death of Peruvian Indians, whose lives are relatively stress free.

In the Abbotts' view our bodies are paying a high price for the materialistic and stressful manner in which we live. Dr. Abbott estimates that about 75% of the physical ailments he treats are psychologically and behaviorally related to stress, and he asserts that most of what he does as a physician that makes a significant difference is psychological in nature rather than medical. According to Abbott, belief in the doctor and in the process and procedures a doctor employs has a great deal to do with curing patients. Taking a blood test, having an X-ray done, getting a shot, and simple conversation with the physician all appear to help patients improve. Indeed, faith healers work on this very principle, embracing the role of belief and its effect on the body.

As discussed in Chapter 4, there is an intimate connection between the body and the mind, and it seems clear that emotional restriction can lead to sickness. However, Brenner (2002) believes it is simplistic to view all illness as caused by ourselves and rejects the idea of self-induced disease: "Responsibility does not mean there is a direct causal relationship between you and your illness, nor does responsibility involve judgment, censure, or blame" (p. 25). Although it may be helpful to assume that we have a part to play in our illness, we need to reject taking blame for our illness.

In our work as counselors, we see evidence of this connection between stress and psychosomatic ailments. We often encounter people who deal with their emotions by denying or repressing them or finding some other indirect channel of expression. Consider Lou's situation, a young man who suffered from occasional asthma attacks. He discovered during the process of therapy that he became asthmatic whenever he was under emotional stress or was anxious. To his surprise, Lou found that he could control his symptoms when he began to express his feelings and talk about what was upsetting him. While continuing to receive medical supervision for his asthma, he improved his physical condition as he learned to more fully explore his emotional difficulties. As Lou let out his anger, fear, and pain, he was able to breathe freely again.

Resilience in Coping With Stress

Some people seem especially resilient, coping with stress with little apparent disruption in their lives. These people not only survive stressful events but thrive and develop resources they did not know existed. **Resilience** is the capacity of individuals to bounce back from major stress events with minimal negative effects. Suzanne (Kobasa) Ouellette (Kobasa, 1979a, 1979b, 1984) provides evidence that personality plays a significant role in helping people resist stress-related illnesses. Her studies addressed the question of who stays well and why. She identified a personality pattern she labeled "hardiness," which distinguishes people who succeed in coping with change without becoming ill. **Hardiness** is characterized by an appetite for challenge, a sense of commitment, a clearly defined sense of self and purpose, and a clear sense of being in control of one's life. Based on her study of high-stress executives who remained healthy, Ouellette (Kobasa 1979b, 1984) identified these personality traits:

▶ **A liking for challenge.** Hardy executives tend to seek out and actively confront challenges. They perceive change as stimulating and as providing them with options for growth. Instead of being riveted to the past, they welcome change and see it as a stimulus for creativity. Less hardy executives tend to view change as threatening.

▶ **A strong sense of commitment.** People who are committed have high self-esteem, a clearly defined sense of self, a zest for life, and a meaning for living. Stress-resistant executives display a clear sense of values, well-defined goals, and a commitment to putting forth the maximum effort to achieve their goals. In contrast, less hardy executives lack direction and do not have a commitment to a value system.

▶ **An internal locus of control**. Individuals with an internal locus of control believe they can influence events and their reactions to events. Such individuals accept responsibility for their actions. They believe their successes and failures are determined by internal factors, such as their abilities and the actions they take. People with an external locus of control believe what happens to them is determined by factors external to themselves such as luck, fate, and chance. Hardy individuals tend to exhibit an internal locus of control, whereas less stress-resistant individuals feel powerless over events that happen to them.

Ouellette's work has been a catalyst for research on the way personality affects health and the ability to tolerate stress, and her studies demonstrate that hardiness is a buffer against distress and illness in coping with the stresses associated with change. Hardiness traits and attitudes have shown up in other related studies, such as those conducted by Salvatore Maddi (2002). Maddi's research shows hardiness to be key to resiliency, not only for surviving but also for thriving under stress. Hardiness enhances performance, leadership, stamina, and physical and mental health by giving people the courage and capability to turn adversity into advantage.

Other researchers have also emphasized the power of resilience. To address the widespread psychological and interpersonal problems faced by military personnel, University of Pennsylvania psychologist Martin Seligman spearheaded the development of the U.S. Army Master Resilience Trainer (MRT) course to teach resilience skills to noncommissioned officers. Drawing from tenets of positive psychology and the Penn Resilience Program curriculum (which was initially designed as a school-based training program for children and adolescents), Seligman and his colleagues created MRT as the foundation for teaching resilience skills to sergeants, who would then teach these skills to soldiers (Reivich, Seligman, & McBride, 2011). MRT is a key component of the Comprehensive Soldier Fitness (CSF) program, which aims to "increase psychological strength and positive performance and to reduce the incidence of maladaptive responses of the entire U.S. Army . . . CSF is proactive; rather than waiting to see who has a negative outcome following stress, it provides ways of improving resilience for all members of the Army" (Cornum, Matthews, & Seligman, 2011, p. 4).

TAKE TIME TO REFLECT

1. What things do you most stress about? _____

_____

_____

2. What have you tried to do to manage these stressors? How well have these strategies worked? _____

_____

_____

3. What are some other steps you could take to more effectively manage your stress?

_____

_____

4. In this chapter we encourage you to assume personal responsibility for the way stress affects your body. How might your life be different if you accepted responsibility for your bodily symptoms (such as stomachaches, headaches, and muscular tension)? _____

_____

_____

5. Having a "hardy personality" can help you stay healthy as you cope with change and stress. What personality characteristics and attitudes do you have that either help or hinder you in dealing with stressful situations? How resilient do you consider yourself to be?

_____

_____

INEFFECTIVE REACTIONS TO STRESS

Reactions to stress can be viewed on a continuum from being effective and adaptive, on one end, to being ineffective and maladaptive, on the other. If our reactions to stress are ineffective over a long period of time, physical and psychological harm is likely. Ineffective ways of dealing with stress include burnout, defensive behavior, and abusing drugs or alcohol.

Burnout as a Result of Continual Stress

Burnout is a state of physical, emotional, intellectual, and spiritual exhaustion characterized by feelings of helplessness and hopelessness. Burnout is a syndrome that can lead to a sense of low personal accomplishment, emotional exhaustion, and depersonalization (Maslach, 2003). It is the result of repeated pressures, often associated with intense involvement with people over long periods of time. Striving for unrealistically high goals can lead to chronic feelings of frustration and failure. People who are burned out have depleted themselves on all levels of human functioning. Although they may have been willing to give of themselves to others, they have forgotten to take care of themselves.

Burnout is a concern for students, and they say that burnout often catches them by surprise. Frequently they do not recognize their hurried lifestyle, nor do they always notice the warning signs that they have pushed themselves to the breaking point. Many students devote the majority of their time to school and work while neglecting their friendships, not making quality time for their families, and not taking time for leisure pursuits. At the end of the semester, they are physically and emotionally exhausted. Consider Doug's situation. By not making self-care a priority, his chance of experiencing burnout is greatly increased.

DOUG'S STORY

In addition to being a full-time student, I have two part-time jobs. I work a graveyard shift as a server at an all-night diner three times a week, and I work a couple of nights as a bartender. The money is decent, and it leaves my days free to take classes and study. I am a psychology major, and to prepare myself for graduate school, I am also volunteering to help a professor with his research. I am preparing for the GRE, so with everything I do, I am lucky to get 5 hours of sleep a day. Sometimes I get so tired that I lose my appetite and forget to eat. Intellectually, I know I need to pace myself so I don't burnout, but how am I supposed to do that when I have to work, go to school, and prepare myself for grad school? I promised myself I would be finished with my PhD by the time I am 30. If I slow down, that's not going to happen.

What can we do when we feel psychologically and physically exhausted? Once we recognize our state of chronic fatigue and low energy and seriously want to change this pattern, we can learn to "work smarter," which means changing the way we approach our work so we suffer less stress (see Chapter 10). Ben-Shahar (2011) believes the real problem lies in a lack of sufficient recovery time following work sessions. Most people can maintain focused intensity at work for up to 2 hours, after which time performance drops. Instead of considering ourselves marathon runners who run long and hard until we drop, Ben-Shahar suggests we operate like sprinters, allowing ourselves recovery time after intensive periods of work. In his view, we need a **multilevel recovery**, which includes recovery on the *microlevel* (punctuating a long day with regular breaks in which we exercise, meditate, listen to music), the *midlevel* (getting adequate sleep at night), and the *macrolevel* (taking a vacation of 1 to 4 weeks every year).

By setting realistic goals and giving ourselves much needed recovery time, we function more productively and reduce our feelings of helplessness, thereby avoiding the frustration and anger that can result in exhaustion and cynicism. We can learn to relax, even for short breaks. Instead of taking personally all the problems we encounter, we can work on ourselves to assume a more objective perspective. Most important, we can learn that caring for ourselves is every bit as important as caring for others.

Although learning coping skills to deal with the effects of burnout is helpful, making better primary choices is the goal. The real challenge is to learn ways to structure our lives so we can prevent burnout. Prevention includes becoming sensitive to our personal signs of burnout and finding ways to energize ourselves. Learning how to use leisure time to nurture ourselves is important. The causes of burnout are complex, and we must all find our own path toward self care that enhances our zest for life.

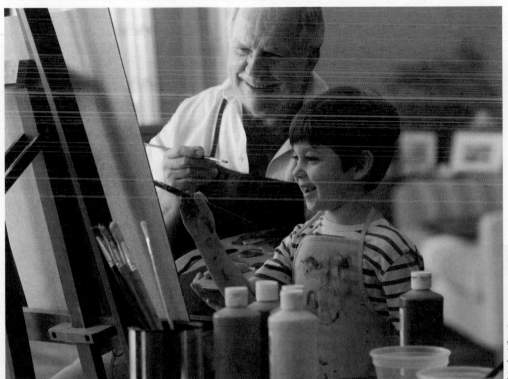

>> Learning how to use leisure time to nurture ourselves is important.

Defensive Behavior

If we experience stress associated with failure in school or work, we may defend ourselves by denying that our actions contributed to this situation. Although defensive behavior does at times have adjustive value and can result in reducing the impact of stress, such behavior increases levels of stress in the long run. If we are more concerned with defending ourselves than with coping with reality, we are not likely to take the steps necessary to resolve a problem. The trouble with relying on defensive behavior is that the more we use defense mechanisms the more we increase our anxiety. When this happens, our defenses become entrenched. This leads to a vicious cycle that is difficult to break and ultimately makes coping with stress more difficult. We suggest that you take time to review the discussion on ego-defense mechanisms in Chapter 2 and reflect on the degree to which you use defense mechanisms to cope with the stresses in your life.

Drugs and Alcohol

Many people take an aspirin for a headache or a tranquilizer when they are anxious, take stimulants to stay awake at the end of a term, and use a variety of drugs to reduce other physical symptoms and emotional stresses. Some time back, I (Jerry) took a bike ride on rough mountain trails. I came home with a headache, a condition that afflicts me only occasionally. Instead of recognizing that I had overexerted myself and needed to take a rest, my immediate reaction was to take aspirin and proceed with my usual work for the day. My body was sending me an important signal, which I was ready to ignore by numbing. Perhaps many of you can identify with this tendency to quickly eliminate symptoms rather than recognize them as a sign of the need to change certain behaviors. Many of us rely too much on drugs to alleviate symptoms of stress rather than looking at the root cause that produces this stress.

We are especially vulnerable to relying on drugs, for drugs offer the promise of freedom from pain. Consider some of the ways we attempt to control problems by relying on both legal and illegal drugs. Because we are troubled with shyness, boredom, anxiety, depression, or stress, we may become chemically dependent to relieve these symptoms. A side effect of drugs is that we numb ourselves physically and psychologically. Instead of paying attention to our bodily signals that all is not well, we engage in self-deception by believing we are in charge of our life. However, once the effects of the drugs or alcohol wear off, we are still confronted by the painful reality we sought to avoid. Because drugs and alcohol can distort reality, these substances prevent us from finding direct and effective means of coping with stress. The problem here is that stress is now controlling us instead of our controlling stress.

When drugs or alcohol are used excessively to escape painful reality, the "solution" to a problem creates another problem. As tolerance is built up for these substances, we tend to take more of them, and addiction can result. Peter, who is now sober, describes how his life revolved around drugs and alcohol for many years.

PETER'S STORY

After many years of abusing alcohol and drugs, I am fortunate to be celebrating 2 years of sobriety. It is a true blessing that I am still alive after putting my body through years of hell. My wake-up call occurred when I had to serve some jail time for a DUI that I got while I was driving on a suspended license. I hit my bottom and realized I didn't like myself and the direction I was headed in. I got involved in AA, found a great sponsor, and attended meetings regularly—and I still do.

I started experimenting with alcohol and drugs when I was 11, and it escalated to full-blown addiction by the time I was 17. My drug of choice was crystal meth. When I was using, I felt invincible. The high was incredible, until I came down from it, so I used more and more. When I wasn't on meth, I was drinking. You might wonder how I hid this from my parents as I was living under their roof. My parents were alcoholics, the kind that spent their evenings at a local bar, where they were considered "regulars." They came home from the bar most nights and went to bed, so I hid my drug addiction from them pretty well. They knew I drank beer, but that was acceptable to them. In fact, most everyone in my family drank. You were considered an outcast if you didn't drink. To this day, my older sister Darcie, who went against the family norm and refused to drink, has almost no contact with any of us. I feel badly about this because I see now how much pain she must have been in to sever ties with the family for the sake of her own self-preservation. I don't think she knows that I am sober now. When I work up the nerve, I am going to e-mail her and see if she'll agree to see me. I need to apologize for awful things I said to her when I was using. I want to have her back in my life. She's my sister, and I love her. We're the only two sober people in the family, and I think—at least, I hope—she will be proud of me for the way I am living my life today.

Because of my history, I know I am vulnerable to stress, so I took the advice of a friend I met in AA and started doing yoga. I practice it religiously, which helps me to feel centered and calm. Between attending meetings, yoga, and watching my diet, I am managing my stress pretty well these days. I used to self-medicate to deal with stress, but I just cannot do that anymore.

Addictions (whether to a drug of choice or to alcohol) become a way of life that can eventually destroy us. As illustrated in Peter's case, they can destroy family relationships as well. Alcohol is perhaps the most widely used and abused drug of all. It is legal, accessible,

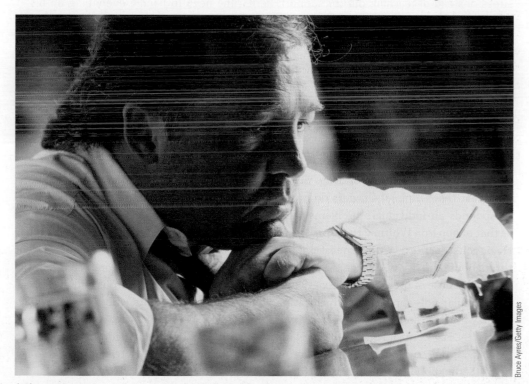

Bruce Ayres/Getty Images

>> Drugs and alcohol can distort reality and prevent one from finding direct and effective means of coping with stress.

and socially acceptable. Alcohol abuse is dangerous and debilitating, and often its effects are not immediately noticeable. Alcoholics organize their existence around drinking more and more to enhance their mood or to numb pain. Those struggling with addictions often substitute using alcohol or drugs for meaningful connection with others and become even more isolated. Many who suffer from alcoholism are trying to gain control of their lives, but they deny the problem inherent in the addiction. Unable or reluctant to engage in either prevention or treatment, they are likely to allow their illness to get to an advanced stage before admitting that they have a problem. Many say they had to hit "rock bottom" before they finally realized that their life had become unmanageable and that they were powerless over alcohol. The many thousands of alcoholics who are in recovery often say that it is necessary to turn their lives over to a higher power and to reach out to others for help in dealing with their illness. Tragically, some alcoholics and addicts are not responsive to help and lose the battle over their addictions as Claire's story illustrates.

CLAIRE'S STORY

My older brother Richard went on a drinking binge and died of alcohol poisoning 5 years ago at the age of 52. It has taken me a long time to come to terms with the choices he made during his life that ultimately led to his untimely death. My parents were both deceased at the time of his death, and a part of me is grateful that they did not see their son spiral out of control and reach the point of no return. When they were alive, they knew he was a heavy drinker, but they rationalized his behavior as being normal for men in the corporate world. He hid from them the fact that he was fired from positions for drinking on the job. My brother was smart and talented, but he did not deal well with stress. Instead of reaching out for support, he felt the need to handle everything on his own so he wouldn't be perceived as weak. He drank to take the edge off of his stress, and oddly enough, his coping mechanism became his downfall.

I have a photograph I hold onto of my brother when he was young, happy, and full of potential. That's the Richard I would like to remember. I'd rather forget the image I have of him shortly before his death when I found him passed out on a urine-soaked sofa surrounded by empty bottles of booze. I can't tell you how excruciating and helpless it feels to see someone you love become a whisper of the person he once was.

As appealing as alcohol or drugs may seem as a way of coping with pain and stress, it is clear that these coping behaviors do not work in the long run. Relying on alcohol or drugs compounds an individual's problems rather than resolving them. In extreme cases, such as that of pop icon Whitney Houston, who publicly battled drug abuse for several years, it has tragic consequences. Without question, prescription drug abuse has become more prevalent throughout our society. Fenton, Keyes, Martins, and Hasin (2010) report an increase in the nonmedical use of prescription anxiety medications, which can be dangerous and even fatal. On a similar note, prescription medication abuse among adolescents who have been diagnosed with attention-deficit hyperactivity disorder (ADHD) is on the increase. "The Office of National Drug Control Policy and the National Institute on Drug Abuse found that, next to marijuana, prescription medications are the most common drugs that teenagers use to get high" (Setlik, Bond, & Ho, 2009, p. 876).

In addition to alcohol and drugs, other problematic behaviors, some of which may be classified as addictions, can be exacerbated by stress. Compulsive overeating, gambling, and shopping are prime examples of this. Although these behaviors may have a self-soothing function, they inevitably perpetuate a vicious cycle.

Many excellent resources are available for people who are suffering from addictions, and treatments that will aid in the healing process are widely available. Part of the treatment involves learning a whole range of new coping strategies. If you are interested in learning more about alcoholism, we suggest the classic book, *Alcoholics Anonymous* (Alcoholics Anonymous World Services, 2001).

POSTTRAUMATIC STRESS DISORDERS

Traumatic incidents, which are extremely stressful, can have a significant impact on us physically, psychologically, socially, mentally, and spiritually. **Posttraumatic stress disorder (PTSD)** is an anxiety disorder resulting from a traumatic event and characterized by symptoms of reexperiencing the trauma, avoidance and numbing, and hyperarousal (American Psychiatric Association, 2000). Many people developed PTSD symptoms as a direct consequence of the terrorist attacks on September 11, 2001, and highly exposed populations showed that PTSD increased over time in a number of specific risk groups including rescue and recovery workers and retired firefighters. "Research conducted in the past decade demonstrates that the burden of 9/11-related PTSD is substantial in both the short and the long term" (Neria, DiGrande, & Adams, 2011, p. 440). On a related note, today's veterans of the Iraq and Afghanistan wars show increased rates of PTSD (Friedman, 2006). Rates of suicide among active duty service members afflicted with PTSD have increased significantly since 2001, which has prompted health care providers to deliver early interventions to promote safety and stabilization and to treat underlying symptoms (Jakupcak & Varra, 2011).

Research has intensified in other areas of posttraumatic stress and other populations as well, a few of which include survivors of major disasters such as Hurricane Katrina (Sprung & Harris, 2010; Wagner et al., 2009), the tsunami that devastated vast regions of Southeast Asia (Hussain, Weisaeth, & Heir, 2011), and tornadoes across the midwestern and southern United States (Houlihan, Ries, Polusny, & Hanson, 2008; Polusny et al., 2011). We also can anticipate research will be done on the aftermath of the devastating earthquake that struck Haiti in 2010 as well as the triple catastrophe that occurred in Japan in 2011 (the earthquake, tsunami, and crisis at the Fukushima Daiichi nuclear facility). Posttraumatic stress is associated with a variety of extremely stressful and traumatic situations involving serious auto, train, and airplane crashes as well. Survivors of assault, violent crimes, child sexual abuse, rape, sexual harassment, domestic violence, abusive parenting, kidnapping, mass shootings, or grievous loss often develop PTSD symptoms. Those who witness death or severe injury are vulnerable to PTSD. Rescue workers, police, firefighters, medical personnel, and other first responders to a crisis have to deal with their reactions to the stress associated with their jobs in various types of disasters. There is no question that traumatic stress can assault the body, mind, and spirit.

Naparstek (2006) indicates that research findings about PTSD have educated us about the syndrome's impact on our physical, emotional, cognitive, and behavioral functioning. She reports that children are more vulnerable to PTSD than adults. The younger the child, the more is the likelihood of developing PTSD and the more severe are the symptoms. Naparstek identifies the following common symptoms of PTSD: intrusive thoughts, reexperiencing the traumatic event in the form of flashbacks and nightmares, alienation, avoidance, agitation, hyperarousal (physiologic signs of increased arousal), emotional numbing, insomnia, concentration problems, panic, disturbed interpersonal relationships, anger and irritability, depression, anxiety, shame, and guilt. Traumatized people tend to shut down on a behavioral and psychological level. Although the frequency and severity of posttraumatic stress symptoms may decline gradually over time, the symptoms are long-lasting in many cases.

In a review of 25 years of research on gender differences in trauma and posttraumatic stress disorder, Tolin and Foa (2006) found that PTSD rates are higher for women even when both genders are compared on the same kind of trauma. These gender differences point to the role that cultural expectations play in explaining why some people develop PTSD and others do not (Knight, 2009). Those who experienced multiple traumas may be more vulnerable to reexperiencing old PTSD symptoms when confronted with new trauma.

Although PTSD is a common reaction to traumatic situations, most people who experience these events do not develop PTSD. However, all survivors of trauma are subjected to stress that affects many aspects of their lives, and at times they may doubt that they can ever trust again or that they can be happy or even wonder if there is a God. The worldview of survivors may change as a result of their experience, and now they may perceive the world as unfair, cruel, unsafe, and unpredictable (Schwartz & Flowers, 2008). Some survivors, like Yallah Kawalla (2011), develop strong defenses in the aftermath of a traumatic experience.

YALLAH'S STORY

The civil war in my country, Liberia, left me totally devastated and traumatized. It paralyzed me and significantly impeded my daily normal functions. For example, I would forget to eat, I did not know where I was when driving, and negative thoughts invaded my mind constantly, reducing me to the point of attempted suicide. I developed some coping methods, but they were unhealthy. For example, I would start an unnecessary argument or debate in a group in order to ward off the traumatic flashbacks. When people who cared about me encouraged me to go to counseling, I responded by putting up a wall that kept everyone and everything else outside. I allowed no one the opportunity to shine any light into my self-made prison. I was afraid to seek counseling because I knew that counselors would want me to bring up the terrible memories that I was trying to bury.

I had devised my own belief or theology of convenience. I was not comfortable in my self-made prison, but it was the only place I believed that I had control over. I fought anyone or anything that tried to get in or get me out. When I finally chose to surrender to counseling, both my counseling experience and my belief in God brought me to a place of amazing healing. My journey to healing was a long and painful process, but it was worth it all. I'm now living in freedom from negative thoughts, fear, anxiety, and terrible memories. The memories are still there, but they no longer have the destructive and paralyzing effects.

I was motivated to get my master's degree in counseling and to write two books, *Concealed by the Light* and *Consoled by the Light*, which are about my experiences that caused the PTSD and my journey to healing.

Anyone who has been subjected to trauma can gain the maximum benefit from healing by seeking professional help as soon possible after being exposed to a traumatic event. Developing PTSD can be greatly reduced for most people if help is available within 24 to 72 hours after the incident (Everly & Mitchell, 1997, 2008). If you wonder about the severity and persistence of symptoms associated with a trauma you have experienced, consider seeking professional help from someone trained to work with trauma situations.

The haunting memories of traumatic experiences often make it difficult to separate past trauma from current reality (van der Kolk, 2008). Under pressure, victims of trauma may feel or act as if they were traumatized over and over. The reenactment of trauma in social relationships is a major problem for many suffering from PTSD. Knight (2009) emphasizes that an adult survivor's past trauma is inextricably linked to his or her present problems. Knight explains the importance of a therapist understanding and connecting a survivor's past pain and present reality. Adult survivors of childhood trauma need to tell their story, and they need to be heard and understood if healing is to occur. Group psychotherapy can be especially powerful in the healing process for adult survivors of trauma. Knight captures this when she states: "Ultimately, the journey of recovery and healing from childhood trauma is a very solitary one; however, sharing the journey with others who have had similar experiences can make it a bit easier and less lonely" (p. 4).

Many treatment programs are available for those dealing with the effects of trauma. A holistic approach that involves focusing on body, mind, and spirit with the goal of restoration of health and well-being is suggested. Some of the resources available include individual psychotherapy, group therapy, support groups, and a variety of crisis intervention programs. Positive psychology is of tremendous value in helping vulnerable populations deal with their exposure to trauma in a way that will lead to growth (Cornum, Matthews, & Seligman, 2011). Positive education and an emphasis on resilience are at the heart of the Comprehensive Soldier Fitness program, which hopes to decrease the number of cases of posttraumatic stress in the U.S. Army (Seligman & Fowler, 2011). For more information on this topic, we recommend *Invisible Heroes: Survivors of Trauma and How They Heal* (Naparstek, 2006), which addresses both understanding and healing trauma.

SEXUAL EXPLOITATION

In the sections that follow we discuss three topics that involve some form of sexual exploitation resulting in trauma: incest, rape, and sexual harassment. In any form of sexual exploitation, power is misused or a trusting relationship is betrayed for the purpose of gaining control over the individual, for degrading, oppressing, coercing, or exploiting a person. Individuals are robbed of choice—except for the choice of how to react to being violated. Incest, date and acquaintance rape, and sexual harassment all entail abusive power, control, destructiveness, and violence. As such, these practices are never justifiable. In all of these forms of sexual exploitation, a common denominator is the reluctance of victims to disclose that they have been wronged. In fact, many victims suffer from undue guilt and believe they were responsible for what occurred. This guilt is exacerbated by segments of society that contribute to the "blaming the victim" syndrome. The victims should not be given further insult by being blamed for cooperating or contributing to the violence that was forced upon them.

More women than men have experienced sexual assault and childhood sexual abuse, but both women and men who are victims of sexual trauma experience psychological suffering and distress (Tolin & Foa, 2006). Knight (2009) reports that childhood trauma, especially if it involves sexual abuse, often results in serious and long-lasting consequences. For women, sexual trauma may cause more psychological suffering and is more likely to result in a PTSD diagnosis than any other kind of trauma. Due to their gender-role socialization, male victims frequently experience barriers in seeking help for the aftermath of sexual trauma. Both women and men who have been traumatized by various forms of sexual exploitation or sexual coercion often carry psychological scars from these experiences that affect the full range of their emotions, their ability to develop relationships, and many other aspects of their lives.

Sexual exploitation continues to be a major threat to the well-being of children and youth in our society. Increased efforts are needed to protect young people from sexual predators. Although the following section focuses on sexual abuse that is perpetrated within the family system, we would be remiss if we did not point out that sexual abuse committed by *any* trusted person or stranger is wrong and can have devastating consequences for the victims.

The Trauma of Incest

Incest involves any form of inappropriate sexual behavior or sexual contact between two people who are related, one of whom is often a child. Incest is one of the world's most widely prohibited sexual behaviors; it occurs at all socioeconomic levels and is illegal regardless of the age of the participants (Crooks & Baur, 2011). Incest is a betrayal of trust and a misuse of power and control. It can never be rationalized away, and the responsibility of the perpetrator can never be diminished.

Children who have been sexually abused by someone in their family feel betrayed and typically develop a mistrust of others who are in a position to take advantage of them. Oftentimes the sexual abuse is only one facet of a dysfunctional family. There also may be physical abuse, emotional abuse, neglect, alcoholism, and other problems. These children are often unaware of how psychologically abusive their family atmosphere really is for all members of the family.

Although females are more often incest victims, males also suffer the effects of incestual experiences. Mother-son incest may be subtle and at times difficult to distinguish from normal mothering behaviors, but men who have been victims of this kind of sexual abuse often experience more trauma than do other sexually abused men (Carroll, 2013). We have worked with some adult men who were incest victims during childhood and adolescence. These men often share the same patterns of dysfunction that are characteristic of women who have experienced the trauma of sexual abuse. Regardless of gender or cultural background, the dynamics of incest are similar, and thus the therapeutic work is much the same for both women and men.

Survivors of incest typically feel burdened with guilt, anger, hurt, and confusion over having been taken advantage of sexually and emotionally. They feel like they are

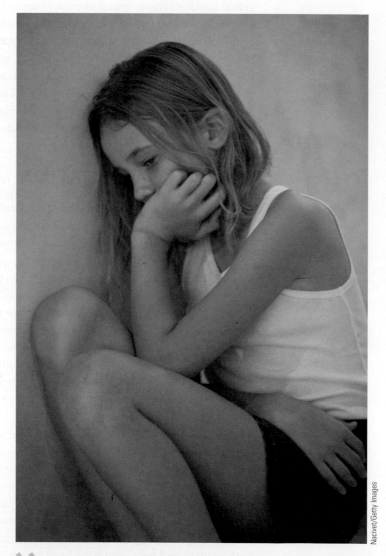

Incest is a betrayal of trust and a misuse of power and control.

victims, but some of them also see themselves as conspirators. Women often experience severe stress over not being able to talk with anyone about their trauma, and many women talk for the first time about how they have been traumatized by incest in their personal psychotherapy. They may believe they were to blame—a belief that is often reinforced by others. They may have liked the affection and love they received even though they were probably repulsed by the sexual component. Because children realize that adults have power over them, they tend to be compliant, even in situations that seem strange. Typically, these experiences happen in childhood or early adolescence; the women remember feeling help-less at the time, not knowing how to stop the perpetrator and being afraid to tell anyone. Some of the reasons children give for not revealing the abuse include not knowing that it was wrong, feeling ashamed, being frightened of the consequences of telling, a sense of self-blame, fearing that others might not believe that such abuse occurred, fear of retali-ation, and fearing the loss of affection from their family and friends. Some survivors of incest seek help only when they fear a younger sibling is threatened (Carroll, 2013). Once survivors of sexual abuse bring out past experiences, intense, pent-up emotions often sur-face and healing can begin.

The reactions to sexual abuse vary among individuals, but sexual abuse has long-lasting effects that may lead to other psychological problems (Carroll, 2013). For now we address the impact of childhood sexual abuse on the woman. The woman's ability to form sexually satisfying relationships may be impaired by events she has suppressed for many years. She may resent and distrust men, associating them with the father or other man who initially abused her. If she could not trust her own father (or grandfather, uncle, brother), then what man can she trust? She may have a hard time trusting men who express affection for her, thinking that they, too, will sexually exploit her. She may keep control of relationships by not letting herself be open and free with men. She may rarely or never allow herself to fully give in to sexual pleasure during intercourse. Her fear is that if she gives up her control, she will be hurt again. Her guilt over sexual feelings and her negative conditioning can prevent her from being open to enjoying a satisfying sexual relationship. She may blame men for her feelings of guilt and her betrayal and victimization. She may develop severe problems with establishing and maintaining intimate relationships, not only with her partner but also with her own children. In adulthood she may marry a man who will later victimize his own chil-dren, which perpetuates the pattern of her experiences growing up. In this way the dynamics from childhood are repeated in adulthood.

Veronika Tracy (1993) studied the impact of childhood sexual abuse on women's sexual-ity, comparing a group of women who were sexually abused with a group of women who had not experienced sexual abuse. She found that the women with a reported history of sexual abuse in childhood tended to have lower self-esteem, a greater number of sexual problems, less sexual satisfaction with a partner, less interest in engaging in sex, a higher propensity for sexual fantasies that involved force, and more guilt feelings about their sexual fantasies. Many of the women who were sexually abused reported that they were not able to achieve orgasm with a partner, but only by themselves. Her research revealed that women who were sexual abuse survivors often blocked out their negative experiences, only to remember the sexual abuse as they became sexually active. Paradoxically, as the women began to feel safer with a partner, their sexual activity often triggered memories, flashbacks, and other symptoms of posttraumatic stress, which tended to interfere with their ability to maintain satisfying intimate relationships.

We have found that it is therapeutic for most women and men who have a history of sexual abuse to share the burden associated with their abuse in a safe environment. In a climate of support, trust, care, and respect, these individuals can begin a healing process that will eventually enable them to move beyond the abuse. A major part of their therapy consists of accepting the reality that they were indeed victims and the trauma they experienced was not of their doing. It is hoped that eventually they can shift the responsibility to the perpetrator, and if applicable, to the silent partner as well. Another aim of treatment is to help victims externalize their feelings of guilt, rage, shame, hurt, fear, and confusion to release them from the heavy burden of responsibility and guilt.

Through personal psychotherapy, the survivor can begin to put these experiences into a new perspective. Although she will never forget these experiences, she can begin the process of letting go of feelings of self-blame and eventually arrive at a place where she is not controlled by these past experiences. In doing so, she is also freeing herself of the power and control that these painful and traumatic experiences have had over her ability to form an intimate relationship with her partner.

If you have been sexually abused in any way, we suggest that you seek counseling. It is not uncommon for people to block out experiences such as sexual abuse, only to have memories and feelings surface at a later time. Counseling can provide you with an opportunity to deal with feelings and unresolved problems that may linger because of earlier experiences. Support groups for incest survivors also can be most beneficial. In addition to counseling or support groups, many fine books deal with sexual abuse, which can be of value. For an excellent book that helps survivors and their partners understand and recover from the effects of sexual abuse, we recommend *The Sexual Healing Journey*, by Wendy Maltz (2001).

Date and Acquaintance Rape

In our contacts with students it has become clear to us that date rape is prevalent on college campuses. **Rape** involves physically or psychologically forcing sexual relations on another person. **Acquaintance rape** is a sexual assault by someone known to the victim. This might involve friends, coworkers, neighbors, or relatives. **Date rape** occurs in those situations where a person is forced to have unwanted intercourse with a person in the context of dating. Rape is an act of aggressive sexuality, or a form of sexual assault or coercion where power is misused to dominate another person. Many people who have been victimized by rape have suffered from symptoms of posttraumatic stress disorder.

Both date rape and acquaintance rape can be considered as a betrayal of trust. Much like in incest, when a person is forced to have sex against his or her will, his or her dignity as a person is violated. Rape often occurs on the part of men assaulting women, but many men experience a sexual assault at some point in their lives. Rape also occurs in same-sex relationships. Clearly, both women and men are potential perpetrators and also potential victims. It is often wrongly assumed that most rapes are committed by strangers. Only a small number of rapes are committed by strangers, whereas over half of all rapes occur in the context of dating relationships (Weiten et al., 2012).

The emotional scars that are a part of date rape are similar to the wounds inflicted by incest. As is the case with incest victims, women and men who are raped by people they know often take responsibility and blame themselves for what occurred, and they are often embarrassed about or afraid of reporting the incident. Some writers consider forcible rape to be one of the most underreported crimes in the United States (Carroll, 2013; Crooks & Baur, 2011). Reasons people do not report rape include thinking that their situation will not be taken seriously, concerns about confidentiality, doubting that anything can be done legally, fearing retaliation, and feeling shame and guilt about the incident (Carroll, 2013). When it is known that a rape has occurred on a college campus, many students report living with panic, extreme stress, and the fear that this could happen to them, especially if the perpetrator is still at large. It is clear that rape is highly stressful and traumatic, and like any kind of trauma, psychotherapy can be a major resource in helping survivors to heal.

Many college campuses offer education directed at the prevention of date rape. The focus of this education is on the importance of being consistent and clear about what you want or do not want with your dating partner, the importance of asking your partner for consent, as well as providing information about factors contributing to date rape. Rape prevention programs are increasing, and these programs are designed for women, men, and both women and men. Programs for women are designed to increase their awareness of high-risk situations and behaviors and to teach them how to protect themselves. Those targeted for men emphasize responsibility and respect for women. Both men and women have a shared responsibility for educating themselves about date rape and for working to prevent sexual violence. Campus preventive programs need to be designed for both women and men. Both women and men can benefit from discussion groups or workshops on rape prevention. In such programs the focus is generally on topics such as interpersonal communication and predicting potential problem areas.

CAITLYN'S STORY

I started college shortly after my 18th birthday and remember being so excited about living in a dorm, meeting new people, and being on my own. I desperately wanted to be independent, and like many teenagers I thought I had it all figured out. During my second semester, I went to a party and got kind of wasted. A guy I had been talking to offered to walk me back to my dorm room across campus, so I let him. He was cute and funny, and I thought we were hitting it off well. I am plagued with guilt now because later that night he raped me. I remember telling him to back off, but because my judgment was impaired that night, I keep wondering if I could have done something else to stop him.

The way I'm describing this, you probably think it happened recently. Well, it didn't. It has been 3 years, yet it feels like it happened yesterday and my guilt feelings won't let up. I can't seem to forgive myself for getting so drunk and losing control. I know intellectually that he should have stopped when I said "no," but I have not yet been able to leave my guilt behind. I am finally seeing a counselor for this, and I hope I eventually find relief.

As unsettling as this may seem, Caitlyn's circumstances occur all too frequently on college campuses. A team of researchers note that "several studies suggest that the frequency of sexual assaults that occur when the victim is unable to consent due to intoxication may be quite high and deserving of special attention" (Lawyer, Resnick, Von Bakanic, Burkett, & Kilpatrick, 2010, p. 453). Their own study showed that drug-related sexual assaults on college campuses occur more often than forcible assaults and are most frequently preceded by voluntary alcohol consumption. This research in no way suggests that the victims of these crimes bear any responsibility for their assaults. No matter how impaired individuals may be to stop an assault, they should never be blamed for having been victimized by a sexual assault.

Sexual Harassment

Sexual harassment is repeated and unwanted sexually oriented behavior in the form of suggestive comments, gestures, humor, or physical contacts. This phenomenon is a major concern in academic settings, in the workplace, and in the military. Women experience sexual harassment more frequently than do men. Sexual harassment is abuse of the power differential between two people. Title VII of the 1964 Civil Rights Act prohibits sexual harassment. A company can be held liable for the coercive actions by its employees.

You may have witnessed, or been the victim of, some of these forms of sexual harassment:

▶ Comments about one's body or clothes

▶ Physical or verbal conduct of a sexual nature

▶ Jokes about sex or gender-specific traits

▶ Repeated and unwanted staring, comments, or propositions of a sexual nature

▶ Demeaning references to one's gender

▶ Unwanted touching or attention of a sexual nature

▶ Conversations tinted with sexually suggestive innuendoes or double meanings

▶ Questions about one's sexual behavior

Men sometimes make the assumption that women like sexual attention, when in fact they may resent being related to in sexual terms. Sexual harassment diminishes choice, and surely it is not flattering. Harassment reduces people to objects to be demeaned, can be traumatic, and is almost always a source of stress. It may seem that sexual harassment is not as shocking or harmful as other forms of sexual coercion, but the impact of harassment on individuals can result in traumatic reactions and can cause long-term difficulties (Carroll, 2013). The person doing the harassing may not see this behavior as being problematic and may even joke about it. Yet it is never a laughing matter. Those on the receiving end of harassment often report feeling responsible. However, as in the cases of incest and date rape, the victim should never be blamed.

Many incidences of sexual harassment go unreported because the individuals involved fear the consequences, such as getting fired, being denied a promotion, risking a low grade in a course, or encountering barriers to pursuing their careers. Fear of reprisals is the foremost barrier to reporting. Not reporting such incidences can result in problems because individuals who are subjected to harassment may not be able to function at their fullest capacity in such a hostile environment.

If you are on the receiving end of unwanted behavior, you are not powerless. Because sexual harassment is never appropriate, you have every right to break the pattern. The initial step is to recognize there is a problem pertaining to sexual harassment. The next step is to make it clear to the person doing the harassing that his or her behavior is unacceptable to you and that you want it stopped. If this does not work, or if you feel it would be too much of a risk to confront this individual, you can talk to someone else. If the offensive behavior does not stop, keep a detailed record of what is taking place. This will be useful in showing a pattern of unwanted behavior when you issue a complaint.

Most work settings and colleges have policies and procedures for dealing with sexual harassment complaints. You do not have to deal with this matter alone if your rights are violated. Realize that the college community does not take abusing power lightly and that procedures are designed to correct abuses. When you report a problematic situation, know that your college most likely has staff members who will assist you in bringing resolution to this situation. As is true for preserving the secret of incest, it will not help if you keep the harassment a secret. By telling someone else, you are breaking the pattern of silence that burdens sexual harassment victims.

VICARIOUS TRAUMATIZATION

If you are preparing to become a helping professional, it is important to protect yourself from the real threat of **vicarious traumatization** (McCann & Pearlman, 1990). As a result of empathic engagement with clients who have been through traumas such as the ones described thus far—sexual abuse, rape, incest, sexual harassment, torture, natural or manmade disasters—you may be vulnerable to experiencing trauma yourself. "[S]ymptoms of vicarious traumatization include anxiety, suspiciousness, depression, somatic symptoms, intrusive thoughts and feelings, avoidance, emotional numbing and flooding, and increased feelings of personal vulnerability" (Culver, McKinney, & Paradise, 2011, p. 34). Trauma victims are often considered the most challenging clients because of their demand for additional time and resources (which already are strained) to process their experiences. Capturing the experiences of mental health professionals who worked with survivors of Hurricane Katrina in affected areas of New Orleans, Culver and her colleagues discovered that the clinicians' perceptions of others and their worldview were negatively affected.

Although this information may initially seem alarming, your training program will equip you with the knowledge and skills you need to handle a range of demanding situations. Reach out for support and consult with your colleagues and supervisors if you find you are feeling overwhelmed. Vicarious traumatization applies not only to counselors but also to a wide range of first responders in crisis situations, such as those who work in public service and safety. You can build your own arsenal of strategies for coping with the stressful aspects of your work by following the ideas presented in the following section on constructive responses to stress.

TAKE TIME TO REFLECT

1. In what ways, if any, do you cope with stress ineffectively? What are you willing to do to change these patterns? _____

_____

_____

2. If you have experienced trauma, how have you handled it? To what extent have you recovered from the trauma? In what ways does it still affect your life and how well you function? _____

_____

_____

_____

3. If someone you know or care about has experienced trauma, how has it affected the way in which they interact with others (including you)? How does this make you feel?

_____

_____

4. If you plan to enter any one of the various helping professions, what are your concerns, if any, about vicarious traumatization? What steps might you take to reduce the potential negative impact of working with trauma survivors? _____

_____

_____

_____

CONSTRUCTIVE RESPONSES TO STRESS

We have talked about ineffective reactions to stress, trauma as a source of stress, various forms of posttraumatic stress disorders, and the stress associated with sexual exploitation and sexual harassment. We now turn our attention to task-oriented constructive approaches aimed at realistically coping with stressful events. Although there are many useful approaches to dealing with stress, it is essential that we understand the basic causes of our stress reactions. Deeper levels of stress management must involve insights and self-discovery if we hope to manage stress in a profound, life-altering manner. With this deeper understanding, it is possible for us to alter some of the basic causes and at the same time utilize a range of constructive coping strategies.

Weiten, Dunn, and Hammer (2012) recommend the following **constructive coping** strategies as behavioral reactions to stress that are judged to be relatively healthful:

▸ Confront the problem directly.

▸ Accurately and realistically appraise a stressful situation rather than distorting reality.

▸ Learn to recognize and manage potentially disruptive emotional reactions to stress.

▸ Learn to exert behavioral self-control in the face of stress.

In addition to these characteristics, three other strategies for constructively coping with stress are identifying and modifying your self-talk, learning to laugh and enjoy humor, and turning stress into strengths. Later in this chapter we discuss other healthy approaches to managing stress, but let's examine these three ideas in more detail now.

Changing Self-Defeating Thoughts and Messages

Your thoughts and what you tell yourself can contribute to your experience of stress. For example, these thoughts about using time often bring about stress: "When I take time for fun, I feel guilty." "I'm constantly feeling rushed, telling myself that I ought to be doing more and that I should be working faster." "If there were more hours in a day, I'd find more things to do in a day and feel even more stressed."

In Chapter 3 we discussed ways to challenge parental injunctions, cultural messages, and early decisions. Those same principles can be effectively applied to coping with the negative impact of stress. Most stress results from beliefs about the way life is or should be. For example, the pressures to perform and to conform to external standards are greatly exacerbated by self-talk such as "I must do this job perfectly." You can use the cognitive techniques described in Chapter 3 to deal with certain faulty beliefs based on "shoulds," "oughts," and "musts." If you can change your self-defeating beliefs about living up to external expectations, you are in a position to behave in ways that produce less stress. Even though it is not always possible to change a difficult situation, you can modify your beliefs about the situation. Doing so can result in decreasing the stress you experience. By monitoring your self-talk, you can identify beliefs that create stress.

From a personal perspective, I (Jerry) know how difficult it is to change certain internalized messages. People who know me well see the following behavior patterns: being wedded to work, impatience, doing several things at once, getting overly involved in projects, meeting self-imposed deadlines, and a desire to control the universe! Over the years I have realized that I cannot cram my life with activities all year, fragmenting myself with many stressful situations, and then expect a "day off" to rejuvenate my system. Even though I am a somewhat slow learner in this respect, a few years ago I recognized the need to find ways of reducing situations that cause stress and to deal differently with the stresses that are inevitable. It has been useful for me to identify my individual patterns, beliefs, and expectations that lead to stress. Furthermore, I am increasingly making conscious choices about my ways of behaving—recognizing that my choices can result in either stress or inner peace. I continue to learn that changing my thinking and behavior is an ongoing process of self-monitoring and making choices. One more thing—some say that I don't have much stress in my personal life; rather, I just cause it for others!

Acquiring a Sense of Humor

Some people take themselves too seriously and have a difficult time learning how to enjoy life. If we are overly serious, there is little room for expressing the joy within us. Laughing at our own folly, our own inconsistencies, and at some of our pretentious ways can be highly therapeutic. Of course, humor should never be directed at belittling others. If we can laugh *with* others, this can enhance our relationships. Taking time for play and laughter can be the very medicine we need to combat the negative forces of stress. If we learn to "lighten up," the stresses that impinge upon us can seem far less pressing. Laughter is a healing force; humor can be a powerful antidote to physical illness and stress.

Humor not only acts as a buffer against stress but provides an outlet for frustration and anger. Humor taps our creativity and spontaneity and can enable us to put our stress into perspective. Hales (2012) points out that humor "is one of the healthiest ways of coping with life's ups and downs. Laughter stimulates the heart, alters brain wave patterns and breathing rhythms, reduces perceptions of pain, decreases stress-related hormones, and strengthens the immune system" (p. 35). Humor can be considered a transformative agent of healing and an approach for putting stressful situations into a new perspective.

Suggestions for Managing Stress

Stress does not have to be a liability. You can transform stress into strength by taking steps to creatively cope with it. Many strategies for stress reduction are based on simple commonsense principles, but actually putting them into action may be more difficult. Nevertheless, your efforts to reduce stress are likely to pay off as they have for these people:

Lynn: "I realized around a year ago that my perfectionism was having a negative impact on my staff because my actions conveyed the message that nothing was ever good

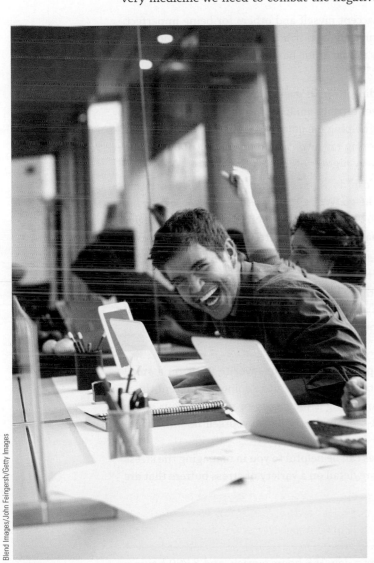

Blend Images/John Feingersh/Getty Images

Laughter is a healing force; humor can be a powerful antidote to physical illness and stress.

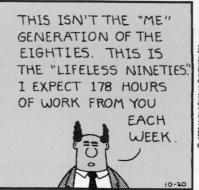
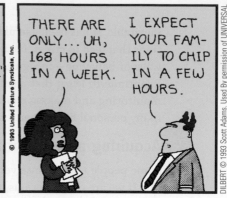

>> Even if it is not always possible to change a difficult office situation, you can modify your beliefs about the situation.

enough. I have made progress in learning to accept myself and others for being imperfect, and in keeping things in perspective. Disputing my own irrational thoughts has been the most useful method of reducing my stress. My new attitude has helped boost morale around the office, and it sure is making my life easier."

Sandra: "I have always struggled with needing to plan everything to excess. Whenever anything deviates from my plan, I tend to feel terribly anxious and out of control. I have sought therapy to work on this issue, which is helping me quite a bit. My therapist gives me homework every week, which includes monitoring my anxiety and journaling about it, and setting aside a little bit of time to meditate every night."

Ethan: "Simple relaxation techniques that I can do wherever I am help to keep me from getting too stressed out. I am constantly on the go. When I am not in a meeting or staring at the computer screen in my office, I am in the car. So there are some relaxation strategies that I can use while I am sitting at my desk that don't draw the attention of my coworkers."

Enrique: "About a year ago, I had to go to the student health center because I had headaches all the time. I started missing class because of the pain I was in, and although I hate going to the doctor, I needed help. My worst fear was that I had a brain tumor, but it turns out that my headaches were a result of stress. This was a wake-up call for me. A friend recommended that I try acupuncture, so I did, and it has helped a lot. I am also trying to manage my stress through diet and exercise."

To put stress-reduction techniques into practice, write your favorite ideas on a small card that you keep with you and can refer to often. Stop what you are doing at different times during the day and ask yourself if what you are doing is increasing or reducing your stress level. At these times you can identify your self-talk and learn to give yourself new and more constructive thoughts.

A wide variety of stress reduction strategies can be helpful to you in managing the stress in your life. The following sections focus in more detail on a variety of stress buffers that are positive ways to deal with stress.

TIME MANAGEMENT

We all have the same amount of time: 24 hours a day, 168 hours a week, and 8,760 hours a year. How people use time varies greatly from individual to individual. Consider time as a valuable resource that enables you to do what you want in your life. The way you choose to use your time is a good indicator of what you value. If you are interested in making better use of your time, a good place to begin is by monitoring it. Once you have identified how you spend your time, you will be able to make conscious choices of where you want to spend it. Keep in mind that there is no one best way to budget your time; you have to find the system that works for you. **Time management** is not an end in itself. If your time management program begins to control you, this is probably a sign that it is best to reevaluate and reset your priorities.

Using time wisely is related to living a balanced life and is thus a part of wellness. Ask yourself these questions:

▶ Am I making the time for taking care of myself in all areas of living?

▶ Do I know where I want to go in the next few months and years?

▶ Am I generally accomplishing what I have set out to do each day? Is it what I *wanted* to do?

▶ Do I balance fun with work? Do I tell myself I do not have time for fun?

▶ Do I feel rushed?

▶ Do I make time for nurturing my significant relationships? If I tell myself that I do not have time for my friends, what is the message in that?

▶ Do I make time for meeting my spiritual needs? Do I allow time for quiet reflection on my priorities in life?

▶ Do I generally like the way I spend my time? What would I like to do more of? What would I like to reduce or cut out in my daily activities?

▶ How would I like to use time differently than I did yesterday? Last week? Last month?

Time management is a key strategy in managing stress. Indeed, much of the daily stress we experience is probably due to our taking on too many projects at once, not using our time effectively, or procrastinating. Putting things off, especially if they need immediate attention, is a direct route to stress. Although there are some short-term gains to procrastination, in the long run it tends to lead to disappointment, feelings of failure, anxiety, and increased stress. If you want to change a pattern, ask yourself if the tasks you are putting off are of value to you. If certain tasks are not meaningful to you, it may be best to drop them.

Here are some suggestions for positive actions you can take to remain in charge of your time:

▶ Reflect on your long-range goals, prioritizing the steps you will take in reaching them. Establish clear and attainable goals. Set goals and reevaluate them periodically.

▶ Break down long-range goals into smaller goals. Develop a plan of action for reaching subgoals. It will help to break down a project into smaller elements that you are willing to complete at a specific time.

▶ Be realistic in deciding what you can accomplish in a given period of time.

▶ Before accepting new projects, think about how realistic it is to fit one more thing into your schedule. Put yourself in the driver's seat, and do not allow others to overload your circuits.

▶ Create a schedule that helps you get done what you want to accomplish. Make use of daily, weekly, monthly, and yearly planners. Make a daily "to do" list to keep yourself from becoming overwhelmed.

▶ Instead of doing everything yourself, ask for help from others and learn to delegate.

▶ You cannot be productive every moment. Make time in your schedule for fun, exercise, journal writing, meditation, socializing, and leisure.

▶ Concentrate on doing one thing at a time as well as you can.

As you learn to organize your time, you will surely meet with obstacles. You may underestimate how long a project will take, unexpected demands may use time you had blocked off for studying, or other external factors may throw off your plans. Be patient with yourself and tolerate some setbacks. Skills in time management take time to acquire as Tony discovered on his path to success in college. You may hear old voices in your head telling you that you never get done what is important to you. Learn to challenge those internal voices that stand between you and your goals.

TONY'S STORY

I am in my second semester of graduate school now, and I say that with a sigh of relief. Although my parents and I never questioned the thought that I would pursue an MBA after graduating from college, I ran into some trouble in the junior year of my undergraduate program that could have ruined my plans. As with many college students who stretch themselves too thin, I had an active social life in college, a full load of classes, and a job. As a high school student, I managed to juggle various activities at the same time, and everything always worked out fine. I procrastinated on assignments, but my grades were good and I maintained a balanced life. So I figured the same would hold true in college. I was mistaken!

My first 2 years of college were a bit of a struggle because I didn't alter my study and work habits, but the consequences weren't that bad. My grades weren't stellar, but they weren't average either, so I didn't feel motivated to change. In my junior year, the pressure increased. There were more demands placed on me academically and socially (I got involved in a fraternity). I thought I could manage well enough, but the truth is that I couldn't. I procrastinated on starting assignments that were due in a few weeks when something more immediate and interesting was happening on campus. More times than I'd like to admit, I put off starting a project so long that I didn't have a moment to spare in meeting the deadline. I was pulling all-nighters just to finish on time.

At that point, the quality of my assignments was the least of my concerns. I just wanted to have something to turn in to the professor. My grades were suffering, and just when I thought it couldn't get worse, it did! I had a major project due in 24 hours, and I was prepared to spend the whole day and night working on it until I got called into work on short notice. I couldn't tell my boss that I couldn't come in to work. So I went to work and ended up getting a low grade on the assignment and in the class. I finally experienced a consequence for my procrastination.

Today, I am very grateful that I was given a second chance. I am a bit more mature now, and I know there is a limit to what I can accomplish in any given time frame. I don't procrastinate nearly as much as I did as an undergraduate, and I am feeling more successful and less stressed. That was a hard lesson to learn!

MEDITATION

Our minds sometimes become cluttered with worries, regrets, negative self-images, memories, reactions, hopes, and fears, which leads to a sense of getting buried deeper and deeper. **Meditation** is a process of directing our attention to a single, unchanging, or repetitive stimulus. This process may include repetition of a word, sound, phrase, or prayer, but its main purpose is to eliminate mental distractions and relax the body. Meditation is a way to sort out the confusion and to bring about tranquility, enabling us to focus on constructive thoughts and to discover positive images of ourselves.

Meditation sharpens our concentration and our thinking power and aims at personal transformation. During much of our waking time, we are thinking and engaging in some form of verbalization or inner dialogue. In fact, many of us find it difficult to quiet the internal chatter that typically goes on inside our heads. We are not used to attending to one thing at a time or to fully concentrating on a single action. Oftentimes we miss the present moment by thinking about what we did yesterday or what we will do tomorrow or next year. Meditation is a tool to increase awareness, become centered, and achieve an internal focus. In meditation our attention is focused, and we engage in a single behavior. The process of meditation keeps our attention anchored in the present moment. Our attention is cleansed of preconceptions and distracting input so that we can perceive reality more freshly. Although we narrow our focus of attention when we meditate, the result is an enlarged sense of being.

Meditation creates a deep state of relaxation in a fairly short time. The meditative state not only induces profound relaxation but also reduces physical and psychological fatigue. Its beneficial effects are numerous, and it has been shown to relieve anxiety and stress-related disease. People who consistently practice meditation show a substantial reduction in the frequency of stress-related symptoms. Some of the physical benefits that can result from the regular practice of meditation include relief from insomnia, lower blood pressure, improved posture, increased energy, and better management of pain (Fontana, 1999). Various studies have shown the benefits of meditation for overall health, but it seems particularly valuable for people with stress-related medical conditions such as heart problems and high blood pressure, and for preventing stress-induced changes in the immune system (Hales, 2012). There are also mental benefits of meditation, such as improved tranquility, patience, concentration and memory, and enhanced understanding and empathy for others. Notice how many of the benefits of meditation are strikingly similar to the benefits of regular exercise discussed in Chapter 4.

There are as many different ways to meditate as there are meditators. Some people allow an hour each morning for silence and internal centering. Others find that they can enter a meditative state while walking, jogging, bike riding, or doing T'ai Chi. You do not have to wear exotic garb and sit in a lotus position to meditate. Sitting quietly and letting your mind wander or looking within can be a simple form of meditation.

It may help to have a mantra to repeat as a way to focus attention. A popular one that I (Jerry) am fond of is the *Om Namah Shivaya* mantra, which I have on an audiotape. The mantra is said very slowly and deliberately, a syllable at a time:

Om — Na — Mah — Shi — Va — Ya

Om Namah Shivaya means "I honor the divinity that resides within me" (see Gilbert, 2006, p. 120). My family finds it quite amusing that sometimes I am able to calm my active grandchildren by having them listen with me to my meditation mantras. Another favorite resource of mine is the prayer of Saint Francis of Assisi (see Chapter 6). For me, slowly and thoughtfully rehearsing each of the lines in this prayer internally is a basis for meditation and personal reflection. Each of us can benefit by finding some way to center ourselves and to promote reflection.

We may convince ourselves that we do not have the time for morning meditation. However, if we do not make time for this centering activity, it is likely that we will be bounced around by events that happen to us throughout the day. To make meditation part of our daily pattern, concerted effort and consistent practice are required. Many writers on meditation recommend a 20- to 30-minute session in the morning. For many of us, this might seem unrealistic. However, if we modify this recommendation to fit our situation, we might discover that devoting some time to centering is beneficial.

It is better to assume a sitting position for meditating rather than lying in bed, and meditating on an empty stomach is recommended for achieving deep meditative states. These exercises must be practiced for at least a month for meditation's more profound effects to be experienced. Several excellent guides to meditation include *Meditation* (Easwaran, 1991), *Going to Pieces Without Falling Apart* (Epstein, 1998), *Learn to Meditate* (Fontana, 1999), *Wherever You Go, There You Are* (Kabat-Zinn, 1994), and *Meditation* (Rinpoche, 1994).

MINDFULNESS

"Multitasking has become a way of life. People talk on a cell phone while commuting to work, or scan the news while returning emails. But in the rush to accomplish necessary tasks, people often lose connection with the present moment" ("Mind Over Matter," 2011, p. 6). Living by the values of accomplishing and producing, we sometimes forget the importance of experiencing the immediate moment unfolding before us. By emphasizing *doing*, we forget the importance of *being*. One answer to our fragmented existence is to practice **mindfulness**, which aims to alleviate our suffering and make our lives rich and meaningful "by attuning us to our moment-to-moment experience and giving us direct insight into how our minds create unnecessary anguish" (Siegel, 2010, p. 5).

Mindfulness keeps us in the here and now, focusing on *what is* rather than on *what if*. If you are living in the present moment, you are not ruminating about the past or worrying about the future. Living in the present allows you to gain full awareness of whatever actions you are engaged in and to be fully present when you are with another person. This is the essence of living mindfully. Thich Nhat Hanh (1992) teaches that we can transform this moment into a wonderful moment if only we stop running into the future, stop fretting about the past, and stop being focused on accumulating things. It is important to realize that living mindfully in the present does not imply getting rid of the past or the future. Nhat Hanh captures this idea nicely: "As you touch the present moment, you realize that the present is made of the past and is creating the future. Touching the present, you touch the past and the future at the same time" (p. 123).

Mindfulness is like meditation in that the aim is to clear our mind and calm our body. It is a state of active attention that involves focusing on here-and-now awareness in a nonjudgmental way. Easwaran (1991) encourages us to slow down if we hope to acquire a mindful approach to living. If we are driven by a hectic, multitasking, hurried pace, we become robotlike with little freedom and no choices. Easwaran believes that if we want freedom of action, good relations with others, health and vitality, and a calm and clear mind, it is essential that we slow down. He teaches that as we acquire the skills of mindfulness, our senses become keener, our thinking patterns become more lucid, and we increase our sensitivity to the needs of others. The ability to observe our physical, emotional, and mental activities with a degree of nonjudgmental detachment enables us to become increasingly aware of what we do and say. Schwartz and Flowers (2008) capture the essence of living mindfully: "When we are mindful, we are engaged in the present, not entangled in the past, not rejecting what is occurring. The result is that we are freer, more alive, more energized, more clearheaded" (p. 104).

Jon Kabat-Zinn (1990) describes some basic attitudes necessary to the practice of mindfulness:

▶ Do not judge. Become aware of automatic judging thoughts that pass through your mind.

▶ Be open to each moment, realizing that some things cannot be hurried.

▶ See everything as if you are looking at it for the first time.

▶ Learn to trust your intuitions.

▶ Rather than striving for results, focus on accepting things as they are.

▶ Develop an accepting attitude.

▶ Let go. Turn your mind off and simply let go of thoughts.

Mindfulness is not limited to periods of formal practice; rather, it is meant to become a way of life and something that we can practice throughout our daily existence.

Two useful books on the subject of mindfulness by Jon Kabat-Zinn are *Full Catastrophe Living* (1990) and *Wherever You Go, There You Are* (1994). Another book we recommend is *The Mindfulness Solution: Everyday Practices for Everyday Problems* (2010) by Ronald Siegel.

DEEP RELAXATION

You don't have to settle for a range of psychophysiological problems such as indigestion, backaches, insomnia, and headaches as part of your life. If you can genuinely learn to relax and take care of yourself in positive and nurturing ways, you will enhance your life and the lives of the people close to you.

One of the best ways to stop our frantic pace is by learning and practicing breathing. Breathing is an effective way to control unhappiness, agitation, fear, anxiety, and anger. Take a few moments right now to become aware of your breathing. Breathing is our most natural instinct, but many of us have forgotten how to breathe properly. Relearning the correct way to breathe can have a significant impact on our well-being and can contribute to our ability to relax. When we are able to breathe properly, we are able to relax more fully.

Devote a few moments to reflecting on how you relax. Do you engage in certain forms of relaxation on a regular basis? What do you consider to be relaxing? What would you be doing if you increased the quantity and quality of your relaxation time?

Progressive muscle relaxation is an approach to deep relaxation that can be practiced in a 10- to 20-minute time frame. To get started, follow these steps:

▶ Get comfortable, be quiet, and close your eyes.

▶ Pay attention to your breathing. Breathe in slowly through your nose. Exhale slowly through your mouth.

▶ Clench and release your muscles. Tense and relax each part of your body two or more times. Clench while inhaling; release while exhaling.

▶ Tense and relax, proceeding through each muscle group.

Herbert Benson (1976, 1984), a Harvard cardiologist, described a simple meditative technique that has helped many people cope with stress. Benson's experiments revealed how it is possible to learn to control blood pressure, body temperature, respiration rate, heart rate, and oxygen consumption through the use of what he called the **relaxation response**. Benson's work demonstrates that it is possible to make use of self-regulatory, noninvasive techniques in the prevention of stress-related illnesses. In his studies participants achieved a state of deep relaxation by repeating a mantra (a word used to focus attention, such as *om*). He described the following three factors as crucial to inducing this state of relaxation, much like a meditative state:

▶ Find a quiet place with a minimum of external distractions. The quiet environment contributes to the effectiveness of the repeated word or phrase by making it easier to eliminate distracting thoughts.

▶ Find an object or mantra to focus your attention on and let thoughts simply pass by. It is important to concentrate on one thing only and learn to eliminate internal mental distractions as well as external ones.

▶ Adopt a passive attitude, which includes letting go of thoughts and distractions and simply returning to the object you are dwelling on. A passive attitude implies a willingness to let go of evaluating yourself and to avoid the usual thinking and planning.

In our complex society, we will inevitably encounter obstacles to full relaxation. All methods of deep relaxation require us to assume a great deal of responsibility. For most of us, it has taken years to build up tension patterns. Realistically, we cannot expect immediate results in acquiring a lifestyle without tensions. It will take effort and perseverance to overcome years of negative mental and physical conditioning. Even if you take a few moments in a busy schedule to unwind, your mind may be reeling with thoughts of past or future events. Another problem is simply finding a quiet and private place where you can relax and a time free from interruptions.

YOGA

Over the past three decades yoga has become quite popular throughout the Western world, and it appeals to a wide range of people, from children to older people, with all levels of abilities. This section on yoga consists of a summary of several different sources: Gilbert (2006), various websites dealing with a guide to popular yoga styles, and a few of the points Feuerstein and Bodian (1993) make about the practice of yoga in their book, *Living Yoga: A Comprehensive Guide for Daily Life*.

Yoga is not simply a form of calisthenics, a system of meditation, or a religion. Like meditation and mindfulness, yoga is a way of life. Yoga, which originated in India, means "union" in Sanskrit. Yoga is often referred to as the union of the body, mind, and spirit. Yoga focuses on breathing, the body, and centering. Gilbert (2006) captures the essence of yoga in these words:

> Yoga is about self-mastery and the dedicated effort to haul your attention away from your endless brooding over the past and your nonstop worrying about the future so that you can seek, instead, a place of eternal presence from which you may regard yourself and your surroundings with poise. (p. 122)

Yoga is about doing the best you can at that day or time, without comparing yourself to others. As a noncompetitive activity, yoga enables you to see the strengths you already have and to build on those strengths.

Those who practice yoga have a personal goal. Some of the goals that motivate people to engage in yoga are to reduce stress, enhance health, expand awareness, deepen spirituality, or provide greater flexibility. Satyapriya, Nagendra, Nagarathna, and Padmalatha (2009) demonstrated through their research that yoga reduces perceived stress and improves adaptive autonomic response to stress in healthy pregnant women. In addition to managing stress, yoga provides numerous health benefits in both prevention and treatment of illnesses. For years Eastern health practitioners have known of the health value of practicing yoga, and now Western doctors are acknowledging the significant health benefits of yoga. Some of these benefits include lowering blood pressure, improving flexibility, enhancing circulation, protecting the joints, strengthening bones and increasing bone density, lowering blood sugar in people with diabetes, and reducing pain in people who are suffering from chronic physical problems (Hales, 2012). Yoga also may benefit those diagnosed with ovarian or breast cancer. One pilot study examined the benefits of a 10-week active relaxation program (a gentle form of yoga) and found that participants experiencing significant improvements in their depression, negative affect, state anxiety, mental health, and quality of life. This small study adds to the growing literature on the benefits of yoga for cancer patients (Danhauer et al., 2008).

Many different styles of yoga are being taught and practiced today. The various styles are based on the same physical postures, or poses, yet each form of yoga has a particular

emphasis. Some kinds of yoga are slow-paced and gentle, providing a good introduction to the basic yoga poses. More vigorous types of yoga match movement to breathing. Another yoga style emphasizes bodily alignments and involves holding poses over long periods rather than moving quickly from one position to the next. Specific types of yoga can work on both internal and external organs as well as on the muscular and skeletal systems. There is no one best yoga style, and selecting a style of yoga depends on your particular goals, personality type, interests, and needs.

As the popularity of yoga has increased and self-teaching videos have proliferated, so have the number of yoga-related injuries. To avoid yoga injuries, beginners are urged to study under a qualified yoga instructor who can supervise them and provide an added degree of safety (Benjamin, 2008). Rather than saying "no pain no gain," a more helpful adage is "no pain no sprain" (p. 11).

If this is a practice you would like to develop, you can probably find yoga classes in your area. To learn more about the value of yoga, we recommend Ana Forrest's (2011) *Fierce Medicine: Breakthrough Practices to Heal the Body and Ignite the Spirit.*

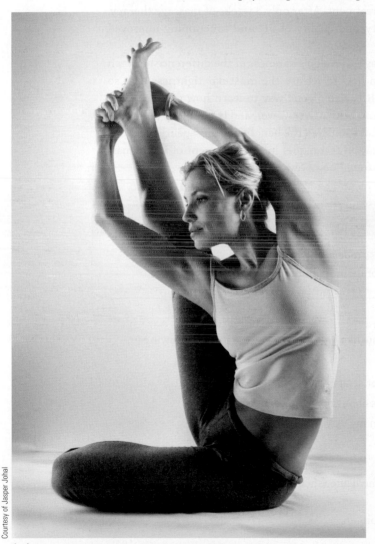

Courtesy of Jasper Johal

Yoga is a path to health and wellness.

THERAPEUTIC MASSAGE

In many European countries, and in Eastern cultures as well, massage is a well-known way to enhance health. In fact, physicians often prescribe therapeutic massage and mineral baths to counter the negative effects of stress. Massage is a positive route to maintaining wellness and coping with stress, but use caution in selecting a reputable practitioner.

Earlier we talked of the need for touch to maintain the well-being of the body and mind, and we also mentioned how the body tells the truth. Massage is one way of meeting the need for touch; it is also a way to discover where and how you are holding onto the tension produced by stressful situations. Practitioners who have studied physical therapy and therapeutic massage say that the body is the place where changes need to be made if long-lasting psychological changes are to result.

Massage therapy can be considered a part of alternative medicine; it can restore us emotionally and physically, and regular massage has many benefits. Sturgeon, Wetta-Hall, Hart, Good, and Dakhil, (2009) assessed the impact of therapeutic massage on the quality of life of breast cancer patients undergoing treatment. After only 3 weeks of massage therapy, the patients' state of anxiety, sleep quality, and quality of life and functioning improved significantly.

Therapeutic massage is an excellent way to develop awareness of the difference between tension and relaxation states and to learn how to release the muscular tightness that so often results when you encounter stress. It is also a good way to learn how to receive the caring touch of another. Massage therapy can be costly, however, and is not likely to be covered by all insurance companies. A study that compared the benefits of therapeutic massage to less expensive methods (such as a relaxation technique) in the treatment of individuals afflicted with generalized anxiety disorder found no noteworthy differences.

TAKE TIME TO REFLECT

1. Humor is believed to be a source of stress relief. To what extent do you find humor in life's ups and downs? How can you incorporate more humor into your life?

_____

_____

2. On a scale of 1 (low) to 5 (high), rate how likely you are to engage in the following stress-reduction practices:

_____ Use more effective time management strategies

_____ Critically evaluate negative thoughts about myself or others

_____ Examine irrational beliefs that get in my way

_____ Practice meditation

_____ Practice mindfulness

_____ Seek out alternative approaches to medicine (such as therapeutic massage and acupuncture)

_____ Practice progressive muscle relaxation

_____ Take a yoga class

_____ Engage in physical exercise on a regular basis

3. This time management inventory can help you recognize your own time traps. Decide whether each statement is more true or more false as it applies to you and place a **T** for true or an **F** for false in the space provided.

_____ I often find myself taking on tasks because I am the only one who can do them.

_____ I often feel overwhelmed because I try to do too much in too little time.

_____ No matter how much I do, I feel that I am always behind and never quite caught up.

_____ I frequently miss deadlines.

_____ I often procrastinate.

_____ I tend to be a perfectionist, and this keeps me from enjoying my accomplishments.

_____ I am bothered by many unscheduled interruptions when doing important work.

_____ I am aware of hurrying much of the time and feeling hassled.

_____ I have a hard time getting to important tasks and sticking to them.

4. What steps are you willing to take to better manage your time? _____
_____
_____

5. What beliefs or attitudes make it difficult for you to cope with stress? In other words, what do you sometimes tell yourself that increases your level of stress?
_____
_____

6. What behaviors are you willing to work on to gain better control over the stressors in your life? _____
_____
_____

Now that you have finished reading this chapter and completed this Take Time to Reflect, consider some of the ways you can manage the stresses you face. Reflect on some of the ways that you can take better care of yourself through a variety of practices. Ask yourself whether your daily behavior provides evidence that you value your physical, psychological, social, and spiritual health. Once you have made this assessment, decide on a few specific areas you would like to improve.

SUMMARY

We cannot realistically expect to eliminate stress from our life, but we can modify our way of thinking and our behavior patterns to reduce stressful situations and manage stress more effectively. The way we process and interpret the stress of daily living has a lot to do with our mental attitude. Stress affects us physically as well as psychologically.

Conquering the negative impact of stress requires a willingness to accept responsibility for what we are doing to our body. We do well to listen to the messages our body gives us. If we are feeling the effects of stress in our body, this is a signal to pay attention and change what we are thinking and doing.

Remember that you are a whole being, which implies an integration of your physical, emotional, social, mental, and spiritual dimensions. If you neglect any one of these aspects of yourself, you will feel the impact on the other dimensions of your being. Reflect on how well you are taking care of yourself in all of these areas. Ask yourself the degree to which you know your priorities and are acting on them.

Ineffective ways of coping with stress include defensive behavior and the use of drugs and alcohol. Traumatic events can lead to posttraumatic stress disorders both for the victims and vicariously for those who come to help them. Not all trauma results in PTSD, but an increasing number of natural and manmade disasters and traumatic events worldwide emphasize our need to learn to cope with stress effectively. Some specific sources of trauma based on sexual exploitation are child sexual abuse, date rape, and sexual harassment. Survivors of sexual coercion and exploitation often are burdened with a constellation of negative feelings about themselves and have great difficulty trusting others. It is essential that they seek sources of help such as therapy to heal their pain.

In this chapter we have described a number of strategies for effectively managing stress. There is no one right way to cope with stress, which means you must devise your own personal approach to handle the stresses of daily life. Be willing to reach out to others and ask for help in more effectively dealing with stress. Although you may not be able to eliminate certain stressors in your life, there is a lot that you can do to manage stress more effectively. You can apply some of the approaches that were described in this chapter to attain your goals of self-care. It is important that you develop your own methods of self-care and consistently work at applying them to a variety of situations in your life.

Where Can I Go From Here?

1. How are you coping with stress? Keep an account in your journal for one week of the stressful situations you encounter. After each entry, note these items: To what degree was the situation stressful because of your thoughts, beliefs, and assumptions about the events? How were you affected? Do you see any ways of dealing with these stresses more effectively?

2. How are you using your time? Take an inventory of how you use your time. Be consistent in recording what you do. Keep a log of your activities for at least 1 week (2 weeks would be better) to see how you have spent your time. Carry a pocket notebook. Write down what you have done a couple of times each hour. After a week, add up the hours you are spending on personal, social, job, and academic activities, then ask yourself these questions:

▸ Am I spending my time the way I want to?

▸ Am I accomplishing what I have set out to do each day? Is it what I wanted to do?

▸ Am I feeling rushed?

▸ Am I spending too much time watching television?

▸ Am I balancing activities that I need to do with ones that I enjoy?

▸ How would I like to use time differently than I did last week?

▸ How well am I currently managing time?

3. List three to five things you can do to feel better when you are experiencing stress (meditate, engage in deep breathing, exercise, talk to a friend, and so forth). Put this list where you can see it easily, and use it as a reminder that you have some ways to reduce stress.

4. Identify some environmental sources of stress or other stresses that are external to you. Finding a parking spot, navigating in rush hour traffic, and noise are all external factors that can put a strain on you. Once you have identified external stressors, write in your journal about how you might deal with them differently. What ways could a change in your thinking or adopting a new attitude change the impact of these external sources of stress?

5. How does stress affect your body? For at least 1 week (2 weeks would be better) record how daily stresses show up in bodily symptoms. Do you have headaches? Are you troubled with muscular aches? Do you have trouble sleeping? Does stress affect your appetite?

6. Consider the constructive ways to cope with stress presented in this chapter. Might some of these stress management strategies help you keep stress from getting the best of you? If you can select even two or three new stress management strategies and begin to practice them regularly (such as relaxation exercises and meditation), your ability to effectively curb the effects of stress are likely to be significantly improved. Write out a plan for practicing these techniques and make a commitment to a friend on what you are willing to do to better deal with your stress.

7. Suggested Readings. The full bibliographic entry for each of these sources can be found in the References and Suggested Readings at the back of the book. For a practical and short book on stress management, see Boenisch and Haney (2004). For a useful discussion on survivors of trauma and the healing process, see Naparstek (2006). For healing from sexual abuse, see Maltz (2001). For guides to meditation, see any of these books: Easwaran (1991), Epstein (1998), Fontana (1999), Kabat-Zinn (1994), and Rinpoche (1994). Useful books on the subject of mindfulness are Kabat-Zinn (1990, 1994) and Siegel (2010).

WEBSITE RESOURCES

Included here are some valuable websites. For access to these websites, video activities, and other supporting materials, visit Cengage Learning's Counseling CourseMate website for *I Never Knew I Had a Choice,* 10th Edition, at **www.cengagebrain.com.**

ADVOCATES FOR SURVIVORS OF TORTURE AND TRAUMA
www.astt.org
Recommended Search Words: "advocates for survivors of torture and trauma"

The mission of this independent, nonprofit organization is to "alleviate the suffering of those who have experienced the trauma of torture, to educate the local, national, and world community about the needs of torture survivors, and to advocate on their behalf." In addition to providing information, the site offers links to other resources for torture survivors.

THE INSTITUTE OF HEARTMATH
www.heartmath.org
Recommended Search Words: "institute of heartmath"

This internationally recognized nonprofit research and education organization is dedicated to helping people reduce stress, regulate their emotions, and build energy and resilience for healthy, productive lives.

AMERICAN INSTITUTE OF STRESS
www.stress.org
Recommended Search Words: "American institute of stress"

This site provides a wealth of information and statistics on stress.

NATIONAL INSTITUTE ON ALCOHOL ABUSE AND ALCOHOLISM (NIAAA)
www.niaaa.nih.gov
Recommended Search Words: "national institute on alcohol abuse and alcoholism"

The NIAAA is a part of the National Institutes of Health and provides this site, which includes resources and references about alcohol abuse and alcoholism. Included are links to publications and databases such as the National Library of Medicine Databases and Electronic Sources, press releases, conferences, and research programs.

JOB STRESS NETWORK
www.workhealth.org
Recommended Search Words: "job stress network"

This site offers information on job strain, projects, risk factors, and outcomes.

APA HELPCENTER
http://apahelpcenter.org
Recommended Search Words: "APA health center"

The American Psychological Association provides this resource for those seeking help in any number of areas of life. The site contains many useful articles about stress and its impact in life domains such as work and school, family and relationships, and health and wellness.

MIND TOOLS™
www.mindtools.com
Recommended Search Words: "mind tools"

Mind Tools is dedicated to "helping you to think your way to an excellent life." This site provides shareware and practical suggestions for problem solving, memory improvement, increasing creativity, mastering stress, time management, goal-setting, links to stress and time management book stores, and much more.

CENTER FOR MINDFULNESS IN MEDICINE, HEALTH CARE, AND SOCIETY
www.umassmed.edu/cfm/index.aspx
Recommended Search Words: "UMass center for mindfulness in medicine"

Housed at the University of Massachusetts Medical School and founded in 1995 by Dr. Jon Kabat-Zinn, this center is a global leader in mind-body medicine. "The Center is an outgrowth of the acclaimed Stress Reduction Clinic—the oldest and largest academic medical center-based stress reduction program in the world." The website offers a great deal of information for anyone interested in mindfulness.

RAPE ABUSE AND INCEST NATIONAL NETWORK
www.rainn.org
Recommended Search Words: "RAINN"

This site offers news, hotlines, a list of local crisis centers, and statistics on the incidence of rape and incest.

NATIONAL CENTER FOR PTSD
www.ptsd.va.gov
Recommended Search Words: "national center for ptsd"

This site, sponsored by the U.S. Department of Veterans Affairs, is devoted to the understanding and treatment of posttraumatic stress disorders. It has well-organized materials for both professionals and the public.

WEBSITES DEALING WITH STYLES OF YOGA
http://ezinearticles.com/?cat=Health-and-Fitness:Yoga
http://yoga.about.com
Recommended Search Words: "ezine articles yoga;" "about yoga;" "types of yoga"

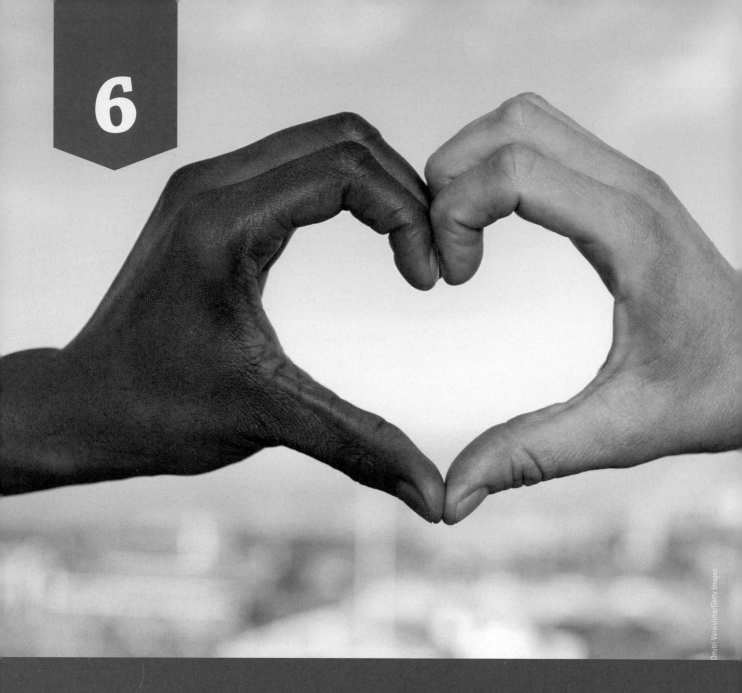

Dmitri Vervsiotis/Getty Images

LOVE

> Where Am I Now?

> Love Makes a Difference

> Learning to Love and Appreciate Ourselves

> Authentic and Inauthentic Love

> Theories of Love

> Barriers to Loving and Being Loved

> Love in a Changing World

> Is It Worth It to Love?

> Summary

> Where Can I Go From Here?

> Website Resources

> *Where there is love, there is no labor; and if there is labor, it is a labor of love.*
>
> —ST. AUGUSTINE

WHERE AM I NOW?

Use this scale to respond to these statements:

4 = I *strongly agree* with this statement.
3 = I *agree* with this statement.
2 = I *disagree* with this statement.
1 = I *strongly disagree* with this statement.

1. My parents showed healthy patterns of love.

2. I have a fear of losing another's love and being rejected.

3. When I experience hurt or frustration in love, I find it more difficult to trust and love again.

4. I reveal myself in significant ways to those I love and am comfortable with intimacy.

5. I am able to express loving feelings toward members of the same sex.

6. I accept the ways that significant others in my life demonstrate their love for me.

7. I realize that allowing myself to love involves both risk and joy.

8. In my loving relationships I experience trust and an absence of fear.

9. I accept those whom I love as they are, without expecting them to be different.

10. I need constant closeness and intimacy with those I love.

There are as many definitions of love as there are people experiencing it, and how people express their love is influenced by cultural norms. Around the world love affects people's lives in myriad ways. In this chapter we speak about love in a way that makes it possible for you to examine your ways of loving even though you may have a very personal definition of it. What meaning does love have in your life? How do you express and receive love? Are love, intimate relationships, and sexuality interrelated? What makes love authentic for you? How capable are you of creating a climate in which love can flourish?

The notion of "falling in love" describes the emotion of love as it is experienced between two people typically feeling a strong physical and emotional attraction. Relationships require loving behavior. In other words, there has to be consistency between my saying "I love you" and how I behave toward you. This kind of love is found in all loving relationships, and the behaviors of love enable the emotion of love to grow and endure. We focus on the behaviors of love because this is the area where relationships either grow or diminish. When we talk of self-love, we focus on appreciating how we are in our world and liking the way we behave toward others, especially those we profess to love. If we do not have this kind of love for ourselves, then in time we will be unable to accept the love, respect, and appreciation of others for us.

There is meaning to be found in actively caring for others and in helping them make their lives better. Love involves commitment, which is the foundation of a genuinely loving relationship. Although commitment does not guarantee a successful relationship, it is perhaps one of the most important factors in setting the stage for nurturing and fostering a relationship.

There are many kinds of loving relationships. There is the love between parent and child, love between siblings, between friends, and romantic relationships. These various types of love have some very real differences, but all forms of genuine love embody the characteristics we have described in one way or another.

One of the purposes of this chapter is to help you clarify your views and values pertaining to love. As you read, try to apply the discussion to your own experience of love, and consider the degree to which you are now able to appreciate and love yourself. As you review your desire for love as well as your fears of loving, do you recognize any barriers within you that prevent you from fully experiencing love?

LOVE MAKES A DIFFERENCE

To fully develop as a person and enjoy a meaningful existence, we need to care for others and have others care for us. Robbins (1996) believes love is the single most important aspect of life: "The measure of our lives and the influence that we have on the world and one another is determined by the degree of love and openness in our hearts" (pp. 145–146). The need for love includes the need to know that our existence makes a difference to someone. Love and intimacy are factors directly linked to our overall health. In Chapter 4 we saw that food, rest, and exercise are basic needs; love is also essential for both physical and psychological well-being. Our physiological responses to those who are close to us demonstrate that the quality of our relationships can affect our health (Brooks, Robles, & Dunkel Schetter, 2011). Giving and receiving love makes a difference in all facets of our lives, including our physiology.

A loveless life is often lived in isolation and alienation. We can harden ourselves so as not to experience a need for love. We can close ourselves off from others; we can isolate ourselves by never reaching out to another; we can refuse to trust others and to make ourselves vulnerable; we can cling to an early perception that we are basically unlovable. In whatever way we do this, we pay a price. When we exclude physical and emotional closeness with others, we create emotional and physical deprivation.

Our love for others or their love for us may enable us to live, even in conditions of extreme hardship. In the concentration camp where he was imprisoned, Frankl (1963) noted that some of those who kept alive the images of those they loved and retained some measure of hope survived the ordeal, whereas those who gave up hope of being united with loved ones succumbed.

Love can be expressed in many different ways. Consider the following statements:

▸ I need to have someone in my life I can actively care for. I need to let that person know he [she] makes a difference in my life, and I need to know I make a difference in his [her] life.

▸ I want to feel loved and accepted for who I am now, not for living up to others' expectations of me.

▸ Although I have a need for connection with people, I also enjoy my time alone.

▸ I am finding out that I have more of a capacity to give something to others than I had thought.

▸ I am beginning to realize that I need to love and appreciate myself more fully, in spite of my imperfections. If I can accept myself for who I am, then maybe I can accept love from others.

▸ There are special times when I want to share my joys, my dreams, my anxieties, and my uncertainties with another person. When I am listened to, I feel loved.

In his popular book *The 5 Love Languages*, Chapman (2010) discusses how love can be expressed through words of affirmation, quality time, gifts, acts of service, and physical

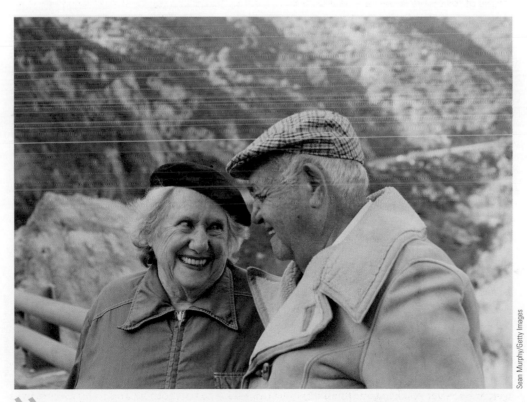

≫ To enjoy a meaningful existence, we need to care about others and have others care about us.

touch. Quite often people differ from each other in terms of their primary love language. Just as an English speaker might have great difficulty understanding someone conversing in Chinese, the same holds true for the person who has a different love language than his or her partner. Ideally, as we grow in love, we learn our partner's love language and can accept the ways he or she gives and receives love.

LEARNING TO LOVE AND APPRECIATE OURSELVES

In our counseling sessions clients are sometimes surprised when we ask them what they like about themselves. They look uncomfortable and embarrassed. They find it easier to talk about how they see themselves in positive ways if we say to them: "If your best friends were here, how would they describe you?" "What characteristics would they ascribe to you?" "What reasons might they give for choosing you as a friend?"

Some have been brought up to think that it is egocentric to talk about self-love. But unless we learn how to love ourselves, we will encounter difficulties in loving others and in allowing them to love us. We cannot give to others what we do not possess ourselves. If we are able to appreciate our own worth, then we are better able to accept love from others. This could even include loving an enemy. Thich Nhat Hanh (1997) speaks about self-love as a prerequisite for loving others: "If you are not yet able to love yourself, you will not be able to love your enemy. But when you are able to love yourself, you can love anyone" (p. 37).

Loving ourselves does not mean having an exaggerated picture of our own importance or placing ourselves above others or at the center of the universe. We must not confuse

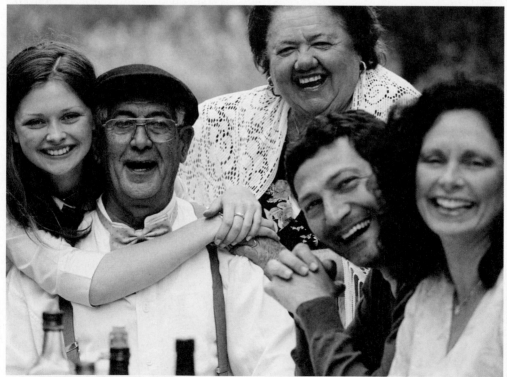

Philip Lee Harvey/Getty Images

>> Active love is something we can choose to share with others.

CHAPTER SIX

self-love with narcissism, a distorted and self-absorbed view of our perfect self (Twenge & Campbell, 2009). Rather, self-love means having respect for ourselves even though we are imperfect. It entails caring about our lives and striving to become the people we want to be.

Many writers have stressed the necessity of self-love as a condition of love for others. In *The Art of Loving*, Fromm (1956) describes self-love as respect for our own integrity and uniqueness and maintains that it cannot be separated from love and understanding of others. We often ask clients who only give to others and who have a difficult time taking for themselves: "Do you deserve what you so freely give to others?" "If your own well runs dry, how will you be able to give to others?" We cannot give what we have not learned and experienced ourselves. Moore (1994) writes that those who try very hard to be loved do not succeed because they do not realize that they have to first love themselves as others before they can receive love from others.

As we learn to treat ourselves with increasing respect and regard, we increase our ability to fully accept the love others might want to give us; at the same time, we have the foundation for genuinely loving them. Caring for ourselves and caring for others are very much connected.

AUTHENTIC AND INAUTHENTIC LOVE

Authentic love enhances us and those we love. Establishing and maintaining loving relationships present a number of challenges, the first of which is being clear about what we want in a long-term intimate relationship. Crooks and Baur (2011) identify what they believe to be the ingredients in a long-term love relationship: self-acceptance, acceptance by one's partner, appreciation of one another, equality in decision making, effective communication, commitment, realistic expectations, shared interests, and the ability to deal with conflict effectively. Compare these criteria with the following positive meanings love has for us.

Love means that I am coming to *know* the person I love. I am aware of the many facets of the other person —not just the beautiful side but also the limitations, inconsistencies, and flaws. I have an awareness of the other's feelings and thoughts, and I experience something of the depth of that person. I can penetrate masks and roles and see the other person on a deeper level. Love also entails making myself known to the other person. Meaningful self-disclosure is essential to establishing loving relationships, especially revealing the deeper facets of ourselves.

Love means that I *care* about the welfare of the person I love and I actively *demonstrate concern* for the other. If my love is genuine, my caring is not a smothering of the person or a possessive clinging. On the contrary, my caring enhances both of us. If I care about you, I am concerned about your growth, and I hope you will become all that you can be. We do more than just talk about how much we value each other. Our actions show our care and concern more eloquently than any words. Each of us has a desire to give to the other. We have an interest in each other's welfare and a desire to see that the other person is fulfilled.

Love means having *respect* for the *dignity* of the person I love. If I love you, I can see you as a separate person, with your own values and thoughts and feelings, and I do not insist that you surrender your identity and conform to an image of what I expect you to be for me. I am not threatened by your ability to stand alone and to be who you are. I avoid treating you as an object or using you primarily to gratify my needs.

Love means having a *responsibility* toward the person I love but not responsibility *for* that person. If I love you, I am responsive to what you need. I am aware that what I am and what I do affects you; I am concerned about your happiness and your sadness. I have the realization that I have the capacity to hurt or neglect you. Authentic love implies accepting another person's weaknesses and bringing patience and understanding to help the person make significant life changes.

Love can lead to *growth* for both the person I love and me. If I love you, I am growing as a result of my love for you. You encourage me to become more fully what I might be, and my loving enhances your being as well. We each grow as a result of caring and being cared for; we each share in an enriching experience that does not detract from our being.

Love means making a *commitment* to the person I love. Commitment to another person involves risks, but commitment is the essential context of an intimate relationship. This means that the people involved have invested in their future together and that they are willing to stay with each other in times of crisis and conflict. Commitment entails a willingness to stay with each other in times of pain, uncertainty, struggle, and despair, as well as in times of calm and enjoyment. A major component of commitment is to give honest feedback to the one we love, even though it may be difficult to give and to hear. Some people have difficulty making a long-term commitment. Perhaps, for some, a fear of intimacy gets in the way of developing a sense of commitment. Loving and being loved is both exciting and frightening, and we may have to struggle with the issue of how much anxiety we can tolerate.

Love means that I am *vulnerable*. Love involves allowing you to matter to me in spite of my fear of losing you. You have the capacity to hurt me as much as I am capable of hurting you. There are no guarantees that our love will endure. My love for you implies that I want to spend time with you and share meaningful aspects of my life with you.

Love means *trusting the person you love*. If I love you, I trust that you will accept my caring and my love and that you will not deliberately hurt me. I trust that you will find me lovable and that you want to be with me. I trust the reciprocal nature of our love. If we trust each other, we are willing to be open to each other and can shed masks and pretenses and reveal our true selves.

Love means *trusting yourself*. In relationships a great deal is made of trusting the person you love, yet the ability to trust yourself is equally important. Indeed, if your trust in yourself wavers, you may not be able to believe or trust in the love another wants to share with you.

Love allows for *imperfection*. Although our love relationship may be strained at times, and we may feel like giving up, we have the intention of riding out difficult times. Authentic love does not imply a perfect state of happiness. We remember what we had together in the past and can envision what we will have together in our future.

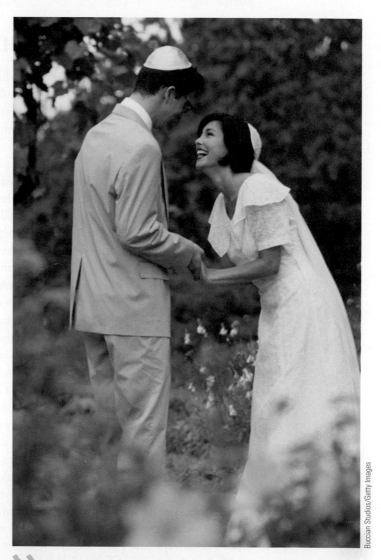

Buccina Studios/Getty Images

» Marriage is one way to make a commitment.

Love is *freely given*. My love for you is not contingent on whether you fulfill my expectations of you. Authentic love does not mean "I'll love you when you become perfect or when you become what I expect you to become." Authentic love is not given with strings attached. There is an unconditional quality about love.

Love is *expansive*. If I love you, I encourage you to reach out and develop other relationships. Although our love for each other and our commitment to each other precludes certain actions on our part with others, we are not totally and exclusively wedded to each other. Only a false love cements one person to another in such a way that he or she is not given room to have other meaningful friendships.

Love means that although I *want* you in my life, I am capable of functioning without you. If life is meaningless without you, it will put a lot of demands on you to be there for me. If I love you and you leave, I will experience a great loss, but I will not be destroyed. If I am overly dependent on you for my meaning and my survival, I am not free to challenge our relationship.

Love means *identifying* with the person I love. If I love you, I can empathize with you, see the world through your eyes, and identify with you. This closeness does not imply a continual togetherness, for distance and separation are part of a loving relationship. Distance can intensify a loving bond, and it can help us rediscover ourselves, so that we are able to meet each other in a new way.

Love involves *seeing the potential* within the person I love. If I love you, I am able to see you as the person you can become, while still accepting who you are now. Goethe's observation is relevant here: "By taking people as they are, we make them worse, but by treating them as if they already were what they ought to be, we help make them better."

Love means *letting go* of the illusion of total control of ourselves, others, and our environment. The more I strive for complete control, the more out of control I am. Loving implies a surrender of control and being open to life's events. It implies the capacity to be surprised.

We conclude this discussion of the meanings that authentic love has for us by sharing the prayer of Saint Francis of Assisi, which to us embodies the essence of authentic love. Born in 1181, St. Francis, the founder of the Franciscan Order, is associated with the love of nature and peace among all people. Maier (1991) cites the prayer of Saint Francis of Assisi as illustrative of a heart that is filled with unconditional love. Regardless of one's possible religious affiliation or spiritual beliefs, there is a deep message in this prayer.

Lord, make me an instrument of your peace.
Where there is hatred, let me sow love;
Where there is injury, pardon;
Where there is doubt, faith;
Where there is despair, hope;
Where there is darkness, light;
Where there is sadness, joy;
O divine Master, grant that I may not
so much seek
To be consoled as to console;
To be understood as to understand;
To be loved, as to love;
For it is in giving that we receive;
It is in pardoning that we are pardoned;
It is in dying that we are born to eternal life.

We have discussed our views on authentic love, and now we turn to an examination of the characteristics of inauthentic love, which has a detrimental effect on those we say we love. This list is not definitive, yet it may give you some ideas to use in thinking about the quality of your love. From our perspective, a person whose love is inauthentic:

▶ Needs to be in charge and make decisions for the other person.

▶ Has rigid and unrealistic expectations of how the other person must act to be worthy of love.

▶ Attaches strings to loving and loves conditionally.

▶ Puts little trust in the love relationship.

▶ Perceives personal change as a threat to the continuation of the relationship.

▶ Is possessive.

▶ Depends on the other person to fill a void in life.

▶ Lacks commitment.

▶ Is unwilling to share important thoughts and feelings about the relationship.

Most of us can find some of these manifestations of inauthentic love in our relationships, yet this does not mean that our love is necessarily inauthentic. For instance, at times you may be reluctant to let another person know about your private life, you may have excessive expectations of another person, or you may attempt to impose your own agenda. It is essential to be honest with yourself and to recognize when you are not expressing genuine love, then you can choose to change these patterns.

TAKE TIME TO REFLECT

1. List some of the meanings love has for you. _____
_____
_____

2. Think of someone you love. What specifically do you love about that person? Then list some ways or times when you fail to demonstrate love for that person. _____
_____
_____

3. What are some specific steps you can take to allow others to love you more fully?
_____
_____

4. What are some steps you can take to demonstrate your love for others? _____
_____
_____

5. Reflect on the prayer of Saint Francis of Assisi, looking for aspects that capture what you consider to be the essence of actively loving others. What personal meaning does this prayer have for you?_____
_____
_____

THEORIES OF LOVE

The question "what is love?" has been addressed by writers, poets, philosophers, theologians, and even reality TV show executives. Not surprisingly, it also has been of interest to psychologists.

Sternberg would undoubtedly respond to this question by describing his **duplex theory of love,** which captures two essential elements of the nature of love (Sternberg & Weis, 2006; Weis & Sternberg, 2008). The first element, which he calls the "triangular subtheory of love," refers to love's structure. According to Sternberg, love is composed of one or more of the following three components: *intimacy*, *passion*, and *decision/commitment*. Intimacy occurs when a loving relationship is characterized by warmth, closeness, and connectedness. Passion refers to one's basic drives that lead to physical attraction, romance, and sexual consummation. Decision/commitment consists of the short-term task of deciding to love someone and the longer-term task of committing to maintain that love. Analogous to a recipe that changes as ingredients are added or subtracted, love can be expressed in different ways depending on the components that are present or lacking in any given relationship. The second part of Sternberg's theory, which he calls the "subtheory of love as a story," refers to love's development. It describes how various kinds of love (triangles composed of some combination of *intimacy, passion,* and *decision/ commitment*) evolve. The love story between two people who have great passion yet lack the other two ingredients (infatuated love) will be very different from the story of a couple who experience all three ingredients (consummate love). Consider Jerilyn's account of her relationships with her ex-husband Marty and her current partner, Wayne.

JERILYN'S STORY

I have been divorced from Marty for 7 years and am now in a committed relationship with Wayne, which I am confident will lead to marriage. Marty and Wayne couldn't be more different, or maybe it's the relationships that were/are so different. Marty and I fell in love almost at first sight. We had a very intense and passionate relationship and eloped after knowing each other for only 4 months. We went to Italy to get married, which seemed like the most romantic thing to do. We had the best time, but when we returned to the "real world," the relationship suffered. As they say, the honeymoon was over!

By contrast, my relationship with Wayne has developed over time. Although the passion may not be quite as intense as it was with Marty, Wayne is a fascinating person, and we get along so well. I can have emotionally intimate conversations with Wayne that I never could have had with Marty. My relationship with Marty was largely based on sex, but my current relationship is based on so much more than that. I feel Wayne really knows me well and would stand by me no matter what. There is a depth to our relationship that was missing in my marriage to Marty.

It took me some time to recover from my divorce, but I see now that Marty and I weren't perfect for each other. I used to be so angry at him for ending our marriage, but perhaps everything turned out for the best.

Another way to respond to the question "what is love?" is to examine the link between love and attachment. Bowlby (1980) and Ainsworth (Ainsworth et al.,1978), both widely regarded as pioneers of attachment theory, paved the path for others to consider the importance of early bonding experiences and attachment styles as the foundation for future interpersonal interactions. Hazan and Shaver's (1987) seminal work on romantic love as an attachment process posited that adults, like infants, can be categorized as *secure, avoidant,* or *anxious-ambivalent*. These ideas have stood the test of time. Results from a recently published longitudinal study (Nosko, Tieu, Lawford, & Pratt, 2011) support Hazan and Shaver's assertion that parent–child relations play an important role in establishing secure attachments in adulthood. In another recent study, researchers found that a secure dispositional attachment style was associated positively with compassionate love for one's romantic partner and, conversely, that an avoidant-dismissing attachment style was negatively associated with this type of love (Sprecher & Fehr, 2011).

What does research suggest about those whose attachment style is anxious-ambivalent? The anxious-ambivalent attachment style was the focus of two studies by Joel, MacDonald, and Shimotomai (2011) that examined the role of ambivalence in the commitment process. In one study, they discovered an association between anxious attachment and greater insecurity in partners' affections and lower satisfaction with relationships. Their second study showed that anxiously attached participants were more inclined to feel dependent on their partners. These two studies combined suggest that anxiously attached individuals experience conflicting pressures on commitment, which may be a source of internal pressure for them. This may help to account for some of their uncertain and confusing relationship behaviors.

As you think about your own life, consider how both attachment theory and Sternberg's duplex theory of love may help to illuminate some of the choices you have made with regard to love and relationships. Reflecting on your early childhood experiences as well as your adult relationships, can you see patterns over time in the way you bond with others? If you had to describe your own attachment style, would you say you were securely attached, avoidant, or anxious-ambivalent like Dylan? What are your stories of love?

DYLAN'S STORY

My friends often comment that my relationship with my partner Joe is like a rollercoaster. I met him at a party 2 years ago, and we've been dating on and off since then. This is the longest relationship I've had, and I am in my late 20s. I live in a state where gay marriage is not legal, and although I support the cause for the sake of all gay couples who want to be married, the truth is that I am glad I am not feeling the pressure to marry Joe. Some of his habits, like smoking and drinking excessively, are not acceptable to me. It creates tension between us, often resulting in temporary breakups. I then go crazy inside wondering if he is sleeping around and start calling him and texting him nonstop until he finally responds. He assures me that he is not cheating on me and just needs some space, but I am so filled with doubt that I make myself sick. Is that healthy? No. I am fully aware of it, but I cannot seem to stop myself. I know I have got to stop this madness and work on my jealousy and dependence on him in therapy, otherwise we are going to continue this destructive cycle.

Whether one chalks it up to having an anxious-ambivalent attachment style or justifies this behavior in another way, many people engage in unhealthy patterns like Dylan and sabotage their relationships with loved ones. If you relate to Dylan's story, you might reflect on behaviors that stifle or harm your relationships. For each behavior that you identify, think of an alternative behavior that would be more constructive and healthy and that has a better chance of leading to a satisfying outcome.

BARRIERS TO LOVING AND BEING LOVED

Myths and Misconceptions About Love

Culture influences our views of connection, love, intimacy, and relationships. We receive messages from our families, friends, and communities that can enhance our ability to give and receive love—and we also receive messages that make it difficult for us to experience love. The media, in particular, plays a significant role in perpetuating myths about love. If we hope to challenge these myths, we must take a critical look at the messages we have received from society about the essence of love. In the following pages we present our views on some common beliefs that we think are worth examining.

The Myth of Eternal Love The notion that love will endure forever without any change is unrealistic because our experience of love changes over time. Your feelings of being in love at the beginning of your relationship may evolve as a result of being together and of creating a history with each other. Love is complex and involves both joyful experiences and difficulties, and the intensity of your love may change as you change. You may experience several stages of love with one person, deepening your love and finding new levels of richness. Conversely, you and your partner may become stagnant and the love you once shared may fade.

The Myth That Love Implies Constant Closeness Betina and Luis dated throughout junior high and high school, and they went to college together because they could not tolerate any separation. They make no new friends, either with the same or opposite sex, and they show extreme signs of jealousy when the other indicates even the slightest interest in wanting to be with others. Rather than creating a better balance of time with each other and time with others, the only alternative they see is to terminate their relationship. The mistaken assumption they are operating on is that if they loved each other they would not have any need for other relationships.

Many of us can tolerate only so much closeness, and at times we are likely to need some distance from others. Another way of looking at it is that we have a dual need for both closeness with others and for solitude. Gibran's (1923) words in *The Prophet* are still timely: "And stand together yet not too near together: For the pillars of the temple stand apart, and the oak tree and the cypress grow not in each other's shadow" (p. 17).

There are times when a separation from our loved one can be beneficial. At these times we can renew our desire for the other person and also become centered again. Consider the case of Martin. He refused to spend a weekend without his wife and children, even though he said he longed for some time for himself. The myth of constant closeness and constant togetherness in love prevented Martin from taking private time. It might also have been that this covered up certain fears. What if he discovered that his wife and children could manage very well without him? What if he found that he could not stand his own company for a few days and that the reason for "togetherness" was to keep him from boring himself?

The Myth That We Fall In and Out of Love A common notion is that we "fall in love" when the right person comes into our life. Buscaglia (1992) contends that it is more accurate to say that we "grow in love," which implies choice and effort:

> We really don't fall out of love any more than we fall into it. When love ceases, one or both partners have neglected it, and have failed to replenish and renew it. Like any other living, growing thing, love requires effort to keep it healthy. (p. 6)

Although the notion of falling in love is popular, most serious writers on the subject deny that it can be the basis for a lasting and meaningful relationship.

People often say "I love you" and at the same time are hard pressed to describe the active way in which they show this love. Words can easily be overused and become meaningless. The loved one may be more convinced by actions than by words. In our professional work with couples, we find that one person may be very verbal about being disillusioned with his or her partner's shortcomings. We often ask, "If the situation is as you describe, what do you imagine keeps you together as a couple?" A standard response is, "I love him (her)," but the person is often unable to describe this love in action. Buscaglia (1996) notes that it is only through action that love can manifest itself. "If we want to love, we must move forward toward love by reaching out to others to love" (p. 138).

The Myth of the Exclusiveness of Love You may believe you are capable of loving only one other person—that there is one right person for you. Indeed, it is common for couples to choose not to have sexual relationships with others because they realize that doing so might interfere with their capacity to freely open up and trust each other. However, their sexual exclusivity does not have to preclude other genuine relationships. One of the signs of genuine love is that it is expansive rather than exclusive. By opening yourself to loving others, you also open yourself to loving one person more deeply.

Jealousy is an emotion that often accompanies feelings of exclusiveness. For example, Drew may feel insecure if he discovers that his wife, Adriana, has friendships with other men. Even if Adriana and Drew have an agreement not to have sexual relationships with others, Drew might be threatened and angry over the fact that Adriana wants to maintain these friendships with other men. He may wrongly reason: "What is the matter with me that Adriana has to seek out these friends? Her friendships with other men must be a sign that something is wrong with me!" In Drew's case, it appears that he is threatened by Adriana's desire to include others in her life. Equally, it is a mistaken notion to equate an absence of jealousy with an absence of love.

The Myth That True Love Is Selfless Lily is a mother who has always given to her children. She never lets them know that she needs anything from them, yet she complains to her friends that the children do not seem to appreciate her. She complains that if she did not initiate visits with them they would never see her. She would never say anything about her feelings to her children, nor would she ever tell them that she would like for them to contact her. If they really loved her, she thinks they would know what she needed without her having to ask for it.

People like Lily are **impaired givers;** that is, they have a high need to take care of others yet appear to have no ability to make their own needs known. They create an inequality; the receivers tend to feel guilty because they do not have a chance to reciprocate. Although these receivers may feel guilty and angry, their feelings do not seem appropriate—how could they have angry feelings toward someone who does so much for them? At the same time, impaired givers may feel resentment toward those who are always taking from them, not recognizing how difficult they are making it to receive.

It is a myth that true love means giving selflessly. Love involves both giving and receiving. If you cannot ask or do not allow others to give to you, then you are likely to become drained or resentful. In giving to others we do meet many of our own needs. There is not necessarily anything wrong in this, as long as we can admit it. For example, a mother who never sets boundaries, and rarely says no to any demands made by her children, may not be aware of the ways she has conditioned them to depend on her. They may be unaware that she has any needs of her own, for she hides them so well. In fact, she may set them up to take advantage of her out of her need to feel significant. In other words, her "giving" is actually an outgrowth of her need to feel like a good mother, not just an honest expression of love for her children. In *Care of the Soul* (1994), Moore addresses this notion of selflessness. One of his clients said, "I can't be selfish. My religious upbringing taught me never to be selfish" (p. 56). Moore observes that although she insisted on her selflessness she was quite preoccupied with herself. Selfless people often depend on others to maintain their feelings of selflessness.

Giving to others or the desire to express our love to others is not necessarily a problem. However, it is important that we recognize our own needs and consider the value of allowing others to take care of us and return the love we show them.

I (Marianne) am finally learning the importance of letting others return favors. It has always been easy for me to show others kindness and take care of them, yet it has been a struggle for me to be on the receiving end. I am very capable of doing things myself and being self-reliant. I would rather not ask for assistance, lest I impose on people. I do see myself as a giver, and that I do not want to change. However, I do not want to create an imbalance of giving and receiving in my life. More often than not, when I do ask for help, I don't get much of a response. I have conditioned people so well that they often act helpless around me. Even capable people act helpless around me! I continue to learn that it takes a concerted effort to challenge ingrained beliefs about being a selfless giver. One way I am able to give to others is by letting others give to me at times.

The Myth That Love and Anger Are Incompatible Many people are convinced that if they love someone they cannot get angry at them. When they do feel angry, they tend to deny these feelings or express them in indirect ways. Anger and love cannot be compartmentalized. It is difficult to feel loving toward others if we are persistently angry at them. These unexpressed feelings tend to negatively affect the relationship and actually create distance. Denied or unexpressed anger can do more damage to the relationship. Anger can be expressed respectfully; it does not have to be judgmental or explosive.

Self-Doubt and Lack of Self-Love

Despite our need for love, we often put barriers in the way of our attempts to give and receive it. One common barrier is the message we sometimes send to others concerning ourselves. If we enter relationships unsure of our lovability, we will give this message to others in subtle ways. We create a self-fulfilling prophecy; we make the very thing we fear come true by being unavailable to others in any kind of loving way.

If you are convinced that no one can love you, your conviction is probably related to experiences you had during your childhood or adolescent years. At one time perhaps you decided that you would not be loved unless you did certain expected things or lived up to another's plan for your life. For example: "Unless I succeed, I won't be loved. To be loved, I must get good grades, become successful, and make the most of my life." Such an assumption can make it difficult to be open to the love that others want to give you.

Jay tried as a child to do whatever it took to meet the expectations of others and to gain their acceptance. He gave his all to please people and to get them to like him, yet he never succeeded. Through his actions of desperately trying to win people over, he pushed them away even more. Although he thought he was doing everything right, people were uncomfortable with the way he was around them. Now he is constantly depressed and complains about how hard life is for him. He seeks sympathy and receives rejection. He

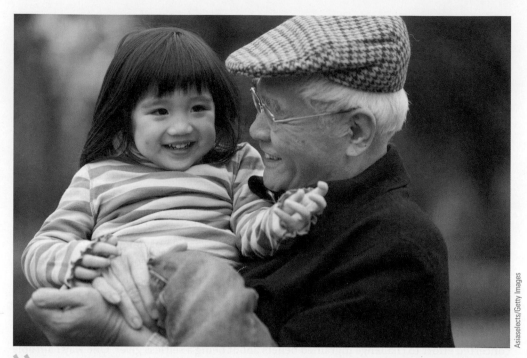

Asiaselects/Getty Images

>> There is an unconditional quality about love.

needs continual reassurance, yet when he does get acceptance and reassurance, he negates it. Eventually people who know him get frustrated and rebuff him. He may never realize that he has created the cycle of his own rejection. In some important ways he continues to live by the theme that no matter what he does or how hard he tries people will still not like him, much less love him. For Jay to make changes, it is essential that he recognize those outside influences on the origins of his beliefs. Our beliefs did not originate in a vacuum. Thus to understand how our early experiences are affecting our present behavior and choices, we need to reflect on these experiences. Once we recognize the sources of the attitudes we hold about love, we are in a position to make new decisions about our thinking and acting.

If you have limited your ability to receive love from others by telling yourself that you are loved primarily for a single trait, it would be healthy to challenge this assumption. For example, if you say to someone, "You only love me because I am attractive," you might try to realize that your attractiveness is only one of your assets. You can learn to appreciate this asset without assuming that it is all there is to the person you are. If you have trouble seeing any desirable characteristics besides your attractiveness, you are not likely to be open to feedback about anything other than your appearance. When you rely exclusively on any one trait as a source of gaining love from others (or from yourself), your ability to be loved is limited to that trait and may not go very deep. This can make it difficult for others to love you.

Our Fear of Love

The Fear of Isolation Despite our need for love, we often fear loving and being loved. Our fear can lead us to deny our need for love, and it can dull our capacity to care about others. In some families relatives have not spoken to one another for years. This act of shunning is generally deliberate and aimed at controlling and isolating those who do not live within the boundaries of acceptable norms. Those who are shunned often feel invisible. Within the Amish culture, the practice of shunning is used to sanction members who violate certain norms and religious values. In its most severe form, shunning almost totally cuts off an individual from interaction within the community. Other members will not eat at the same table with those who are shunned, will not do business with them, and will not have anything to do with them socially (Good & Good, 1979).

The fear of isolation as a result of being cut off emotionally is so overwhelming that many would not even think of going against their cultural norms. The need for love and acceptance may be far stronger than giving expression to your own individual desires. Have you ever faced an emotional cutoff? If so, what was it like? Have you sometimes felt isolated because others that you cared about shunned you or treated you as though you were invisible?

The Fear of Being Discovered Some of us are afraid that if we get too close to others they will certainly discover what we are really like. We may think that at the deepest level there is nothing to us. We may question the positive reactions we receive from others and have difficulty believing that others really value us. We wear masks so that others will not discover who we are. This sets up a dilemma for us. If others love us with our mask, we will likely conclude that they really don't love the person behind the mask, and therefore, we cannot trust their love. We have heard a partner in a relationship complain, "I no longer recognize the person I originally met. He is a very different person." He might not be himself out of fear that others would not like what they see.

The Uncertainty of Love Love does not come with guarantees. Buscaglia (1996) reminds us that we may wait forever if we wait to love until we are certain that we will be loved in return. We cannot be sure that another person will always love us, and we do lose loved ones. If we open ourselves to love, we are vulnerable to getting hurt. Our loved ones may die or be injured or become seriously ill, or they may simply leave us. We cannot eliminate the possibility that we will be psychologically wounded if we choose to love. However, avoiding the experience of love can lead to another kind of pain: A loveless existence is very painful!

Most of the common fears of risking in love are related to rejection, loss, the failure of love to be reciprocated, or uneasiness with intensity. Here are some of the ways these fears might be expressed:

▸ I have been so badly hurt in a love relationship, I'm not willing to take the chance of loving again.

▸ I fear allowing myself to love others because of the possibility that they will be seriously injured, contract a terrible illness, or in some way leave me. I don't want to care that much; that way, if I lose them, it won't hurt as much.

▸ I'm afraid of loving others because they might want more from me than I'm willing to give, and I might feel suffocated.

▸ I'm afraid that I'm basically unlovable and that when you really get to know me you'll want little to do with me.

▸ If people tell me they care about me, I feel I've taken on a burden, and I'm afraid of letting them down.

▸ I've never really allowed myself to look at whether I'm lovable. My fear is that I will search deep within myself and find little for another to love.

LOVE IN A CHANGING WORLD

This is the age of social media and reality TV and texting and constant connection. What impact has this had on how people demonstrate their love for one another? In certain respects, technology is a wonderful tool that enhances our communication with others. For example, I (Marianne) never dreamed that I would be able to sit at my computer and use Skype to talk with my relatives in Germany or with my grandchildren. In other respects, technology can easily be used as a barrier to forming meaningful relationships with others.

Texting, tweeting, and checking e-mail on your smart phone can become a full-time occupation that prevents you from connecting with the person right in front of you. If you often engage in these behaviors, consider how others around you might feel when you are preoccupied with communicating with someone who is not physically present. If you are frequently with others who are distracted by technology, how connected to them do you feel? Although not problematic in all circumstances, these devices can be a barrier to intimacy in relationships that really matter to you.

Emotional intimacy can easily be avoided when these tools are used to replace communicating face to face with close friends, partners, and family members. As one therapist noted, "I hear clients talk about feeling hurt that their family members don't call them or talk to them in person during crucial periods . . . but only text or send a Facebook message . . . avoiding any real contact or intimacy."

We like to stay in touch with our grandchildren, yet often when we call them on the phone we don't reach them. When we complained about this to our 7-year-old grandchild, she said we could always text her and reach her that way. When we told her that we did not know how to text, she replied: "Oh, that's easy; I can teach you." So far we resist texting and prefer talking on the phone because we see this as a more intimate way of communicating.

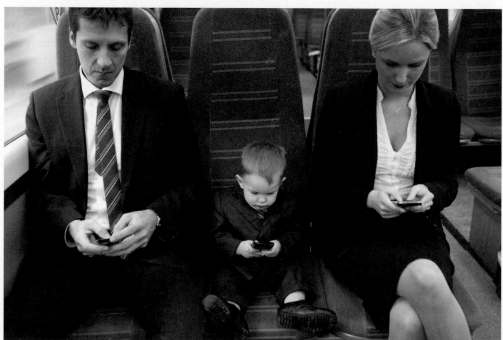

Peter Cade/Getty Images

≫ Technological advances are extraordinary and have the potential to enhance relationships, but they can also become a barrier to meaningful connections.

1. What did you learn about love in your family of origin? What have you learned about love through other sources such as the media? _____

_____

_____

2. How do you express your love to others? _____

_____

_____

3. How do you let another person know your own need to receive love, affection, and caring?

_____

_____

4. List some specific fears you have concerning loving others. _____

_____

_____

5. How do you make it difficult for others to love you? _____

_____

_____

6. List some qualities you have that you like. _____

_____

_____

7. What are some specific ways in which you might become a more lovable person?

_____

_____

8. What are some ways that love has played a positive role in your life?

_____

_____

IS IT WORTH IT TO LOVE?

Often we hear people say, "Sure, I need to love and to be loved, but is it *really* worth it?" Underlying this question is a series of other questions: "Is the risk of rejection and loss worth taking?" "Are the rewards of opening myself up as great as the risks?"

It would be comforting to have an absolute answer to these questions, but each of us must struggle to decide for ourselves whether it is worth it to love. Our first task is to decide whether we prefer isolation to intimacy. Of course, our choice is not between extreme isolation and constant intimacy; surely there are degrees of both. But we do need to decide whether to experiment with extending our narrow world to include significant others. We can increasingly open ourselves to others and discover for ourselves what that is like for us; alternatively, we can decide that people are basically unreliable and that it is better to be safe and go hungry emotionally.

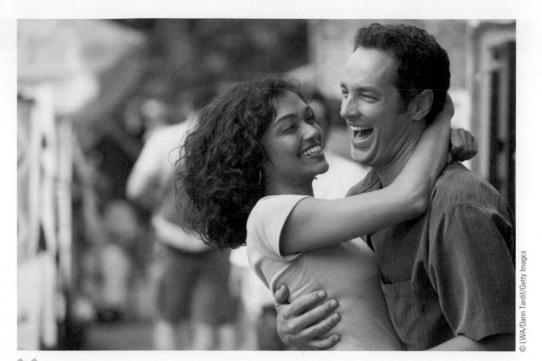

© LWA/Dann Tardif/Getty Images

》 We cannot love others if we are not capable of loving ourselves.

Perhaps you know very little about love but would like to learn how to become more intimate. You might begin by acknowledging this reality to yourself, as well as to those in your life with whom you would like to become more intimate. In this way you can take a significant beginning step.

In answering the question of whether it is worth it to you to love, you can challenge some of your attitudes and beliefs concerning acceptance and rejection. You can ask yourself: "Is being rejected any worse than living a life without experiencing love?" Being rejected is not a pleasant experience, yet we hope this possibility will not deter you from allowing yourself to love someone. If a love relationship ends for you, it is worthwhile to honestly evaluate your part in contributing to this situation without being overly self-critical. Identify some ways in which you would like to change and learn from this experience. Elana had to learn to trust again after being deeply hurt in a relationship.

ELANA'S STORY

I had a mutual loving bond with Monte, yet most of my friends had a hard time understanding why I continued in this relationship. I guess I had an idealized picture of Monte and made excuses for his insensitive behavior. I became extremely dependent on Monte and preoccupied with trying to please him at all costs, even if it meant sacrificing my own happiness to keep peace with him. My friends let me know of their concern and tried to convince me that I deserved better treatment. My response was to cut myself off from my friends so I would not have to deal with their feedback. Eventually, Monte betrayed me, which led to a crisis. I ended my relationship with Monte, but I was quite fearful of loving again, and old wounds were reopened each time I met a new man. I approached new relationships with fear and distrust, which made it difficult to open myself to love again.

With concerted work on her part, Elana became aware of how clinging to her past hampered her ability to receive love and develop friendships. Elana's immediate impulses were to flee from getting close, yet she challenged her fears with the realization that the risk of rejection did not have to keep her helpless and guarded.

As adults we are not helpless; we can do something about rejection and hurt. We can choose to challenge relationships or even leave them. We can learn to survive pain, and we can realize that being rejected does not mean we are beyond hope. We can choose to love again and again throughout our lives—and be open to the joy of loving and being loved.

SUMMARY

We have a need to love and to be loved, but there are many barriers to meeting these needs. Being convinced of our unworthiness can be a major roadblock to loving others and receiving their love. Those who experience deep-seated feelings of unworthiness, and even self-loathing at times, may have had inadequate bonding experiences with their first caregivers and may have developed avoidant or anxious-ambivalent attachment styles in response to these early experiences. Learning to give love to others and to receive love from them is contingent upon having a secure attachment style and loving and appreciating ourselves. We cannot love others if we are not capable of loving ourselves. How can we give to others something we do not possess ourselves?

Our fear of love is another major impediment to loving. Although most of us would like guarantees that our love for special people will last as long as they live, the reality is that there are no guarantees. It helps to realize that loving and the anxiety surrounding uncertainty go together and to accept that we are faced with learning to love despite our fears.

Myths and misconceptions about love make it difficult to be open to giving and receiving love. A few of these are the myth of eternal love, the myth that love implies constant closeness, the myth of the exclusiveness of love, the myth that true love is selfless, and the myth of falling into eternal love. Although genuine love results in the growth of both persons, some "love" is stifling. Not all that poses as real love is authentic, which is evidenced by the way love is depicted in reality TV shows. One of the major challenges is to decide for ourselves what authentic love means to us. By recognizing our attitudes about loving, we can increase our ability to choose the ways in which we behave in our love relationships. As technological advances and social media have added many new ways to communicate and to connect instantly with others, our ability to establish bonds of caring with those we love is both enhanced and challenged.

Where Can I Go From Here?

1. Think about some early decisions you made regarding your own ability to love or to be loved. Have you ever had any of these thoughts?

▶ I'm not lovable unless I meet others' expectations.

▶ I am worth loving because of the person that I am.

▶ I won't love another because of my fears of rejection.

▶ Love is what makes life worth living.

Write down some of the messages you have received and perhaps accepted uncritically. What messages have you received from your family of origin? How has your ability to feel loved or to give love been restricted by these messages and decisions?

2. For a period of at least a week, pay close attention to the messages conveyed by the media concerning love. What picture of love do you get from television? What do popular songs and movies portray about love? What messages are conveyed about love through social networking and websites? Make a list of some common myths or misconceptions regarding love that you see promoted by the media.

3. Do you agree with the proposition that you cannot fully love others unless you first love yourself? What does this mean to you? In the journal pages at the end of this chapter write some notes to yourself concerning situations in which you do not appreciate yourself. Also record the times and events when you do value and respect yourself.

4. What do you think of Sternberg's duplex theory of love and his ideas about love? What are your thoughts about the importance of attachment style as the foundation of future love relationships? If you were asked to create your own theory of love, what would you emphasize?

5. Suggested Readings. The full bibliographic entry for each of these sources can be found in the References and Suggested Readings at the back of the book. For a classic work on love, see Fromm (1956). For useful books on love, see Buscaglia (1972, 1992) and Sternberg and Weis (2006).

WEBSITE RESOURCES

Included here are some valuable websites. For access to these websites, video activities, and other supporting materials, visit Cengage Learning's Counseling CourseMate website for *I Never Knew I Had a Choice,* 10th Edition, at **www.cengagebrain.com.**

ASSOCIATION FOR TREATMENT AND TRAINING IN THE ATTACHMENT OF CHILDREN
www.attach.org
Recommended search words "association for attachment"

This association is dedicated to providing information about healthy attachment as well as attachment disorders. The site offers resources such as publications and book recommendations.

INTERNATIONAL ASSOCIATION FOR THE STUDY OF ATTACHMENT
www.iasa-dmm.org
Recommended search words "international association for attachment"

IASA is a multidisciplinary association of mental health professionals who are interested in advancing the study of attachment. This site contains information about attachment across the life cycle.

THE 5 LOVE LANGUAGES
www.5lovelanguages.com
Recommended search words "5 love languages"

This is the official website of Gary Chapman's internationally renowned book, *The 5 Love Languages.* In addition to information about the love languages, the site offers a blog and self-assessments so you can identify your own love language.

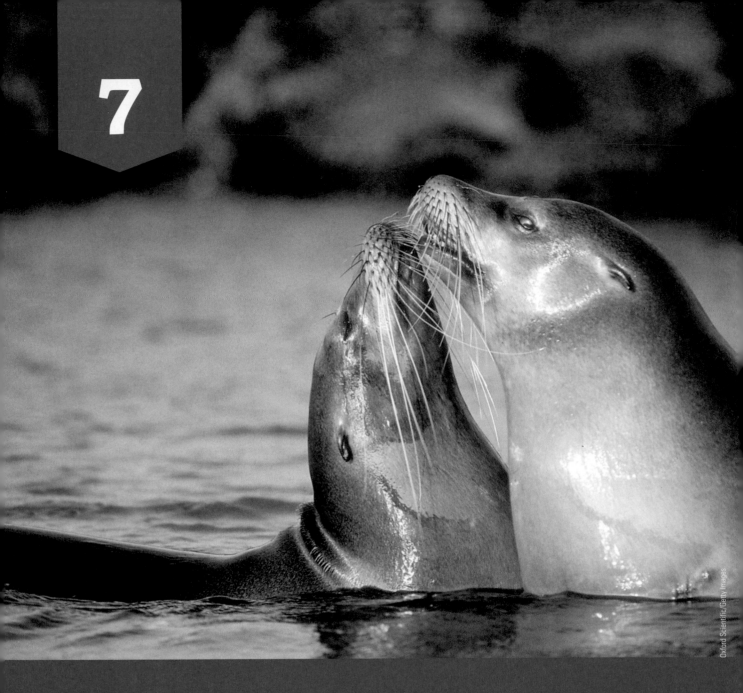

7

RELATIONSHIPS

› Where Am I Now?

› Types of Intimacy

› Meaningful Relationships: A Personal View

› Anger and Conflict in Relationships

› Dealing With Communication Barriers

› Relationships in a Changing World

› Gay and Lesbian Relationships

› Separation and Divorce

› Summary

› Where Can I Go From Here?

› Website Resources

Oxford Scientific/Getty Images.

It takes both imagination and effort to think of ways to revise our relationships so that they will remain alive.

WHERE AM I NOW?

Use this scale to respond to the following statements:

4 = I *strongly agree* with this statement.
3 = I *agree* with this statement.
2 = I *disagree* with this statement.
1 = I *strongly disagree* with this statement.

1. I consider the absence of conflict and crisis to be a sign of a good relationship.

2. It is difficult for me to have several close relationships at the same time.

3. I consider my communication skills to be a strength in my relationships.

4. I believe the mark of a successful relationship is that I enjoy being both with and without the other person.

5. I prefer to communicate with people through social media or text messaging rather than in person.

6. At times, wanting too much from another person causes me difficulties in the relationship.

7. I feel confident in what I have to offer in a relationship.

8. I am comfortable with the amount of energy I spend in my relationships.

9. I feel satisfied with my connection with others.

10. I can be emotionally intimate with another person without being physically intimate with that person.

Relationships play a significant role in our lives. In this chapter we deal with a range of relationships—friendships, marital relationships, intimacy between people who are not married, dating relationships, relationships between parents and children, and a variety of other meaningful personal relationships. Love is very much a part of intimate relationships, and the ideas discussed in Chapter 6 are linked to our discussion of relationships in this chapter.

Whether you choose to marry or not, whether your primary relationship is with someone of the same or the opposite gender, you will face many similar relationship challenges. In this chapter we invite you to reflect on what you need from your relationships and to examine the quality of them. All relationships experience times of growth, meaningfulness, and challenges. Use the ideas presented in this chapter as a catalyst as you rethink what is important to you in relationships and clarify your choices.

TYPES OF INTIMACY

Forming intimate relationships is the major task of early adulthood (Erikson, 1963). Being able to share significant aspects of yourself with others, understanding the barriers to intimacy, and learning ways of enhancing intimacy can help you better understand the many different types of relationships in your life.

The intimacy shared with another person can be emotional, intellectual, physical, spiritual, or any combination of these. It can be exclusive or nonexclusive, long term or brief. For example, many of the participants in the personal-growth groups we conduct develop genuine closeness with one another, even though they may not keep in touch after the termination of the group. This closeness does not come about automatically. The participants create a strong connection with one another by interacting in a more open way. Instead of keeping their thoughts, feelings, and reactions to themselves, they share them in ways that they typically have not done before. The cohesion comes about when people discover that they have similar feelings and when they are willing to share their pain, anger, frustration—and their joys. We hope that those who participate in these therapeutic groups are able to translate what they learned about creating intimacy into their outside relationships.

In avoiding intimacy, we deprive ourselves of relationships that can potentially enrich our lives. We may pass up the chance to get to know neighbors and new acquaintances because we fear that someone will move and that the friendship will come to an end. We may avoid intimacy with sick or dying persons because we fear the pain of losing them. Although such fears may be well founded, too often we deprive ourselves of the uniquely rich experience of being truly close to someone. We can enhance our lives greatly by caring about others and fully savoring the time we spend with them.

We can choose the kinds of relationships we want. By spending time reflecting on how we might want to revise some of our interactions with others, we can bring new life to our relationships. Throughout this chapter we ask you to think about how you view your relationships and what role you play in making them meaningful. If you want to improve your relationship with another, making changes in yourself is more likely to be successful than insisting that the other person change.

As you read the remainder of this chapter, spend some time thinking about ways you experience intimacy in your life. Are you involved in the kinds of relationships that satisfy you? What are you willing to do to improve your relationships? The following Take Time to Reflect exercises provide an opportunity for you to address these questions and clarify what you are doing in your relationships.

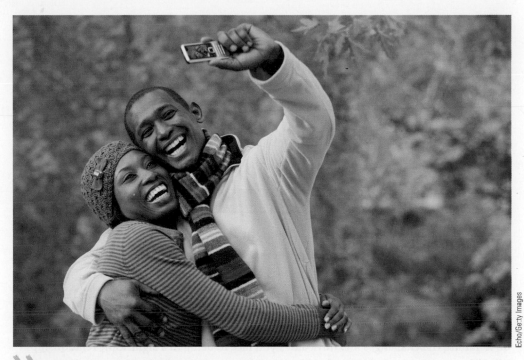

Echo/Getty Images

>> The challenge of forming intimate relationships is the major task of early adulthood.

TAKE TIME TO REFLECT

1. What attracts you to a person you would like to form an intimate relationship with? Score each item using the following scale:

1 = This quality is *very important* to me.

2 = This quality is *somewhat important* to me.

3 = This quality is *not very important* to me.

_____ intelligence

_____ character (a strong sense of values)

_____ physical appearance and attractiveness

_____ financial success

_____ prestige and status

_____ strong sense of identity

_____ sense of humor

_____ caring and sensitivity

_____ emotional stability

_____ independence

_____ quiet demeanor

_____ outgoing personality

_____ decisive

_____ willing to make decisions cooperatively

_____ dependable

_____ strong work ethic and self-discipline

_____ playful

_____ similar or compatible value system

Now list the three qualities that you value most in a person when you are considering an intimate relationship. _____

_____

_____

2. What attracts people to you? List some of those qualities. _____

_____

_____

3. Identify the kinds of intimate relationships you have chosen so far in your life. What have you learned from them? If you are not now involved in an intimate relationship, what stops you? _____

_____

_____

4. What are the challenges and difficulties you face in being in a significant relationship? What do you get from being involved in a significant relationship? _____

_____

_____

MEANINGFUL RELATIONSHIPS: A PERSONAL VIEW

In this section we share some of our ideas about the characteristics of a meaningful relationship. Although these guidelines pertain to couples, they are also relevant to other personal relationships. For example, one guideline is, "The persons involved are willing to work at keeping their relationship healthy." Parents and children often take each other for granted, rarely spending time together. Either parent or child may expect the other to assume the major responsibility for the relationship. The same principle applies to friends or to partners in a primary relationship. As you look over our list, adapt it to the different relationships in your life, keeping in mind your particular cultural background. Your culture plays an influential role in your relationships, and you may need to adapt our ideas to better fit your core values. As you review our list, ask yourself what qualities are most important to you.

We see relationships as most meaningful when they are dynamic rather than fixed. Any relationship may have periods of joy and excitement as well as times of pain and distance. As long as the individuals in a relationship are willing to accept this, their relationship has a chance to change as well. The following qualities of a relationship seem most important to us.

▶ *Each person in the relationship has a separate identity.* Long-term relationships have a better chance for success when people balance their times of separateness and togetherness. If there is not enough togetherness in a relationship, people typically feel isolated and do not share feelings and experiences. If there is not enough separateness, they are apt to give up a sense of their own identity and control, devoting much effort to becoming what the other person expects.

▶ *Each is able to give and receive honest and respectful feedback.* Both people openly express grievances and let each other know the changes they desire. They ask for what they want rather than expecting the other to intuitively know what they want. Assume that you are not satisfied with how you and your mother spend time together. You can take the first step by letting her know, in a respectful way, that you would like to talk more personally. Rather than telling her how she is, you can focus more on telling her how you are in your relationship with her. Instead of focusing on what you don't want with your mother, you can tell her what you would like with her.

▶ *Each person assumes responsibility for his or her own level of happiness and refrains from blaming the other when unhappy.* In a close relationship or friendship, the unhappiness of the other person is bound to affect you, but you should not expect another person to make you happy, fulfilled, or excited. Although the way others feel will influence your life, they do not create the way you react to them. Relying on others for your personal fulfillment and confirmation as a person can have a negative influence on your relationships. The best way to build solid relationships with others is to work on developing your own self. Ultimately, you are responsible for defining your goals and your life, and you can exercise choice in taking steps to enhance your life. You have a great deal of control when it comes to changing your attitudes about situations in which you find yourself unhappy.

▶ *Both people are willing to work at keeping their relationship healthy.* To keep a relationship vital, we must reevaluate and revise our way of being with each other from time to time. Consider how this guideline fits your friendships. If you take a good friend for granted and show little interest in doing what is necessary to maintain that friendship,

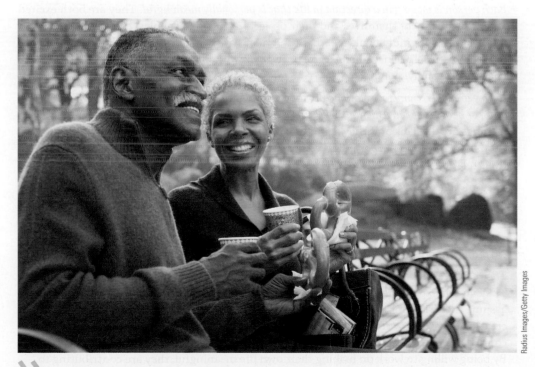

»In a meaningful relationship, the people involved work to keep their relationship alive.

that person may soon grow disenchanted and wonder what kind of friend you are. We sometimes keep old patterns alive by bringing them into our current relationships. These old habits can create strain in our relationships.

▶ *Both people are able to have fun and to play together; they enjoy doing things with each other.* Sometimes we do not take time to enjoy those we profess to love. One way of changing unfulfilling relationships is to determine what gets in the way and what prevents us from having a more enjoyable life together. Again, think of this guideline as it applies not only to your intimate relationships but also to your friendships.

▶ *If the relationship contains a sexual component, each person assumes responsibility for the enjoyment of the relationship.* Although sexual partners may experience different degrees of intensity in an ongoing relationship, they can continue to create a climate of romance and closeness. In their lovemaking they are sensitive to each other's needs and desires; at the same time, they are able to ask each other for what they want and need. Their sex life can be a barometer of their relationship.

▶ *The two people are equal in the relationship.* People who feel that they are typically the "givers" and that the other person is usually unavailable when they need him or her might question this imbalance. In some relationships one person may feel compelled to assume a superior position relative to the other—for example, to be very willing to listen and give advice yet unwilling to go to the other person and show his or her own vulnerability. Both parties need to be willing to look at aspects of inequality and demonstrate a willingness to negotiate changes.

▶ *Each person finds meaning and sources of nourishment outside the relationship.* Sometimes people are very possessive in their friendships. A sign of a healthy relationship is that each avoids assuming an attitude of ownership toward the other. Although they may experience jealousy at times, they do not demand that the other person deny his or her feelings for others.

▶ *Each person is moving in a direction in life that is personally meaningful.* They are both excited about the quality of their lives and their projects. Applied to couples, this guideline implies that both individuals feel that their needs are being met within the relationship, but they also feel a sense of engagement in their work, play, and relationships with other friends and family members.

▶ *If they are in a committed relationship, they maintain this relationship by choice, not out of duty, or because of convenience.* They choose to keep their connection with each other even if things are difficult or if they sometimes experience pain in the relationship. Because they share common purposes and values, they are willing to look at what is lacking in their relationship and to work on changing undesirable situations.

▶ *They are able to deal with conflict in their relationship.* Couples often seek relationship counseling with the expectation that they will learn to eliminate conflict, which is an unrealistic goal. More important than the absence of conflict is being able to deal with conflict constructively. Finding effective ways of addressing conflict and anger is also extremely important in family relationships and friendships.

▶ *They do not expect the other to do for them what they are capable of doing for themselves.* They do not expect the other person to make them feel happy, take away their boredom, assume their risks, or make them feel valued and important. Each is working toward creating his or her own identity. Consequently, neither person depends on the other for confirmation of his or her personal worth; nor does one walk in the shadow of the other. By being willing to work on making their own life meaningful, they are contributing to each other's happiness.

▶ *They encourage each other to become all that they are capable of becoming rather than trying to control the other person.* People often try to keep those with whom they are intimately involved from changing. Out of their fear, they try to control their partner and thus make it difficult for their partner to be his or her authentic self. Acknowledging this fear is the first step toward relinquishing control of others.

Sam's story highlights how his failure to identify his control issues led to the breakup of an important relationship in his life.

SAM'S STORY

My girlfriend of 5 years broke up with me about 10 months ago. During this time, I have been trying to assess what went wrong. I seriously thought Kate was the woman I was going to marry, so it was shocking when she told me she didn't want to see me anymore. I am trying to come to terms with this so I can move on and not make the same mistakes in my next relationship. Kate often argued that I was too controlling, and I repeatedly told her that she was overreacting. Kate wanted to go to graduate school to pursue her MBA, but I thought a better plan would be for us to take some time off after college to travel. Why couldn't she postpone her graduate studies until after we spent some quality time together traveling and possibly until after we got married and had a family? At the time I didn't see anything wrong with this point of view, but I see things differently now. It was important to Kate for me to support her in pursuing her dreams, not my dreams for her. For some reason, I was afraid to deviate from my life plan, but what I neglected to consider were Kate's ambitions and dreams. I had to learn the hard way. Kate is dating someone else now. Although it's too late for us to get back together, I am determined to do a better job in my next relationship by being more supportive and encouraging.

Sam's control issues did not lead to physical violence in his relationship with Kate, but these kinds of issues have the potential to escalate to abuse. We address the topic of using power and control to dominate and terrorize one's partner in the section on intimate partner violence later in the chapter.

Creating and maintaining friendships, especially intimate relationships, is a major interest for many college students. There is no single or easy prescription for success; developing meaningful relationships entails the willingness to make commitments. Some students say that they do not have enough time to maintain their friendships and other relationships. If this fits you, realize that your relationships and friendships are likely to suffer when you neglect them. You can make choices that will increase your chances of developing lasting friendships:

▶ Be accepting of differences between your friends and yourself.

▶ Learn to become aware of conflicts and deal with them constructively.

▶ Be willing to let the other person know how you are affected in the relationship.

▶ Stay in the relationship and talk even though you may experience a fear of rejection.

▶ Check out your assumptions about others instead of deciding for them what they are thinking and feeling.

▶ Be willing to make yourself vulnerable and to take risks.

▶ Avoid the temptation to live up to others' expectations instead of being true to yourself.

John Gottman, cofounder and codirector of the Gottman Relationship Institute, has conducted extensive research to determine what factors are associated with successful marital relationships. In *The Seven Principles for Making Marriage Work*, John Gottman and Nan Silver (1999) describe some key characteristics of a successful relationship:

Intimate familiarity: Couples know each other's goals, concerns, and hopes.

Fondness and admiration: Couples who feel honor and respect for one another can more easily revitalize their relationship.

Connectedness: When individuals honor each other, they are generally able to appreciate each other's perspective.

Shared sense of power: When couples disagree, they look for common ground rather than insisting their way has to be supreme.

Shared goals: Partners incorporate each other's goals into their concept of what their intimate relationship is about.

Open communication: Each person in the relationship can talk fully and honestly about his or her convictions and core beliefs.

Are there gender differences regarding what people look for in an intimate relationship? According to Carroll (2013), women often report that promising financial prospects and a good career are very important; men often report that physical attractiveness is important. However, good looks and financial stability are qualities that both women and men look for in their partners. People tend to like and love others who are similar to themselves, who reciprocate expressions of affection, and who are physically attractive.

Developing meaningful intimate relationships requires time, work, and the willingness to work through difficult times. Further, to be a good friend to another, you must first be a good friend to yourself, which implies knowing yourself and caring about yourself. In this Take Time to Reflect, we ask you to focus on some of the ways you see yourself as an alive and authentic person, which is the foundation for a meaningful relationship.

TAKE TIME TO REFLECT

1. Identify some ways in which you see yourself as evolving in your relationships.

_____

_____

2. Are you resisting change by sticking with some old and comfortable patterns, even if they don't work? What are these patterns? _____

_____

_____

3. How is the person with whom you are most intimate changing or resisting change?

_____

_____

4. If you are involved in a committed relationship, in what ways do you think you and your partner are growing closer? In what ways are you going in different directions?

_____

_____

5. Are you satisfied with the relationship you have just described? If not, what would you most like to change? Would you be willing to talk to your partner about it?

_____

_____

6. Would you be satisfied if you had a marriage or committed relationship very similar to that of your parents? Explain. _____

_____

_____

7. To what extent do you have an identity apart from the relationship? How much do you need (and depend on) the other person? Imagine that he or she is no longer in your life, and describe the ways your life would be different. _____

_____

_____

A suggestion: If you are involved in a relationship, have the other person respond to these questions on a separate sheet of paper. Then compare your answers and discuss areas of agreement and disagreement.

ANGER AND CONFLICT IN RELATIONSHIPS

"We have never had a fight!" some people proudly say of their long-term relationships. Perhaps this is true, but the reasons couples do not fight can be complex. Anger is a powerful emotion. Passion is the driving force for life, and it can also be the impetus for anger. Take a moment to think about how you view anger. How did you see anger expressed when you were a child? Who got angry and what typically occurred? Did dealing with conflict and anger bring people closer together or move them farther apart? How do you deal with anger today? What do your friends tell you about your anger? How does the way you deal with anger affect the quality of your relationships? How often do you use anger to avoid feeling hurt?

Dealing Constructively With Anger, Conflict, and Confrontation

Expressing anger or dealing with situations involving conflict may be difficult for you because of what you have experienced and the messages you have heard about anger, conflict, and confrontation. You may have been told not to be angry. You may have observed harmful and destructive anger and made an early decision never to express these emotions (see the discussion of injunctions and early decisions in Chapter 3). Perhaps you have experienced mostly negative and frightening outcomes in situations involving conflict. If so, it may be necessary for you to critically evaluate some of the messages you received from your family of origin about feeling and expressing anger.

It is generally helpful to express persistent annoyances rather than to pretend they do not exist. Once you have expressed your anger, it is important to put it aside and not become attached to it. Ideally, sources of anger are best recognized and expressed in a direct and honest way. To be able to express your anger, however, there must be safety in the relationship that will enable you to share and deal with your feelings. If you cannot trust how your reactions will be received, chances are that you will not be willing to open yourself to the other person. To us, a sign of a healthy relationship is that people are able to express feelings and thoughts that may be difficult for the other to hear, yet the message is delivered in such a way that it does not assault the other person's character.

For many people the expression of anger becomes a reflex behavior that is easily escalated. It happens without thinking, and it takes considerable effort to change this pattern. You may have learned that anger leads to withdrawal of a person's love. One of our colleagues talks about the violence of silence, which is a form of destructive anger. Dealing with anger by growing silent generally does not help the situation; rather, both parties tend to pay a price for withholding their feelings. Avoiding dealing with anger may appear to work in the short term, but over time it typically erodes the relationship. In fact, Gottman and Silver (1999) consider *stonewalling*—remaining silent and offering no feedback to one's partner— to be a sign that a marriage is in trouble and may be headed for divorce.

Without a doubt, one of the major challenges for people involved in close relationships is learning how to deal with anger in realistic and appropriate ways. When you avoid being judgmental and avoid being emotionally or physically abusive, anger does not have to rupture the relationship. Once conflict is recognized and dealt with appropriately, healing is possible. This opens communication pathways that can deepen the relationship.

Ask yourself how you and your partner deal with anger and conflict. Recognizing signs of trouble may be the first step in bringing about change. Do you recognize yourself or your partner in any of these statements?

▸ What you say and what you feel are not congruent. For instance, you tell the other person that you are fine, yet you are feeling angry.

▸ You overreact to what is said to you when the message is difficult to hear.

▸ You typically walk away from conflict situations.

▸ You respond without thinking and often have regrets later about what you said.

▸ You often have physical symptoms such as headaches and stomachaches.

▸ You know you hurt the other person, yet you are unwilling to acknowledge that.

▸ You rarely resolve a conflict, assuming that time will take care of everything.

▸ You focus on the other person's flaws and rarely on your own shortcomings.

▸ During altercations, you bring up a litany of old grievances.

▸ You hold onto your anger or grudges and are unwilling to forgive.

It is difficult to change that which you are not aware of. However, with awareness you can catch yourself in familiar behavior patterns and begin to modify what you say and do. If some of these strategies are no longer working for you, reflect on and consider implementing these guidelines.

▸ *Recognize that conflict can be a healthy sign of individual differences and an integral part of a good relationship*. Both people in a relationship can be strong. When this leads to differences of opinion, it is not necessarily true that one is right and the other is wrong. Two people can agree that they see an issue differently.

▸ *See confrontation as a caring act, not an attack on the other person*. Confront a person if you care and do it in a caring way. Rather than being an attack, confrontation can be a conversation about some aspect of the relationship. Even though the tendency is to get defensive and attempt to fault the other person, strive to really listen and understand what the other person is saying. Deliver your message in a way that you would want it delivered to you. Respectful delivery makes for good listening. You may not be feeling loving at the moment, but a respectful confrontation is love in action.

▶ *Resist the temptation to plan your next response while the other person is speaking to you.* Learning to manage conflict situations is not about one person winning and another person losing. Successfully working through conflicts allows all the parties involved to retain their dignity.

▶ *If you do confront a person, identify your motivation.* Are you doing so out of concern? Are you expecting change in the way you deal with each other? Is your motivation to get even? Are you hoping to enhance your relationship?

▶ *Clarify your intentions when you are confronting someone and encourage this person to seek clarification from you.* People tend to get defensive when they perceive they are being attacked. If you need to express concerns to a person about something he or she has said or done, try to present your case with as much clarity and sensitivity as possible. If you are on the receiving end of a confrontation, ask about the confronter's purpose in directing his or her anger or frustration at you if you are unsure.

▶ *Accept responsibility for your own feelings.* Be aware of wanting to blame others for how you feel. At times it is easy to lash out at someone close to you simply because he or she is there. Be willing to examine the source of your feelings. Even though others may elicit your feelings in a situation, this is very different from making them responsible for how you feel.

▶ *In confronting another, try not to make dogmatic statements about the other person.* Instead of telling others how they are, say how their behavior affects you. It is easy for us to judge others and focus on all that they are doing. It is more difficult to focus on ourselves and what we are doing.

▶ *Tell others how you are struggling with them.* Too often we leave out all the information that leads to a particular reaction. Instead, we give only the bottom line. We might say, "You are insensitive and uncaring." Let the other person know your thoughts and feelings that led up to that statement. When you say all that led up to your bottom line, you are more likely to be heard.

▶ *Don't walk away from conflict.* Walking away from conflict does not solve the problem. However, when emotions are very highly charged and you are unable to resolve a conflict, it may be best to ask for a time-out and agree to resume discussing this issue at a later time. Do not pretend that the situation is resolved. Make a commitment to continue talking about the differences that may be separating you at a later time when both of you are able to listen to each other.

▶ *Recognize the importance of forgiving those who have hurt you.* If you desire intimacy with an individual, holding onto grudges and pain will inhibit intimacy. Letting go of old grievances and forgiving others is essential in maintaining intimacy. Forgiveness does not imply that you have forgotten what was done to you. However, you no longer harbor feelings of resentment, nor do you seek to get even. Forgiveness is an emotion-focused coping strategy that can reduce health risks and promote health resilience (Worthington & Scherer, 2004), and it is associated with enhanced personal adjustment and well-being (McCullough & Witvliet, 2002). Forgiveness is not a one-time event; rather, it is a process that involves experiencing successive stages of healing.

For Jampolsky (1999), the purpose of forgiveness is to release us from the past and the grievances we hold toward others. He writes: "We can look upon forgiveness as a journey across an imaginary bridge from a world where we are always recycling our anger to a place of peace" (p. 18). He adds that through forgiveness we can let go of fear and anger. The process of forgiving heals the wounds associated with past grievances.

▶ *Recognize that it is essential to forgive yourself.* Sometimes others are willing to forgive us for causing them hurt, yet we may fail to forgive ourselves for our wrongs. It is not just other people that we need to forgive—we need to forgive ourselves. As Jampolsky (1999) states, "I believe with all my heart that peace will come to the world when each of us takes the responsibility of forgiving everyone, including ourselves, completely" (p. 123). Macaskill (2012) found *self-unforgiveness* to be associated with higher anger, anxiety, shame, life dissatisfaction, and poorer mental health.

▶ *Seek forgiveness from others for your wrongdoings.* As imperfect human beings, there will be times when we make mistakes and hurt others' feelings. Although forgiveness often focuses exclusively on the perspective of the victim, Reik (2010) underscores the importance of also thinking about forgiveness from the perspective of the transgressor. His research shows that "seeking forgiveness is more likely to occur when a perpetrator is close to the victim, perceives their offense as severe, feels responsible for the offense, and/or has spent time ruminating about the event" (p. 251). He adds that shame and guilt tend to differentially influence forgiveness-seeking behavior. Whereas guilt serves as the impetus to seek forgiveness, shame may lead people to avoid the offended party. Reflect on times when you have hurt someone's feelings. How easy was it for you to work up the nerve to ask for forgiveness? Did you avoid the person hoping that all would be forgotten over time, or did you actively seek the person's forgiveness? As Sir Elton John captured so beautifully through his lyrics, "sorry seems to be the hardest word."

Clearly, recognizing and expressing anger can be valuable in relationships, but we must include the caveat that it also can be destructive or dangerous. On a daily basis we see evidence that misdirected anger and rage are harmful and destructive. Expressing anger in relationships is not always safe, nor does it always bring about closeness. Some people may be incapable of handling even the slightest confrontation, no matter how sensitively you deliver your message. In the following section, we address a problem of critical importance that can have a devastating impact on those affected—intimate partner violence, also referred to as "domestic violence."

Anger, Power, and Control Gone Wild: Intimate Partner Violence and Abuse

We all have a need to feel we are in control of our life in some ways. Some people, and a disproportionately higher percentage of men, are inclined to expand this concept to include exerting power and control over others. **Intimate partner violence** or **domestic abuse** poses a grave problem for many families and threatens the well-being of family members. Domestic abuse can take the form of physical, sexual, emotional, psychological, or economic abuse (U.S. Department of Justice, 2011). You may be in an abusive relationship, if you answer "yes" to some of the following questions.

Does your partner:

▶ humiliate or yell at you?

▶ criticize you and put you down?

▶ treat you so badly that you're embarrassed for your friends or family to see?

▶ ignore or put down your opinions or accomplishments?

▶ blame you for their own abusive behavior?

▶ see you as property or a sex object, rather than as a person?

- ▸ act excessively jealous and possessive?
- ▸ control where you go or what you do?
- ▸ keep you from seeing your friends or family?
- ▸ limit your access to money, the phone, or the car?
- ▸ constantly check up on you?
- ▸ have a bad and unpredictable temper?
- ▸ hurt you, or threaten to hurt or kill you?
- ▸ threaten to take your children away or harm them?
- ▸ threaten to commit suicide if you leave?
- ▸ force you to have sex?
- ▸ destroy your belongings? (Smith & Segal, 2011)

If you believe you are in an abusive relationship in which the outcome of anger is most often destructive, you need to exercise great caution in how you interact with that person. In such situations, it may never be safe for you to express your true feelings to this person.

Many people wonder why victims of domestic abuse stay with their abusers. Victims may rationalize their choice to stay by saying that their situation is not really so bad and that it is likely to improve. They often excuse their partner's behavior and find fault with themselves for bringing about the abuse. The perpetrator of the abuse might well demonstrate regret for hurting the partner and make promises to reform. However, soon afterward the same cycle repeats itself, and the victimized partner feels trapped, humiliated, and worthless. He or she often becomes numb and is cautious about trusting anyone. Many times people stay in this kind of relationship because they do not know where to go, nor do they know who can help them. Moreover, they may have legitimate concerns for their safety and the safety of their loved ones if they leave. See the web resources at the end of the chapter for links to websites that may be useful in the event that you or someone you care about is in an abusive situation.

Because abusers use tactics that are intended to increase their victim's dependence on them, victims of intimate partner violence often feel isolated from others. If you know someone who is being abused by their partner, an important first step is to express your concern, listen, and be supportive without imposing advice. If you recognize that domestic abuse is a problem in your life, we urge you to seek protection and professional help, but do so discreetly. Remember to consider your safety and, if applicable, the safety of your children or other dependents first. Many organizations—college counseling centers, community agencies, and hotlines, to name a few—offer a range of services to assist victims of intimate partner abuse.

TAKE TIME TO REFLECT

1. What changes would you like to make, if any, in the manner in which you deal with conflicts in your relationships? _____

_____

_____

2. What importance do you place on forgiveness as a way to enhance significant relationships?

_____

_____

3. To what degree are you able to forgive yourself for any of your past transgressions or regrets? How does this influence your ability to establish meaningful connections with others? _____

_____

_____

4. If you or someone you know is in an abusive relationship, what steps are you willing to take at this time? If you have reservations about taking action, what are they?

_____

_____

DEALING WITH COMMUNICATION BARRIERS

Effective communication is basic to sound and healthy relationships, and many relationship problems stem from misunderstandings and inadequate communication. A number of barriers to effective communication can inhibit developing and maintaining intimate relationships. Here are some common communication barriers:

▶ Failing to really listen to another person

▶ Selective listening—that is, hearing only what you want to hear

▶ Being overly concerned with getting your point across without listening to the other's point of view

▶ Silently rehearsing what you will say next as you are supposedly listening

▶ Becoming defensive, with self-protection being your primary concern

▶ Attempting to change others rather than first attempting to understand them

▶ Stereotyping people instead of trying to understand them

▶ Telling others how they are rather than telling them how they affect you

▶ Being blinded by prejudice

▶ Hanging onto old patterns and not allowing the other person to change

▶ Overreacting to a person

▶ Failing to state what your needs are and expecting others to know them

▶ Making assumptions about another person without checking them out

▶ Using sarcasm and hostility instead of saying directly what you mean

▶ Avoiding responsibility by using accusatory phrases such as "You manipulate me!"

These barriers make it difficult to have authentic encounters in which both people are open with themselves and each other, expressing what they think and feel and making genuine contact. When barriers exist between people who are attempting to communicate, they typically create distance.

Carl Rogers (1961), a pioneer in the humanistic approach to counseling, has written extensively on ways to improve personal relationships. For him, the main barrier to effective communication is our tendency to evaluate and judge the statements of others. He believes that what gets in the way of understanding another is the tendency to approve or disapprove, the unwillingness to put ourselves in the other's frame of reference, and the fear of being changed ourselves if we really listen to and understand a person with a viewpoint

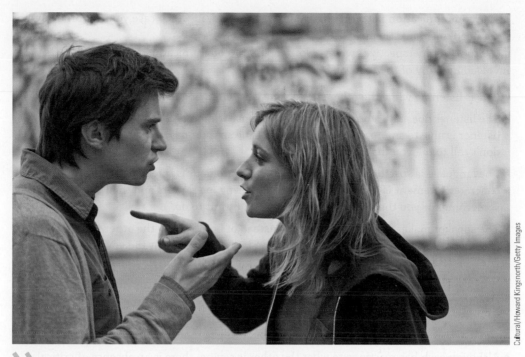

Cultura/Howard Kingsnorth/Getty Images

Many relationship problems stem from misunderstandings and inadequate communication.

different from our own. Rogers suggests that the next time you get into an argument with your partner, your friend, or a small group of friends, stop the discussion for a moment and institute this rule: "Each person can speak up for himself only after he has restated the ideas and feelings of the previous speaker accurately, and to that speaker's satisfaction" (p. 332).

Carrying out this experiment requires that you strive to genuinely understand another person and achieve his or her perspective. Although this may sound simple, it can be extremely difficult to put into practice. It involves challenging yourself to go beyond what you find convenient to hear, examining your assumptions and prejudices, not attributing unintended meanings to statements, and not coming to quick conclusions based on superficial listening. If you are successful in challenging yourself in these ways, you can enter the subjective world of the significant person in your life; that is, you can acquire empathy, which is the necessary foundation for all intimate relationships. Rogers (1980) contends that the sensitive companionship offered by an empathic person is healing and that such a deep understanding is a precious gift to another.

Effective Personal Communication

Your culture influences both the content and the process of your communication. Some cultures prize direct communication; other cultures see this direct style of behaving as being insensitive. In certain cultures direct eye contact is as insulting as the avoidance of eye contact is in other cultures. Harmony within the family is a cardinal value in certain cultures, and it may be inappropriate for even adult children to ever confront their parents. To do so could have detrimental consequences such as being physically and emotionally cut off. As you read the following discussion, recognize that variations do exist among cultures. Our discussion has a European-American slant, which makes it essential that you adapt the communication style we present to your own cultural framework. You might well be satisfied with most of the communication patterns that you have acquired, in which case you will probably not see a need to change them.

From our perspective, when two people are communicating meaningfully, they are involved in many of the following processes:

▸ One is listening while the other speaks; one is listening in order to understand.

▸ The listener does not rehearse his or her response while the other is speaking. The listener is able to summarize accurately what the speaker has said. ("So you're hurt when I don't call to tell you that I'll be late.")

▸ The language is specific and concrete. (A vague statement is "I feel manipulated." A concrete statement is "I don't like it when you bring me flowers and then expect me to do something for you that I already told you I didn't want to do.")

▸ The speaker makes personal statements instead of bombarding the other with questions. (A questioning statement is "Where were you last night, and why did you come home so late?" A personal statement is "I was worried and scared because I didn't know where you were last night.")

▸ The listener takes a moment before responding to reflect on what was said and on how he or she is affected. There is a sincere effort to walk in the shoes of the other person. ("I'm sorry. It didn't even cross my mind to call you. I will be more sensitive next time.")

▸ Although each has reactions to what the other is saying, there is an absence of critical judgment. (A critical judgment is "You never think about anybody but yourself, and you're totally irresponsible." A more appropriate reaction would be "I appreciate it when you think to call me, knowing that I may be worried.")

▸ Each of the parties can be honest and direct without insensitively damaging the other's dignity. Each makes "I" statements rather than second-guessing and speaking for the other. ("Sometimes I worry that you don't care about me, and I want you to know that, rather than assuming that it's true.")

▸ There is respect for each other's differences and an avoidance of pressuring each other to accept a point of view. ("I look at this matter very differently than you do, but I understand that you have your own thoughts on it.")

▸ There is congruence (or matching) between the verbal and nonverbal messages. (If the speaker is expressing anger, he or she is not smiling.)

▸ Each person is open about how he or she is affected by the other. (An ineffective response is "You have no right to criticize me." An effective response is "I'm disappointed that you don't like the work I've done.")

▸ Neither person is being mysterious, expecting the other to decode his or her messages.

These processes are essential for fostering any meaningful relationship. You might pay attention to yourself while you are communicating and take note of the degree to which you practice these principles. Decide if the quality of your relationships is satisfying to you. If you determine that you want to improve certain relationships, it will be helpful to begin by working on these skills.

Communicating With Your Parents

It is important to recognize the present influence your parents are having on you and to decide the degree to which you like this influence, as well as any changes you may want to make. Rather than expecting your parents to make the first move, it may be more realistic for you to take the first step in bringing about the changes you desire. For example, if you hope for more physical signs of affection between you and your parents, you might initiate it. If you want more time with your mother and are disappointed with the quality of your time with her, ask yourself what is stopping you from asking for it. Too often people withdraw quickly when their expectations of others are not immediately met. If you desire intimacy with your parents, put aside your need to remake them, and instead, be willing to be patient with them.

Our experience with our therapeutic groups has taught us how central our relationship with our parents is and how it affects all of our other interpersonal relationships. We learn from our parents how to deal with the rest of the world. We are often unaware of both the positive and negative impact our parents had, and perhaps continue to have, on us. Our groups consist of people of various ages, sociocultural backgrounds, life experiences, and vocations, yet many of the members have present struggles with their parents. It is not uncommon to have a 60-year-old man and a 20-year-old woman both expressing their frustration over not being supported by their parents. They both desire the parental approval that they have yet to experience. We find that there are also people who did get parental approval and support, yet who failed to recognize or accept it. Rather than being able to recognize what their parents did give them, they discount any positive aspects of the relationship. In our practice, we often encounter parent blaming, and it seems to be a challenge for many to come to terms with the fact that their parents are human. By accepting the fallibility of their parents, they make it possible to get beyond their grievances and open the channels of communication with their parents. Donald's story illustrates his struggle to come to terms with what his father can offer him.

DONALD'S STORY

My father seems uncaring, aloof, and preoccupied with his own concerns. I deeply wish to be physically and emotionally closer to my father, but I have no idea how to bring this about. I decided to talk to my father and tell him how I feel and what I want. My father appeared to listen, and his eyes moistened, but then without saying much he quickly left the room. I am pretty hurt and disappointed that my father wasn't more responsive when I talked to him. I just don't know what else I can do.

Donald missed the subtle yet significant signs that his father had been touched and was not as uncaring as he had imagined. His father may be every bit as afraid of his son's rejection as Donald is of his father's rebuffs. Donald will need to show patience with his father if he is really interested in changing the way they relate to each other.

Sometimes barriers to effective communication with one's parents are a result of differing levels of acculturation and assimilation. As in Annie's case, language barriers also affected the dynamics in her relationship with her parents.

ANNIE'S STORY

My family has been in the United States for 10 years, so I have spent a good portion of my life growing up in American culture. My parents are very traditional and insist that my brother and I speak our native language, Mandarin Chinese, at home. They have relied on my uncle, who lives with us, to help them communicate with others. At times this is a major problem because my uncle travels overseas a lot for business. Then me and my brother, who are both teenagers, have the responsibility of translating everything for our parents. I am pretty obedient, so I don't take advantage of my parents like my brother does. For example, when the school sent home a memo to my parents, my brother made up something that worked in his favor. I see how he manipulates them because he has the advantage of speaking English. I don't have the heart to tell my parents that he is doing that because I think they would feel even more powerless than they do now and also feel hurt and disrespected. I wish they would learn English, but I doubt they will. So that leaves me with the responsibility to look out for them. Even though I am just a teenager, it feels like I am in the parental role when my uncle is overseas, which feels strange.

RELATIONSHIPS IN A CHANGING WORLD

In Chapter 6, we addressed the topic of love in a changing world. Here we expand on that discussion and explore how advances in technology are shaping the way people meet, develop relationships, and communicate with one another.

Relationships and Social Networking

The social networking phenomenon has truly changed what it means to have "friends." Today, it is not uncommon for people to have a large number of Facebook or MySpace friends all over the world. Clearly, there are advantages to communicating in this manner. You can connect with people you already know, rekindle relationships from your past such as former classmates or childhood friends, and communicate with others who share your special interests (Weiten et al., 2012). Many organizations and institutions also have Facebook pages to foster a sense of community among their employees, clients, or consumers. If you find in-person contact difficult, you may find it is easier or more comfortable to establish connections with others online.

Although many people have embraced social media, you need to be aware of the level of risk you are incurring by disclosing personal information through these connections. Violations of online privacy are a concern of which we must all be aware. Even though resources are invested in keeping your information secure, nothing is foolproof. In addition, college admissions personnel and prospective employers are increasingly finding invaluable information on these sites about people they are considering admitting to their institutions or hiring. It is important to be mindful of these other users as you make choices about how much to self-disclose online.

Online communication is more easily misunderstood by the receiver because he or she doesn't have access to nonverbal cues such as the tone of the sender's voice or facial expressions (Weiten et al., 2012). Suppose you post a seemingly innocuous comment on someone's Facebook page, such as "I saw you at the store the other day. Nice haircut!" If the person feels insecure about the new hairstyle or does not trust your intentions, this comment may be interpreted as being sarcastic and attacking. Think about times when you questioned the tone of someone's post or message. What thoughts crossed your mind? Did you try to clarify the intended meaning or avoid bringing it up?

Online Dating

Reality television shows such as *The Bachelor*, *The Bachelorette*, and *Temptation Island* have escalated dating to a competition that only the very attractive can win. Although designated "reality television," these shows hardly represent reality as most of us know it.

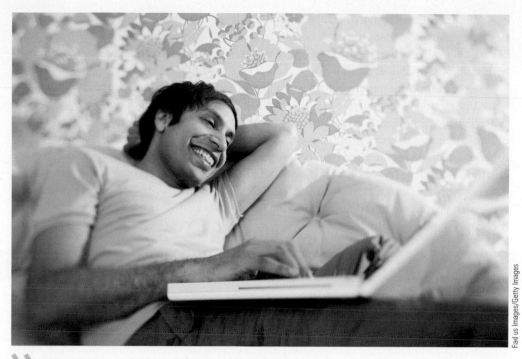

>> Online dating has become a popular way to meet people.

Increasingly, people are drawn to online dating sites such as eHarmony and Match.com in an effort to narrow their search and find a mate. Instead of meeting someone the old fashion way, users of online dating sites can search the Internet for prospective partners who meet criteria that they specify. A potential advantage of using an online service is that it offers a mechanism for matching for compatibility, which may reduce if not altogether eliminate the experience of a "bad date." "[R]elationships that develop online often move successfully to the offline realm" (Whitty, 2011, p. 192).

In some online relationships, intimacy is developed more rapidly than in face-to-face relationships, resulting in *hyperpersonal relationships* (Whitty, 2011). In online communication, people can take more time to construct a message and edit it before sending, thereby managing others' impressions of them. They can present themselves as more likable than they are in person. A potential downside of the development of hyperintimacy is that the relationship may be idealized by one or both people. As Whitty suggests, "having people respond more positively to this more, well crafted, likable self, could be more appealing than the more mundane self of everyday life" (p. 193). When these individuals ultimately decide to meet in person, will they recognize their potential mate? Will they be able to allow themselves to be authentic with each other? What happens when each person gets to know the other's real self?

Internet Infidelity: An Alarming Trend

Some people develop affairs in cyberspace that they keep separate from the outside world. Using the defense mechanism of splitting, they may see the object of their affection as all good, which can be contrasted with their offline relationship. "The online relationship can potentially cater to an unfettered, impotent fantasy that is difficult to measure up to in reality" (Whitty, 2011, p. 193). Whitty speculates that people engage in online affairs for some of the same reasons that others engage in offline affairs: they may have certain personality characteristics that predispose them to cheat, or they may have relationship problems (such as a partner who sexualize others, who is extremely jealous and possessive, or who is condescending, withholds sex, or abuses alcohol).

Two examples of unfaithful acts that occur online are cybersex (sexual gratification while interacting with someone online) and hot chatting (erotic talk that progresses beyond cyberflirting). Emotional infidelity can be just as painful a betrayal as sexual infidelity, and online affairs can destroy your offline relationship. Infidelity dating sites have been established for people in committed relationships who are open and honest about wanting to have an affair. According to Wysocki and Childers (2011), "AshleyMadison.com, whose tag line is 'Life is short . . . Have an affair,' states it has 6,095,000 members" (p. 223). In our counseling work with people, we find that participating in activities such as these can contribute to the breakup of a relationship.

TAKE TIME TO REFLECT

1. What are the barriers to effective communication in your relationships? What can you do to address these barriers? _____
_____
_____

2. To what extent do you rely on technology to communicate with people? How careful are you about protecting your privacy online? _____
_____
_____

3. In what ways does technology enhance your relationships with others? _____
_____
_____

4. In what ways does technology detract from or harm your relationships with people?
_____
_____

GAY AND LESBIAN RELATIONSHIPS

Common factors underlie all forms of intimate relationships: gay, lesbian, and bisexual relationships are basically no different from heterosexual relationships. Despite these similarities, people in same-gender relationships are subjected to discrimination and oppression that people in heterosexual relationships typically do not face in daily life.

Some states have granted the right to marry to same-sex couples, but same-sex marriage has generated strong opposition in other states. Likewise, rules regarding adoption of children by same-sex couples also vary from state to state. "[A] handful of states explicitly bar same-sex partners from adopting jointly as well as disallowing second-parent adoptions by gay partners" (Goldberg & Smith, 2011, p. 140). Until recently, the U.S. "Don't Ask, Don't Tell" policy on gay and lesbian people serving in the military prohibited closeted individuals from being discriminated against, but it barred openly gay, lesbian, and bisexual individuals from serving. This policy was repealed in 2011. We cannot provide a comprehensive discussion of such a complex issue here, but we can dispel some of the myths and examine some of the prejudices toward people based on their sexual orientation.

The guidelines for meaningful relationships presented earlier can be applied to relationships between couples who are married or unmarried, gay or straight. The term **sexual orientation** refers to the gender or genders that a person is attracted to physically, emotionally, sexually, and romantically. Matlin (2012) defines some key terms pertaining to sexual identity:

▶ **Heterosexism** is a bias against gay males, lesbians, and bisexuals; it is a belief system that values heterosexuality as superior to homosexuality.

▶ A **lesbian** is a woman who is psychologically, emotionally, and sexually attracted to other women.

▶ **Gay men** are psychologically, emotionally, and sexually attracted to other men.

▶ **Bisexual** individuals are psychologically, emotionally, and sexually attracted to both women and men.

The following discussion is designed to assist you in thinking about your views, assumptions, values, and possible biases and prejudices pertaining to sexual orientation.

Psychological Views of Homosexuality

How sexual orientation is established is still not understood. Some experts argue that sexual orientation is at least partly a function of genetic or physiological factors, and others contend that homosexuality is entirely a learned behavior. Some maintain that both an internal predisposition and an environmental dimension come together to shape one's sexual orientation. And there are those who assert that sexual identity is strictly a matter of personal choice. Many gay men, lesbians, and bisexuals report that they did not actively choose their sexual orientation anymore than they did their gender. Some will say that where choice enters the picture is in the choice of keeping who they are a secret or of "coming out" by claiming and disclosing their sexual identity.

Only when scientists critically evaluated the assumption that homosexuality is a sickness was progress made in understanding homosexuality (Carroll, 2013). The American Psychiatric Association in 1973 and the American Psychological Association in 1975 stopped labeling homosexuality as a mental disorder, ending a long and bitter dispute. Along with these changes came the challenge to mental health professionals to modify their thinking and practice to reflect a view of homosexuality as being normal and healthy, rather than a manifestation of arrested psychosexual development and unresolved conflicts. Although decades have passed since the decision to no longer consider homosexuality a form of psychopathology, there is still a good deal of social prejudice, social stigmatization, and discrimination here and in many countries around the world (Pardess, 2005).

Some heterosexual counselors see their role as actively trying to change gay couples or gay individuals to a heterosexual orientation, even if these clients do not present their sexual orientation as a problem. Some counselors automatically attribute an individual's problems to his or her sexual orientation (Pardess, 2005). Such practices are unethical and clinically ineffective.

Today most therapists practice **gay-affirmative therapy,** helping individuals accept their sexual identity and learning strategies to deal with those in society who harbor prejudice toward them. This shift in therapeutic focus is significant because it locates the problem with society's negative attitudes toward homosexuality rather than in people who are homosexual (Crooks & Baur, 2011).

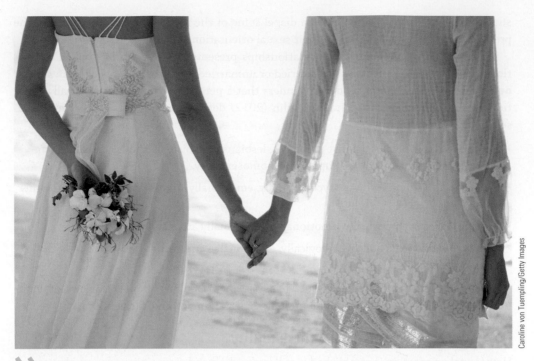

Caroline von Tuempling/Getty Images

>> Same-gender sexual orientation can be regarded as another style of self-expression.

Gay individuals and couples are not interested in changing their sexual orientation but seek counseling for many of the same reasons straight people do. Examples of the personal concerns they bring to therapy include identity issues, relationship difficulties, and coping with crisis situations. In addition to these concerns, gay, lesbian, and bisexual individuals are often faced with dealing with the effects of prejudice, oppression, and discrimination. The task of the counselor is to help these individuals explore the problems that most concern them. We see the counselor's responsibility as helping clients clarify their values and deciding for themselves what course of action to take. We strongly oppose the notion that counselors have the right to impose their values on their clients, to tell others how to live, or to make decisions for them.

Prejudice and Discrimination Against Homosexual Teens and Adults

In the past many people felt ashamed and abnormal because they had homosexual feelings. Heterosexuals frequently categorized gay and lesbian people as deviants and as sick or immoral. Cross-cultural attitudes toward homosexuality range from condemnation to acceptance; in our society there are many who have negative attitudes toward homosexuality (Crooks & Baur, 2011). Pardess (2005) points out that negative views of homosexuals and opposition to homosexuality have been part of the culture of many religious traditions (Christianity, Judaism, and Islam), and in most religious settings homosexuality is considered to be morally wrong and a sin. Some more progressive churches that welcome gay clergy have endured fierce resistance from parishioners who vow to leave the church if gay people are ordained. According to Pardess, antigay prejudices are not limited to any specific cultural, social, or educational group. These prejudices exist across religions, professions, institutions, and cultures. For these and other reasons, many gay, lesbian, and bisexual individuals conceal their sexual identity, perhaps even from themselves.

Lesbian, gay, and bisexual people frequently are confronted with interpersonal discrimination, heterosexual biases, verbal harassment, and physical assaults (Matlin, 2012).

Hate crimes often include assault and murder and are directed against a victim because he or she is of a certain race, ethnic group, religion, or sexual orientation. **Homophobia**—the irrational fear of homosexual people and strong negative attitudes about homosexuality—is at the root of many hate crimes. Homophobia is a prejudice much like racism that often results in discrimination and oppression. Currently, 33 states have hate crime laws that prohibit antigay violence (Crooks & Baur, 2011).

It is disheartening to hear about hate crimes directed at homosexual adults, but it is even more unsettling to know that gay teens are often tormented by their peers and classmates. Bullying is a serious offense whether it happens in real space or cyberspace, and whether it happens to people who are straight or gay. But gay teens are particularly vulnerable to such attacks. Some teens who have been bullied are driven to commit suicide as did Ryan Patrick Halligan in 2003. This 13-year-old boy from Vermont was relentlessly harassed about his sexual identity and threatened by middle school classmates both in person and online. In 2010 Tyler Clementi, an 18-year-old Rutgers University student, jumped off a bridge after a roommate allegedly uploaded a video of his sexual activities with another man on the Internet. Many young gay men and lesbians have been casualties of hate and intolerance, and the emotional pain these young people must endure can be overwhelming.

Today, the gay pride movement is actively challenging the social stigma attached to sexual identity, and those with same-sex partners are increasingly asserting their rights to live as they choose. A special issue that lesbians, gay men, and bisexuals often bring to counseling is the struggle of concealing their identity versus "coming out." Just as gay men, lesbians, and bisexuals had won some rights and were becoming more willing to disclose their sexual identity, the AIDS crisis arose, once again creating animosity, fear, and antipathy toward the gay population. Some heterosexuals perpetuate the myth that the gay population is responsible for this crisis, which is not true. Despite widespread efforts to promote tolerance, many people continue to cling to stereotypes, prejudices, and misconceptions regarding behavior between same gender couples.

Dealing with other family members is of special importance to gay couples. They may want to be honest with their parents, yet they may fear alienating them. Ann and Berit, friends of ours from Norway, wrote this personal account of the development of their relationship.

ANN AND BERIT'S STORY

We met when we were in our early 20s while attending a teacher education program in Norway. Over the years we became close friends and spent more and more time together. Even though neither of us ever married, both of us had various relationships with men, which for the most part were not very satisfying.

Our families and friends often expressed concern and disapproval about the closeness of our relationship, which didn't appear "natural" or "normal" to them and which, they thought, might interfere with our "settling down with a good man" and starting a family. We kept our feelings for each other a secret for fear of rejection.

At one point, our relationship became a sexual one, a fact that brought out many of our self-doubts and vulnerabilities and the concern that, should we become separated, being sexually involved would make the parting even more difficult. The burden of pretending to be other than we were became increasingly heavy for us. We felt insincere and dishonest both toward each other and toward our families and friends, and we found the need to invent pat answers when others asked us why we were still single. Had we been honest, we would have said, "I'm not interested at all in a traditional marriage. I have a significant other, and I wish I didn't have to hide this very important part of my life."

Ann and my relationship was very anxiety producing, and I developed severe panic attacks. I saw a therapist, and my symptoms decreased. I never felt a need to explore my preference for women, but I did spend a good deal of time on the conflict between my need to do what I thought was right for me and my need to give in to external pressure to be "normal."

At the age of 40, we made the decision that we could no longer live with the duplicity. Either we would go separate ways, or we would share a life and acknowledge our relationship. After years of struggling, we were finally able to face ourselves, each other, and then the other significant people in our lives. Much to our surprise, when we did disclose the truth about our relationship, most of our relatives and friends were supportive and understanding, and some even told us that they knew of our "special" relationship. We felt a great burden had been lifted from us and began to experience a new sense of peace and happiness.

Just last year we got married. Ann's mother's first reaction to this was somewhat negative, probably because of her concern over what the neighbors and other relatives would think. However, when Ann's mother experienced nothing but positive reactions from her friends and family, her attitude changed and she accepted our marriage. My parents acted as if the marriage never took place. No remarks were ever made about the event, but they continued to treat both of us with respect, friendliness, and hospitality.

We got married first and foremost to protect each other financially. However, we are convinced that marriage overall has been an important aspect in our lives. It has made us feel more confident being the "number one" in each other's lives. It also makes a difference in how others view us as a couple. We are both happy to live in Norway, a country that allows people of the same sex to marry.

Ann and Berit's story illustrates the struggle that many couples go through as they decide how they will live. Many of the issues that concerned Ann and Berit are the same interpersonal conflicts that any couple will eventually face and need to resolve. However, they must also deal with the pressure of being part of a segment of society that many consider unacceptable. Thus being involved in a gay or lesbian relationship is not simply a matter of sexual preference; it involves a whole spectrum of interpersonal and practical issues. In categorizing relationships as heterosexual or homosexual, we sometimes forget that sex is not the only aspect of a relationship. It is important that you define yourself, that you assume responsibility and accept the consequences for your own choices, and that you live out your choices with peace and inner integrity.

According to Goldberg and Smith (2011), "lesbians and gay men experience many of the same life transitions as heterosexuals, but the stresses of these transitions may differ due to their sexual orientation or, more specifically, to their exposure to heterosexism" (p. 139). The transition to parenthood may be especially difficult for many same-gender couples to navigate. "The experience of being 'recognized' as a gay-parent family may be particularly disconcerting for individuals who are not comfortable with their sexuality and who also live in communities that are intolerant of sexual minorities—whose members may respond to their family status with hostile stares, remarks, or outright discrimination" (p. 147).

All the concerns about friendships, heterosexual relationships, and traditional marriage that we explore in this chapter apply to gay and lesbian relationships as well. Indeed, barriers to effective communication are found in every kind of intimate relationship. The challenge is to find ways of removing the blocks to honest communication and intimacy. The media and entertainment industry play a substantial role in shaping attitudes and in educating the public about lesbian, gay, and bisexual issues. By airing TV shows such as the critically acclaimed comedy *Modern Family*, which depicts a gay couple who have adopted a Vietnamese baby, perhaps progress will be made in challenging heterosexist assumptions.

TAKE TIME TO REFLECT

1. Are you aware of any prejudice toward people who have same-gender sexual orientations?
_____
_____

2. What are your views concerning the gay liberation movement? Should people who openly admit they are gay have rights equal to those of heterosexuals? _____
_____
_____

3. Do you think anyone should be denied any specific job because of his or her sexual orientation alone? _____
_____
_____

4. How do you react when you hear others making disparaging remarks about gay, lesbian, or bisexual individuals? _____
_____
_____

5. What are your thoughts about the many religions that view homosexuality as a sin?
_____
_____

SEPARATION AND DIVORCE

The principles we discuss here can be applied to separations between people who are friends, to unmarried people involved in an intimate relationship, or to married couples who are contemplating a divorce. The fear of being alone often keeps people from dissolving a relationship, even when they agree that there is little left in that relationship. People may say something like this: "I know what I have, and at least I have somebody. So maybe it's better to have that than nothing at all." Because of fear, many people remain in stagnant relationships.

When to Separate or Terminate a Significant Relationship

Ending a relationship can be an act of courage that makes a new beginning possible, and sometimes it is the wisest course. But how do two people know when a separation is the best solution? No categorical answer can be given to this question. However, before two people decide to terminate their relationship, they might consider these questions:

▶ *Has each of you sought personal therapy or counseling?* Self-exploration would lead to changes that may allow you and your partner to renew or strengthen your relationship.

▶ *Have you considered seeking relationship counseling?* Perhaps relationship counseling could lead to changes that would allow you and your partner to renew or strengthen your relationship. If you do get involved in relationship counseling of any type, it is important that both of you be committed to it.

▶ *Are you both interested in maintaining your relationship?* Perhaps you are no longer interested in keeping the old relationship, but you both at least want time together. We routinely ask both partners in a significant relationship who are experiencing difficulties to decide whether they even want to preserve their relationship. Here are some of the responses people give: "I don't really know. I've lost hope for any real change, and at this point I find it difficult to see a future together." "I'm sure that I don't want to live with this person anymore; I just don't care enough to work on improving things between us. I'm here so that we can finish the business between us and do what is best for the children." Another might say, "Even though we're going through some turmoil right now, I would very much like to care enough to make things better. Frankly, I'm not too hopeful, but I'm willing to give it a try." Whatever your response, it is imperative that you both know how the other feels about the possibility of renewing the relationship or terminating it.

▶ *Have you each taken the time to be alone, to focus, and to decide what kind of life you want for yourself and with others?* Few couples in troubled relationships arrange for time alone with each other. It is almost as if couples fear discovering that they really have little to say to each other. This discovery in itself might be very useful, for at least you might be able to do something about the situation if you confronted it; but many couples seem to arrange their lives in such a way as to prevent any possibility for intimacy.

▶ *What do you each expect from the dissolution of the relationship?* Sometimes, problems in a relationship are reflections of inner conflicts within one or both of the partners. In general, unless there are some changes within the individuals, the problems they experience may not end by simply ending the relationship. In fact, many who end a relationship with the expectation of finding increased joy and freedom discover instead that they are still lonely, depressed, and anxious. Lacking insight into themselves, they may soon find a new partner very much like the one they left and repeat the same dynamics. Thus, a woman who finally decides to leave a man she thinks of as weak and passive may find a similar man to live with again unless she comes to understand why she aligns herself with this type of person. Or a man who contends that he has "put up with" his partner for more than 20 years may find a similar person unless he understands what motivated him to stay with his first partner for so long. It is essential, therefore, that you come to know as clearly as possible why you are terminating a relationship and that you look at the changes you may need to make in yourself as well as in your circumstances.

Sometimes one or both members of a couple identify strong reasons for separating but say that, for one reason or another, they cannot do so. This kind of reasoning is worth examining; an attitude of "I couldn't possibly leave" will not help either partner make a free and sound choice. Here are some of the reasons people give for refusing to call an end to their relationship:

▶ I have too many years invested in this relationship.

▶ I'm afraid to break off the relationship because I might be even more lonely than I am now.

▶ I'm concerned that I have not given us a fair enough chance to make a go of it.

▶ I would lose my immigration status.

- I'm dependent financially and am concerned that I won't be able to support myself.
- I fear the judgment of my family and friends.
- My religion does not condone divorce.
- My culture prohibits me from divorcing.
- I can't leave because of the children. I would feel very guilty.

When there are children involved, the decision to divorce entails considering ways to minimize the impact of the divorce on the children's well-being. Philip Stahl (2007), author of *Parenting After Divorce*, provides some practical guidelines for raising children of divorce in a healthy way. Stahl emphasizes the importance of parents making a commitment to the well-being of their children. Often there is turmoil and change associated with a divorce, which can cause great stress for children. Because parents are caught up in their own turmoil, they may not listen to their children or understand what is going on in their world. For those who are interested in a realistic perspective on divorce and its effects on children, we recommend Stahl's book. We also recommend Bruce Fisher's (2005) book, *Rebuilding: When Your Relationship Ends*, as a useful resource for finding new ways of being in relationships.

Coping With Ending a Long-Term Relationship

When a long-term relationship comes to an end, a mixture of feelings ranging from a sense of loss and regret to relief may be present. Betty, an unmarried college student in her mid-20s, is going through some typical reactions to the breakup of a 3-year relationship with her boyfriend Isaac.

BETTY'S STORY

At first I felt abandoned and was afraid of never finding a suitable replacement. I kept wondering who was at fault. I switched back and forth between blaming myself and blaming Isaac. I was depressed, and I wasn't eating or sleeping well. Then I began to withdraw from other relationships too. I felt worthless and inadequate. Because my relationship with Isaac didn't work out, it proves that I'm a failure and unlovable and that I won't be able to establish and keep any other relationships. It is a sure sign that I'll never get along with any man. Isaac found me undesirable, and I don't think I can stand the pain of this rejection.

Internal dialogue such as this kept Betty from taking any action that could change her situation. It was not the breakup itself that was causing Betty's reactions; rather, her beliefs about and her interpretations of the breakup were giving her trouble.

There are no easy ways to ending a long-standing relationship. A breakup or loss of a friend or significant other can lead to feelings of pain, anger, and grief. If you find yourself in such a situation, there are some attitudes you can assume and some behaviors you can choose that are likely to help you work through these feelings. Here are some suggestions for dealing effectively with the termination of a meaningful relationship:

- *Allow yourself to grieve.* You are likely to experience a range of feelings, including sadness, anger, guilt, loss, pain, joy over certain memorable times, and relief. Although grieving can be both overwhelming and painful, the alternative of denying your feelings will keep you from being able to move on and could cause you to have intimacy problems later.

- *Give yourself time.* Some say, "Time heals all wounds," but in reality it is what you do with that time that helps you heal. However long or short it takes, it is important to permit yourself to grieve based on being true to your own self and not because others feel you should be over it by now.

- *Express your anger.* Sometimes breakups leave us feeling angry and bitter. Anger is a normal reaction, but if unexpressed or overindulged in, anger can cause serious problems later, especially if the anger keeps you from expressing hurt.

- *Depersonalize your partner's actions.* Often, when one person ends a relationship, the other is left feeling rejected as though the failure was of his or her making. A person's decision to end a relationship with you may say more about that person than it does about you.

- *Take responsibility for your own part in the relationship.* It may be easier to find fault in the other person, but exploring your own behaviors can be helpful to your healing process. The point is not to find blame but to gain insight into how you relate to people in both negative and positive ways.

- *Find a support network.* Whether you are shy or social, having people to support you can provide you with some level of stability in a time of loss and change. Seek counseling or professional help if you feel that you cannot cope with the loss on your own. Many universities offer free student counseling.

- *Write in your journal.* Writing can help you release emotions even if you are not able to talk to others about how you are feeling. Later, it can be useful to read what you wrote to see how you processed your pain.

- *Make amends.* Making amends and forgiving both yourself and your partner can free you from carrying the pain and anger into future relationships. Remember, your anger can hurt and burden you more than anyone else. You must be ready to make amends; this is not something that should be hurried.

- *Get closure.* Coming to some type of closure is essential to moving forward. Closure does not mean it never happened, rather it means you have decided to live. To one person it may mean forgiveness, and for another it may include some type of a ritual or final letter. You may not be able to deal directly with a partner who is abusive, but you can find other ways to move forward.

- *Love and learn.* At some point you will find that it can be freeing to reflect on what you have learned from the experience. Even the most abusive or unhealthy relationship can teach you something about yourself and the types of relationships you want to have.

TAKE TIME TO REFLECT

Complete the following sentences by writing down the first response that comes to mind. Suggestion: Ask your partner or a close friend to do the exercise on a separate sheet of paper; then compare and discuss your responses.

1. To me, intimacy means _____

2. The most important thing in making an intimate relationship successful is _____

3. The thing I most fear about an intimate relationship is _____

4. What I like most about an intimate relationship is _____

5. One of the reasons I need another person is _____ finances _____

6. One conflict that I have concerning intimate relationships is _____ know as 100% they are the one _____

7. In an intimate relationship, it is unrealistic to expect that _____ continues and passion _____ with other persons.

8. To me, commitment means _____

9. I have encouraged my partner to grow by _____

10. My partner has encouraged me to grow by _____ spending time around friends _____

SUMMARY

We have encouraged you to think about what characterizes a growing, meaningful relationship. It is our hope that the topics in this chapter will assist you in assessing the present state of your intimate relationships and also in improving the state of your relationships. The themes we explored can be applied to all intimate relationships, regardless of one's sexual orientation. Although same-sex relationships are not well accepted by some people in our society, it is important to realize that all couples share many common challenges.

A major barrier to developing and maintaining relationships is our tendency to evaluate and judge others. By attempting to change others, we typically increase their defensiveness. A key characteristic of a meaningful relationship is the ability of the people involved to listen and to respond to each other. They are able to communicate effectively, and they are committed to staying in the relationship even when communication is difficult. It is important to pay attention to both cultural and gender differences that make up our conversational style. Many misunderstandings are due to the different ways women and men express their thoughts and feelings. At times people decide that a relationship has reached an end, and they give serious consideration to separating. This may be a solution for some; others may decide to work together to resolve the issues that are divisive and have caused the conflicts.

Maintaining a relationship entails dedication and hard work. It takes both imagination and effort to think of ways to keep our relationships vital. With the widespread popularity of social networking sites and other technologies, we have greatly expanded our opportunities for communicating with each other. Of course, we also have a growing number of ways in which our communications can be misunderstood.

Where Can I Go From Here?

Some of these activities can be done on your own; others are designed for partners in an intimate relationship. Select the ones that mean the most to you and consider sharing the results with the other members of your class.

1. In the journal pages at the end of this chapter write down some reflections on your parents' relationship. Consider these questions:

▸ Would you like the same kind of relationship your parents have had?

▸ What are some of the things you like best about their relationship?

▸ What are some features of their relationship that you would not want in your own relationships?

▸ How have your own views, attitudes, and practices regarding intimacy been affected by your parents' relationship? Would you marry a woman like your mother? A man like your father? Why or why not?

2. How much self-disclosure and honesty do you want in your intimate relationships? Reflect in your journal on how much you would share your feelings concerning each of the following with your partner.

- Your need for support from your partner
- Your angry feelings
- Your dreams
- Your friendships and past intimate relationships with other persons
- Your ideas on religion and your philosophy of life
- The times when you feel inadequate as a person
- The times when you feel extremely close and loving toward your partner
- The times in your relationship when you feel boredom, anger, or detachment

Now think about how open you want your partner to be with you. If your partner were doing this exercise, what answers do you wish he or she would give for each of the items?

3. Over a period of about a week, do some writing about the evolution of your relationship and ask your partner to do the same. Consider why you were initially attracted to each other, and how you have changed since then. Do you like these changes? What would you most like to change about your life together now? List the best things about your relationship and also some problem areas you need to explore. After you have each written about these and any other questions

that are significant for you, read each other's writing and discuss it. This activity can stimulate you to talk more honestly with each other and can also give each of you the chance to see how the other perceives the relationship.

4. If you tend to rely heavily on technology to connect with others, give yourself a "technology time out" for a day or two (perhaps on a weekend). Record your reactions in a journal. Reflect on both the positive and negative aspects of this experience, and write about what you learned during your time out.

5. Suggested Readings. The full bibliographic entry for each of these sources can be found in the References and Suggested Readings at the back of the book. For a book based on extensive research to determine what factors are associated with successful marital relationships, see Gottman and Silver (1999). For a practical book on forgiveness, see Jampolsky (1999). For a discussion of conversational styles in communication in intimate relationships, see Tannen (1987, 1991). For a treatment of parenting after divorce, see Stahl (2007). For a useful resource on finding new ways of being in relationships, see Fisher (2005).

WEBSITE RESOURCES

Included here are some valuable websites. For access to these websites, video activities, and other supporting materials, visit Cengage Learning's Counseling CourseMate website for *I Never Knew I Had a Choice*, 10th Edition, at **www.cengagebrain.com.**

THE GOTTMAN RELATIONSHIP INSTITUTE
www.gottman.com
Recommended Search Words: "Gottman institute"
Cofounded by Dr. John Gottman and Julie Schwartz Gottman, this institute "applies leading-edge research on marriage in a practical, down-to-earth therapy and trains therapists committed to helping couples. No other approach to couples education and therapy has relied on such intensive, detailed, and long-term scientific study of why marriages succeed or fail." The site offers research on parenting,

gay and lesbian relationships, and marriage and couples.

RELATIONSHIPS: THE COUNSELING CENTER, UNIVERSITY AT BUFFALO
http://ub-counseling.buffalo.edu/relationship.shtml
Recommended Search Words: "relationships university of buffalo"

The counseling center at the University at Buffalo offers information on topics such as starting and ending relationships, communication, rape and surviving, and about men and women and lesbian, gay, bisexual, and transgendered people.

UNIVERSITY OF DENVER CLINIC FOR CHILD AND FAMILY PSYCHOLOGY
www.du.edu/psychology/child_and_family_clinic/couplesclinic.html

Recommended Search Words: "University of Denver prevention and relationship enhancement program"

This website offers information about a research-based education program for couples called the Prevention and Relationship Enhancement Program.

DIVORCE CENTRAL
www.divorcecentral.com

Recommended Search Words: "divorce central"

Divorce central provides information and advice on legal, emotional, and financial issues for individuals who are considering or going through a divorce. You can use all of their services and can become a member of their online community for free. Links to other divorce-related sites are also available here.

THE UNITED STATES DEPARTMENT OF JUSTICE: OFFICE ON VIOLENCE AGAINST WOMEN
www.ovw.usdoj.gov/domviolence.html

Recommended Search Words: "department of justice domestic violence"

This government website offers a wealth of resources, including links to local hotlines and agencies devoted to assisting victims of domestic violence.

HELPGUIDE.ORG
www.helpguide.org

Recommended Search Words: "helpguide"

At this website you will find educational materials and resources to help you improve your emotional well-being and make more informed health decisions. Topics include domestic violence, abuse and bullying, and relationship help.

PARTNERS TASK FORCE FOR GAY AND LESBIAN COUPLES
http://buddybuddy.com/partners.html

Recommended Search Words: "buddybuddy"

This is a national resource for same-sex couples, supporting the diverse community of committed gay and lesbian partners through a variety of media. This frequently updated website contains more than 200 essays, surveys, legal articles, and resources on legal marriage, ceremonies, domestic partner benefits, relationship tips, parenting, and immigration.

THE GAY-STRAIGHT ALLIANCE NETWORK
http://gsanetwork.org

Recommended Search Words: "gay straight alliance"

Gay-Straight Alliance clubs have been established in schools and universities throughout the nation. This website offers guidance to those interested in starting clubs, as well as news and an array of resources.

SEXUAL ORIENTATION: SCIENCE, EDUCATION, AND POLICY
http://psychology.ucdavis.edu/rainbow/html/facts_mental_health.html

Recommended Search Words: "psychology UC Davis rainbow"

This site builds on the work of Dr. Gregory Herek, focusing on sexual orientation, antigay violence, homophobia, and other concerns of gay, lesbian, and bisexual individuals.

HUMAN RIGHTS CAMPAIGN
www.hrc.org

Recommended Search Words: "human rights campaign"

This organization focuses on securing equal rights for lesbians and gay men. The site provides news updates on legislation related to gay rights and descriptions of public education programs.

8

BECOMING THE WOMAN OR MAN YOU WANT TO BE

> Where Am I Now?

> Male Roles

> Female Roles

> Alternatives to Rigid Gender-Role Expectations

> Summary

> Where Can I Go From Here?

> Website Resources

Michael Rougier/Getty Images

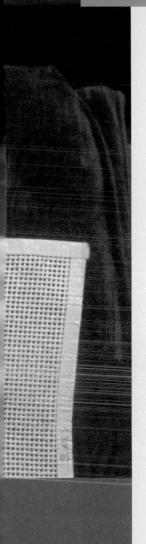

When gender transcendence occurs, people can be just people.

—BASOW

WHERE AM I NOW?

Use this scale to respond to the following statements:

4 = I *strongly agree* with this statement.
3 = I *agree* with this statement.
2 = I *disagree* with this statement.
1 = I *strongly disagree* with this statement.

1. It is important to me to be perceived as feminine [masculine].

2. I have a clear sense of what it means to be a man [woman].

3. It is relatively easy for me to be both logical and emotional, tough and tender, objective and subjective.

4. I have trouble accepting women who show masculine qualities and men who show feminine qualities.

5. It is difficult for me to accept in myself traits that are often associated with the other gender.

6. I welcome the change toward more flexibility in gender roles.

7. I think I am becoming the kind of woman [man] I want to become, regardless of anyone else's ideas about what is expected of my gender.

8. I am glad that I am the gender that I am.

9. I feel discriminated against because of my gender.

10. My parents provided good models of what it means to be a woman [man].

We are all products of our cultural conditioning to some extent. Behavior depends not on gender but on prior experience, biology, learned attitudes, cultural expectations, sanctions, opportunities for practice, and situational demands. We learn behavior that is appropriate for our gender by interacting in society. **Gender-role socialization** is a process of learning those behaviors (norms and roles) that are expected of people in a particular society, and it begins in one's family of origin. Learning about gender differences does not cease with childhood; rather, it is a lifelong process.

In this chapter we ask you to examine the experiences that have directly and indirectly influenced your gender-role identity. We describe some of the detrimental effects and costs for women and men who feel they must live in accordance with prescribed gender roles. **Sexism** is a bias against people on the basis of their gender. People tend to make clear distinctions between women and men, and they divide the world into two categories, male and female. Because women and men are viewed as being both biologically and psychologically different, people react differently to them (Matlin, 2012).

Ask yourself these questions: "What did I learn about gender roles from my parents?" "What attitudes prevailed in my home about gender roles, and how does this influence the woman or man I am today?" "How were my parents' views of gender roles shaped and reinforced by their culture?" "What have I learned about gender roles from the media?" "Do I hold biases toward individuals based on gender?" "Has the way I've been socialized enhanced or hindered the manner in which I live?" With increased awareness, you can assess the effects your gender-role socialization is having on all aspects of your life. You can decide what changes, if any, you want to make. You can think critically about gender-role stereotypes and form your own standards for the woman or man you could be and want to be. This assessment requires patience and an appreciation of the difficulties involved in overcoming ingrained attitudes, but the real challenge is to translate the new attitudes that you may acquire into new behaviors.

As you read this chapter, reflect on the models that have influenced your views of what it means to be a woman or a man and on the choices that you have made about your gender-role identity. Societal norms provide you with a set of standards, but you can decide to live by these standards or to modify them to be more congruent with the personal values you have developed. Personalize the chapter by reflecting on these questions and answering them for yourself:

▶ To what degree have you made conscious choices regarding gender-role identity?

▶ What changes may you want to make? What are the consequences of making these changes?

▶ What kind of support, or lack of support, do you expect you would get if you went against your socialization?

▶ Who and what has influenced your gender identity?

MALE ROLES

An increasing number of men are giving expression to both masculine and feminine dimensions of their personalities. However, many men in our society still live according to a traditional masculine model of what it is to be a man. Many men have put all their energy into maintaining an acceptable male image at a cost to themselves. Traditional male roles certainly pose problems for those men who are not in agreement with what is now considered to be truly "masculine" in our society. Ethnic or racial differences, socioeconomic differences, and geographical or regional differences all influence how gender roles are defined. What is considered traditional in one cultural context may not be considered traditional in another.

If you are a man, ask yourself to what degree you have accepted your socialization regarding expected male patterns. What costs and what benefits do you experience in striving to live up to what is expected of you as a man? Now might be a good time to reevaluate your gender-role identity and to consider in what ways, if any, you may want to alter your picture of what it means to be a man.

Gender-role socialization begins early in life. According to Root and Denham (2010), parental attitudes about gender roles and the encouragement of gender-typed behaviors influence what children believe about gender and the way they are supposed to behave. In addition to receiving direct messages about appropriate ways of handling emotions based on gender, children are influenced by observing others: "The expression of emotion within the family unit affords children with the opportunity to witness others' emotional expressions and evaluate the responses others receive after the display of specific emotions" (Root & Denham, 2010, p. 3).

Throughout childhood in Western cultures, boys are socialized to reject anything that makes them appear feminine. Orr (2011) claims that boys continue to be encouraged to participate in gender-typed activities such as interactive games, physical play, sports, and spending time outdoors. She adds that "boys are exposed to an often rigid set of expectations that require them to be, among other things, active, tough, aggressive, competitive, in control, unemotional, independent, and in charge" (p. 281). Expressing a similar view, in his discussion of society's messages to boys, Terrance Real (1998) states that boys learn early on that they should have fewer emotional needs than girls. While girls are encouraged to fully develop connection and relationship, boys are discouraged from developing their relational, emotional selves. Boys are encouraged to develop their assertive selves, while girls are discouraged from developing assertive skills and independence. According to Real, boys and men need social connection to the same degree as girls and women. Boys and men will not heal from their wounds of disconnection until they learn to place themselves inside relationships rather than outside them.

As toddlers, boys are pressured to leave their close relationship with their mother so they can begin to become independent and self-reliant little men. William Pollack (1998) suggests that the sadness and disconnection men often experience stems from the loss of this relationship. Men sometimes have fears about commitment in long-term relationships. The fear of getting too close in adult relationships may be grounded in their reaction to this earlier loss of the maternal relationship. The move from the female world of nurturance and love to the male world of independence and competition can be drastic for some boys. The pain of this loss is often repressed, yet it may surface in an intimate relationship, especially in relationships with women.

Pollack (1998) asserts that when boys feel ashamed of their vulnerability they often mask their emotions and ultimately their true selves. Because society's prevailing myths about boys do not allow for emotions such as feeling alone, helpless, and fearful, it is common for boys to feel that they do not measure up. Eventually, their sensitivity is submerged until they eventually become desensitized and "tough" in the way society expects them to be. The result of this socialization process is an emotional straightjacket. Pollack argues that boys should be encouraged to show *all* of their emotions. Boys need to know that both their strengths and their vulnerabilities will be celebrated. In short, boys need to hear the message that all of their feelings, not just anger, are normal and "masculine." Because vulnerability requires the most courage, boys are strongest when they can be vulnerable.

Roles That Alienate Men

Some men are caught in rigid roles, and they may be sanctioned if they deviate from those roles or display characteristics that are not associated with their gender. People often become so involved in their roles that they become alienated from themselves. They no longer know what they are like within because they put so much energy into maintaining an acceptable image. This was certainly the case for Gabriel who learned traditional male attitudes and behaviors from his father.

GABRIEL'S STORY

My father was hard-working, distant with us children, stoic, and prized himself for being a self-reliant individual. I learned from my father what a man is supposed to be and what behaviors are acceptable, and these attitudes were reinforced in school and by society. For a long time I did not even realize I was being restricted psychologically by these expectations, but then I faced a crisis in midlife. My father had a heart attack, and I was shocked to realize the toll that living by traditional roles had taken on him.

I began to look at the impact my definition of maleness was having on all aspects of my life, and I decided to make some changes. I realized that I had never questioned my attitudes about gender-role behavior and that I was behaving unconsciously and automatically rather than by choice. I wanted to become more expressive, but I had to struggle against years of conditioning that restricted the range of my emotional responses. I did increase my level of consciousness intellectually through reading and personal counseling, but I seem to be having trouble catching up emotionally and behaviorally. It is more difficult than I thought it would be to turn these insights into new behaviors.

Both Gabriel and his father suffer from **gender-role strain** (Pleck, 1995). Societal norms for gender ideals are often contradictory, inconsistent, and unattainable. When men are unable to live up to these unrealistic societal expectations, they are subject to many psychological problems. Men who experience gender-role conflict and stress are more likely to be depressed, anxious, express hostility in interpersonal behaviors, have poor self-esteem, harbor anger, misuse substances, and engage in high-risk behavior (Mahalik, 1999a). In a review of 25 years of research, O'Neil (2008) concluded that gender-role conflict "significantly relates to dysfunctional patterns in men's relationships, including interpersonal restrictions, attachment problems, and marital dissatisfaction" (p. 393). Furthermore, gender-role conflict has been linked to negative attitudes toward women, gay people, and racial minorities.

Both straight and gay men endorse traditional masculinity, and many gay men deride the effeminate behavior of some gay men (Sánchez, Westefeld, Liu, & Vilain, 2010). In evaluating the differences between gay and lesbian or straight couples, more strengths were revealed in the same-sex relationships, including using humor during disagreements, remaining positive after disagreements, and displaying less belligerence, fear, and domineering behavior with each other (Gottman et al., 2004). According to Crooks and Baur (2011), "researchers speculate that the greater strengths of same-sex couples may be due to the lack of gender-role conflicts that are inherent in heterosexual relationships" (p. 272). "[I]n regard to gender roles, a homosexual relationship may well be more flexible than a heterosexual one in our society" (p. 271).

The next section considers some of the aspects of the traditional masculine ideology, examining stereotypes of males and identifying messages that men are given about appropriate role behavior. It is difficult to describe traditional male roles and male stereotypes without further stereotyping men, and we remind you that these general categories are based on the literature and do not apply universally to all men.

Stereotypical View of Males

Gender stereotypes—widely accepted beliefs about females' and males' abilities, personality traits, and behavior patterns—are common fare in American culture. It is true that some behavioral differences exist between the genders, but gender stereotypes are not entirely accurate (Weiten, 2013). The findings on gender and behavior are complex and confusing, with both biological and environmental factors contributing to gender differences in behavior. For example, men are considered to be higher in **agency** (concern with self-interests, such as competition and independence), and women are considered to be higher in **communion** (concern for one's relationship with other people). These general beliefs have remained fairly consistent throughout recent decades (Matlin, 2012).

Some people live restricted lives because they have uncritically accepted these societal messages about what it means to be male or female. Although biological and environmental factors strongly influence our behavior, we still have a range of choices when it comes to how we relate to expectations based on gender.

The limited view of the traditional male role that many men have accepted, to a greater or lesser degree, is characterized by the traits various writers have identified in the following list. Keep in mind that these characteristics represent a *stereotypical* view of males, and certainly many men do not fit this narrow characterization.

▶ *Emotional unavailability.* A man tends to show his affection by being a "good provider." Frequently, he is not emotionally available to his female partner or to his family. Because of this, she may complain that she feels shut out by him. He also has a difficult time dealing with her feelings. If she cries, he becomes uncomfortable and quickly wants to solve the problem so she will stop crying, or he will label her as overly emotional.

▶ *Independence.* A man is expected to be mainly self-reliant. Rather than admitting that he needs anything from anyone, he must lead a life of exaggerated independence. He should be able to do by himself whatever needs to be done, and he finds it hard to ask for emotional support or nurturing.

▶ *Power and aggressiveness.* A man is told that he must be powerful physically, sexually, intellectually, and financially. He must take risks, be adventurous, and resort to violence if necessary. He must be continually active, aggressive, assertive, and striving. He views the opposites of these traits as signs of weakness, and he fears being seen as soft.

▶ *Denial of fears.* A man is told that it is important to hide his fears, even in situations where he is frightened. He has the distorted notion that to be afraid means that he lacks courage, so he hides his fears from himself and especially from others. He does not see that being frightened is a necessary part of courage. He fears being ashamed or humiliated in front of other men or being dominated by stronger men (Kimmel, 1996, 2010).

▶ *Protection of his inner self.* With other men he keeps himself hidden because they are competitors and in this sense potential enemies. He does not disclose himself to women because he is afraid they will think him unmanly and weak if they see his inner world. A woman may complain that a man hides his feelings from her, yet it is probably more accurate to say that he is hiding his feelings from himself. A man's tendency to protect his inner self begins when he is a boy and learns to hide his true self with an image of toughness, stoicism, and strength (Pollack, 1998).

▶ *Invulnerability.* He cannot make himself vulnerable, as is evidenced by his general unwillingness to disclose much of his inner experience. He will not let himself feel and express sadness, nor will he cry. He interprets any expression of emotional vulnerability as a sign of weakness. To protect himself, he becomes emotionally insulated and puts on a mask of toughness, competence, and decisiveness.

▶ *Lack of bodily self-awareness.* Common physical stress signals include headaches, nausea, heartburn, muscle aches, backaches, and high blood pressure, but men often ignore these stress symptoms, denying their potential consequences and failing to address their causes. For example, it is well known that heart disease and cardiovascular disease death rates are significantly higher in men than women. According to Real (1998), men die early because they do not take care of themselves. They are slow to recognize when they are sick, take longer to get help, and even after getting treatment tend not to cooperate with it as well as women do. Too often a man will drive himself unmercifully and treat his body as some kind of machine that will not break down or wear out. He may not pay attention to his exhaustion until he collapses from it.

▶ *Remoteness with other men.* Although he may have plenty of acquaintances, he rarely confides in male friends. It is not uncommon for men to state that although they have male friends, intimacy is lacking. He can talk to other men about things but rarely is he personal by sharing emotional concerns. When men talk to each other, it is often about planning what they are going to do.

▶ *Driven to succeed.* A man is told that it is important to win, to be competitive, and to gain recognition, respect, and status. A man is socialized with the message that work is the most important part of his identity; thus failure in his work attacks the core of his masculinity (Zunker, 2012). He measures his worth by the money he makes or by his job status. A chief burden a man carries is his need to continually prove his masculinity to himself and to others. He puts much of his energy into external signs of success through his achievements at work. Thus, little is left over for his wife and children, or even for leisure pursuits.

▶ *Denial of "feminine" qualities.* Men are frequently shut off from their emotional selves because they see the subjective world of feelings as being essentially feminine. From infancy through adulthood men are socialized to give short shrift to their emotions (Rabinowitz & Cochran, 1994). Some psychologists who have studied the traditional male role (Levant, 1996; Pleck, 1995) consider anti-femininity to be the key theme associated with the male gender role. A man believes the message that he should always be in full control of his emotions. He cannot be a man and at the same time possess (or reveal) traits usually attributed to women. Therefore, he is highly controlled, cool, detached, objective, rational, worldly, competitive, and strong, and he shuts out much of what he could experience, resulting in an impoverished emotional life.

▶ *Avoidance of physical contact.* A man has a difficult time touching freely or expressing affection and caring for other men. He thinks he should touch a woman only if it will lead to sex, and he fears touching other men because he does not want to be perceived as effeminate or homosexual. A man finds it difficult to express warmth and tenderness or to publicly display tenderness or compassion to either females or males.

▶ *Rigid perceptions.* A man tends to view gender roles as rigid categories. Women should be dependent, emotional, passive, and submissive; men are expected to be independent, logical, active, and aggressive.

▶ *Loss of the male spirit and experience of depression.* Because he is cut off from his inner self, he has lost a way to make intuitive sense of the world. Relying on society's definitions and rules about masculinity rather than his own results in a lack of clear gender identity. The secret legacy of male depression is a silent epidemic in men, a condition they hide from their family, friends, and themselves to avoid the stigma of "unmanliness" (Real, 1998). Recovery from depression entails the willingness of a man to face his pain and learn to cherish and take care of himself. Not until a man captures his own spirit will he be able to value and care for others.

This picture is not an accurate portrayal of the way *most* men are or should be, but in our society men hear messages like these that reinforce how they should think, feel, and act. Masculine identity and gender-role socialization of males in the United States cannot be accurately portrayed without considering the cultural context. A range of factors need to be understood and challenged if men are to make choices about how they want to change certain aspects of their masculine identity. Men have the task of defining who they want to be for themselves, whether that involves conforming to or rejecting traditional gender roles.

The Price Men Pay for Remaining in Traditional Roles

What price does a man pay for denying aspects of himself and living up to an image that is not true of him? First, he loses a sense of himself because of his concern with being the way he thinks he *should* be. Many men find it difficult to love and be loved. As we have seen, they hide their loneliness, anxiety, and hunger for affection, making it difficult for anyone to love them as they really are. Part of the price these guarded males pay for remaining hidden is that they must always be alert for fear that someone might discover their inner feelings and what lies beneath the image.

Second, adhering to a rigid model of what it means to be a man keeps men looking for others to make them happy. In this process men avoid knowing themselves and appreciating the richness of life. The principal costs to men of remaining tied to traditional gender roles are excessive pressures to succeed, becoming strangers to their emotional lives, and sexual difficulties (Weiten et al., 2012). Other costs include early death, illnesses, alcoholism, a tendency to take excessive and sometimes reckless risks, depression, and workaholism.

Challenging Traditional Male Roles

Are the traditional notions of what a man is supposed to be really changing in our society? Weiten and colleagues (2012) believe gender roles are changing, but that this change process is very slow. Age-old gender-roles stemmed from a need for a division of labor in society. Because these roles no longer make economic sense, traditional gender roles are being questioned and modified.

Some men are recognizing how lethal some of the messages they received are—not only for themselves but also for their relationships—and many others are challenging their childhood conditioning and are struggling to overcome stereotypes and to redefine what it takes to be a man. In the modern male role, "masculinity is validated by economic achievement, organizational power, emotional control (even over

© Christopher Robbins

Men are challenging traditional male roles.

anger), and emotional sensitivity and self-expression, but only with women" (Weiten et al., 2012, p. 354). In our work, we continue to encounter men who are willing to break out of the rigid patterns of masculine behavior they had adopted to conform to society's view and embrace a new and different set of behavioral norms. Change may be slow, but we see signs of change happening. Leroy is one man who is challenging his conditioning.

LEROY'S STORY

To me, life was a constant struggle, and I could never slow down. I was a driving and driven man, and my single goal in life was to prove myself and become a financial and business success. Life was a series of performances that involved me pleasing others and then waiting for the applause to come. But the applause was never enough, and I felt empty when the applause would die down. So I continued to push myself to give more performances, and I worked 70 to 90 hours a week. I was on my way to becoming the president of a corporation, and I was thinking that I had it made. When I got my W-2 form, I became aware that I had made more money than was in my plan for success, yet I had had a miserable year.

Then one day I became ill, landed in the hospital, and almost died. I began to look at my life and slow down, and I realized there is a world out there that does not solely involve my work. I decided that I wanted to experience life, to smell more flowers, and to not kill myself with a program I had never consciously chosen for myself. I decided to work no more than 50 hours a week. With that extra time, I decided to smell life—there are a lot of roses in life, and the scent is enticing and exciting to me. I'll thrive on it as long as I can breathe.

At age 54 Leroy showed the courage to reverse some of the self-destructive patterns that were killing him. He began deciding for himself what kind of man he wanted to be rather than living by an image of the man others thought he should be.

Like Leroy, many men are showing a clear interest in men's consciousness-raising workshops. There is a great increase in the number of conferences, workshops, retreats, and gatherings for men. Some key books have provided impetus for the men's movement. One is the poet Robert Bly's (1990) best-selling book, *Iron John*. According to Bly, men suffer from "father hunger," which results in unhappiness, emotional immaturity, and a search for substitute father figures. Bly writes and talks about the ways that having an absent, abusive, or alcoholic father results in the wounding of the children. Bly says that many mothers look to their sons to meet their own emotional needs, which are often denied to them by their husbands, and that boys feel ashamed when they are not able to psychologically fill their mothers' longing.

Some men expect the women in their lives to heal their boyhood wounds caused by their fathers, but the wounded must be the ones who do the healing. One of the bases of men's gatherings is to share common struggles, reveal their stories, and find healing in the men's collective. The fact that men from all walks of life are becoming interested in talking about their socialization from boyhood to manhood indicates that many men are examining the steep price they have paid for subscribing to traditional role behavior.

Traditional gender roles are not completely unhealthy for everyone, but we want to promote the notion of individual choice in determining what aspects of these roles you may want to retain and what aspects you may choose to modify. To make this choice, you need first to be aware of how you have been influenced by your gender-role socialization.

Traditional males should not be told that they *must* change if they hope to be healthy and happy; indeed, many aspects of traditional roles may be very satisfying to some men. However, other men are reinventing themselves without discarding many of the traits traditionally attributed to them. We suggest that you look at the potential costs associated with your gender-role identity, and then decide if you like being the way you are. The Take Time to Reflect exercises may help you discover some areas in your life that you most want to change.

TAKE TIME TO REFLECT

1. The following characteristics have been identified as gender stereotypes, some associated with women and others with men. Describe the degree to which you see each trait as a part of yourself. If you do not have this trait, explain why you would or would not like to incorporate this trait into your personality.

▸ Emotional unavailability _____

▸ Independence _____

▸ Dependence _____

▸ Aggressiveness _____

▸ Denial of fears _____

▸ Emotional expressiveness _____

▸ Passivity and submissiveness _____

▸ Lack of bodily awareness _____

▸ Drive to succeed _____

▸ Avoidance of physical contact _____

▸ Rigid perceptions _____

▸ Devotion to work _____

2. How does accepting traditional roles affect your life? _____
_____
_____

3. What are some specific qualities associated with each gender that you would most like in yourself? _____
_____
_____

4. What did your father teach you about being a man? A woman?_____
_____
_____

5. What did your mother teach you about being a man? A woman?_____
_____
_____

6. What did your culture teach you about being a man? A woman? _____
_____
_____

The Value of Men's Groups

Participating in a therapy group provides a unique opportunity for men to express themselves in unique ways. However, men often view therapy as something foreign to the male psyche: disclosing oneself to an authority figure (a therapist who is a stranger), revealing failures and insecurities, and revealing family and personal matters (Schwartz & Flowers, 2008). Rabinowitz and Cochran (2002) note that a men's group can counteract the negative side of male gender-role socialization, with its emphasis on competition, control, and stoicism in the face of pain. In the safe environment that a therapy group can provide, men can modify some of the ways in which they feel they must live and restructure some of the beliefs they have long held. As trust builds within the therapeutic group, these men become increasingly willing to share their personal pain and longings, and they struggle to accept this dimension of themselves. As they become more honest with women, they typically discover that women are more able to accept, respect, and love them. The very traits that men fear to reveal to women are the characteristics that draw others closer to them. This often results in removing some of the barriers that prevent intimacy between the genders.

Groups for men offer some unique advantages in assisting men in clarifying their gender roles and helping them cope with life's struggles. All-male groups provide men with the support they need to become aware of the restrictive rules and roles they may have lived by and provide them with the strength to question the mandate of the masculine role. The group helps men to confront their disappointments and losses and to express a wide range of emotions, from anger to tenderness. Rather than denying past hurt and wounding, members are invited to openly share and explore these experiences and feelings. In a supportive *and* challenging climate, men are able to face their fears of the unknown and to take risks. Although each man must decide what, when, and how to risk, he knows that the group will accept him regardless of the choices he makes (Rabinowitz & Cochran, 2002).

Fredric Rabinowitz (personal communication, September 23, 2007) has conducted men's groups for more than 21 years in his private practice and has observed the following recurrent themes and topics:

▸ What it means to trust other men

▸ How our relationships with parents and siblings affect our current relationships

▸ What it means to be a father

▸ What we hide from ourselves and others in everyday work environments

▸ How we deal with the loss, depression, and existential anxiety that accompany aging

▸ How our bodies carry the weight of our unexpressed emotions and desires

▸ How our inner judge keeps us from being satisfied with our lives

▸ How the fear of abandonment keeps us from taking risks

▸ Healthy ways to deal with frustration and anger

▸ How we can decide for ourselves what it means to be a man

FEMALE ROLES

Women today are questioning many of the attitudes they have incorporated and are resisting the pressures to conform to traditional gender-role behaviors. They are pursuing careers that in earlier times were closed to them, and more women are working. They are advocating to receive equal pay for equal work. Women are increasingly considering their career priorities and are challenging the traditional feminine working roles. For many women who aspire to a career outside of the home, the new order of preference is a career first and marriage later. Although women now have greater opportunities to expand their career choices, there are still barriers to the changing role of women in the working world. Gender stereotyping is a significant barrier in the workplace that needs to be removed to allow for shared work roles (Zunker, 2012).

Many women are making the choice to postpone marriage and child rearing until they have established themselves in careers, and some are deciding not to have children. Many are balancing both child rearing and a career, and more. Although in the past single women were pressured to give up their single life, choosing a single life is now an acceptable option. Single women are generally well adjusted, and they frequently report being quite satisfied with their single life (Matlin, 2012). Women are increasingly assuming positions of leadership in government and business, and more women are choosing to leave stifling or abusive relationships. In dual-career marriages, responsibilities previously allocated to one gender or the other are now often shared.

Despite these changes, women have not achieved equality with men in American society. For example, the woman's role in family life still places a great share of the responsibility on her. Women tend to be blamed for the breakdown of family solidarity and may be accused of abandoning their children and destroying their family by considering their own needs first. Even when both the woman and man work full time outside the home, the majority of household labor generally falls on the woman (Matlin, 2012). When other family members participate in house work, they still tend to believe they are "helping" the woman with a responsibility that should primarily be hers (McGoldrick et al., 2011b). Women's lives have always required great improvisation, but never more than today.

Like men, women in our society have suffered from gender stereotypes. According to Matlin (2012), gender stereotypes can affect cognitive processes, behavior, and gender identity. People tend to adapt their behavior to fit gender-role expectations, and women have been encouraged to lower their aspirations for achievement in the competitive world. Many women are concerned that they will be perceived as unfeminine if they strive for success with too much zeal. Women pay a price for living by narrowly defined rules of what women should be. Typically, women who achieve career success continue to carry the major responsibilities in juggling three roles—spouse, parent, and worker (Weiten et al., 2012).

Traditional Roles for Women

Traditional gender stereotypes categorize women as passive, dependent, and unaccomplished. But women also operate outside these narrow limits. As is the case for traditional roles for men, the following discussion about stereotypic views of females certainly does not fit every woman. As you examine these stereotypic characteristics of the traditional portrait of femininity, think about your own assumptions about and expectations of women.

▶ *Women are warm, expressive, and nurturing.* In their relationships with other women and men, women are expected to be kind, thoughtful, and caring. Women are so attuned to giving that they often do not allow themselves to receive nurturance or consider their own needs. Until recently, women's development was defined by the men in their lives. Their role was defined by their position in another's life, such as mother, daughter, sister, or grandmother. Rarely has there been acceptance of the notion of a woman having a right to a life for herself (McGoldrick et al., 2011b).

▶ *Women are not aggressive or independent.* If women act in an assertive manner, they may be viewed as being hard, aggressive, and masculine. If women display independence, men may accuse them of trying to "prove themselves" by taking on masculine roles. Those women who are independent often struggle within themselves over being too powerful or not needing others.

▶ *Women are emotional and intuitive.* Women who defy their socialization may have trouble getting their emotional needs recognized. But women can be emotional and rational at the same time. Having an intuitive nature does not rule out being able to think and reason logically.

▶ *Women must not deviate from their female role.* If women venture beyond the boundaries of their expected gender roles and act in a way that is regarded as "unfeminine," they may encounter negative attitudes from men as well as from other women.

▶ *Women are more interested in relationships than in professional accomplishments.* Rather than competing or striving to get ahead, women are expected to maintain relationships. Many women are concerned about the quality of their relationships, but at the same time they are also interested in accomplishing goals they set for themselves.

Some of the problems associated with the traditional female role include diminished career aspirations, juggling multiple roles, and ambivalence about sexuality (Weiten et al., 2012). Just as subscribing to traditional male roles stifles creativity in men, unthinkingly accepting traditional roles can result in greatly restricting women. Indeed, women can be both dependent and independent, give to others and be open to receiving, think and feel, and be tender and firm. Women who are rejecting traditional roles are embracing this complex range of characteristics.

If you are a woman, ask yourself to what degree you are tied to your socialization regarding expected female patterns. What potential conflicts might this create in your life? Now might be a good time to reevaluate your gender-role identity and to consider whether you want to alter your picture of what it means to be a woman.

If you are a man, reflect on the way you think and behave in relation to women and whether you may want to make any changes to your behavior. Consider the flexibility you might gain if women had a wider range of traits and behaviors available to them.

Challenging Traditional Female Roles

Gender stereotypes influence societal practices, discrimination, individual beliefs, and sexual behavior itself. Gender stereotypes are powerful forces of social control, but role expectations that are oppressive and that limit women's achievement can be challenged. Sensitizing ourselves to the process

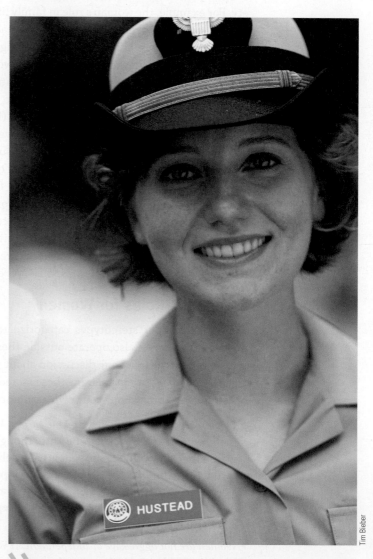

Tim Bieber

》 Women are challenging gender-role stereotypes.

of gender-role development can help us make choices about modifying the results of our socialization. Women are beginning to take actions that grow out of their awareness.

The changing structure of gender relations in recent generations has altered what women expect of themselves and of the role men play in women's lives. A young woman's expectations today may vary significantly from those of her mother or grandmother. As change continues, subsequent generations will look to the women of today for the pattern of their gender relations. Who might those role models be—women who have questioned the status quo and rejected traditional roles or those who walk a different path? Jocelyn describes how she has managed to critically evaluate traditional roles despite her upbringing within a patriarchal family structure.

JOCELYN'S STORY

My dad definitely prided himself on being the breadwinner and problem solver of the family, and my mother seemed to take pride in maintaining a very clean and orderly home. She was expected to be a housewife and take care of my brother and me without developing her own career interests. My parents' roles never seemed to overlap, and I could tell from a young age that my dad had the power in our family and that my mother did not. I never said this out loud, but I remember thinking as a child that I did not want to be like my mother. I didn't want to be subservient to a man; I wanted to have a career so I could have control over my life.

Now as an adult with a professional degree and a career, I often wonder how my mother felt as she catered to my dad's needs. I know she felt angry at him sometimes, but she rarely complained. In some respects, I think my parents found comfort in having such well-defined roles. I would not want to be in my mother's shoes, but I sometimes wish gender roles were a little bit less confusing today. Don't get me wrong. I am grateful that I have more options than women in my mother's generation, but sometimes the expectations get a little fuzzy. For example, my boyfriend, Rob, will soon be earning his law degree, and we are talking about getting married. He wants us to relocate to a bigger city so he will have better job prospects, but I have a well-established veterinary practice in this town. Rob and I talk about being equals, yet it seems that his needs are eclipsing my needs in this regard. Is it unreasonable for me to expect him to find a job at a local law firm when we get married? My mother had to deal with a different kind of pressure than I do, but I am finding that new problems and issues bring their own pressures. I have more of a voice in the family than my mother had, but having a voice can be a source of conflict as Rob and I are finding out when we each want our own way.

Women and Work Choices

A large number of women, even mothers of small children, are now employed in the workplace. Many women work not out of choice but out of necessity. In today's world, few families can afford to have children unless both partners have paid work (McGoldrick, 2011). Some women feel the pressure of taking care of the home and holding down an outside job to help support the family. Women who are employed in satisfying occupations are as healthy and psychologically well adjusted as women who do not work outside the home. Employed women may experience role strains from conflicting responsibilities, but several studies have demonstrated that women's lives are enhanced by employment (Matlin, 2012).

Changes in women's choices are influencing the attitudes of both women and men with respect to work, marriage, family, home, and children.

Single parents often face tremendous pressures in providing for their families and have no viable option other than working. Consider the case of Deborah, who after her divorce said, "I know I can survive, but it's scary for me to face the world alone. Before, my job was an additional source of income and something I did strictly out of choice. Now a job is my livelihood and the means to support my children."

Today women are working in virtually all areas of the economy, but their numbers are still small in jobs traditionally performed by men. Women in traditionally male, high-prestige professions often face discrimination, sexist attitudes, and patronizing behavior (Matlin, 2012). The message is that they are not really equal to men in the same positions. Although women and men should receive equal pay for equal work, this is still not the case. Salary discrimination is a reality for women, and in 2010 U.S. women earned only 77% of the median annual salary of men (National Committee on Pay Equity, 2010).

Increasing numbers of women are postponing marriage and children so they can pursue an education and a career. It appears that homemakers and workers of both genders are returning to school or to work after their 20s to launch new careers. Other women find their fulfillment primarily through the roles of wife, mother, and homemaker, having chosen not to pursue a career and to devote their time to their family. Women who have chosen one path or the other are at times critical of one another. For example, those who decide to be homemakers are often critical of women who work outside the home. Likewise, women who have chosen a career outside the home and who break with the traditional role of women sometimes negatively judge those women who choose homemaking as their primary career.

One woman we know, Valerie, talks about the importance of accepting her choice, despite reactions from others that she should not settle for being "merely" a mother. Valerie and her husband, Phil, had agreed that after they had children both would continue working.

VALERIE'S STORY

When our first child was born, I continued to work as planned. What I had not foreseen was the amount of energy and time it took to care for our son, Dustin. Most important, I hadn't realized how emotionally attached I would become to him. My work schedule was extremely demanding, and I was only able to see Dustin awake for one hour a day.

Phil was being Mr. Mom in the evening until I returned home, which eventually strained our marriage. I felt torn. When I was working, I felt I should be at home. I began to feel jealous of the babysitter, who had more time with Dustin than I did.

When our second son, Vernon, was born, I quit my job. Because we primarily depended on Phil's income, we thought it best that I stay home with our children. Some of my friends are pursuing a career while they take care of a family. For me, it was too difficult to manage both to my satisfaction. It means a lot to me to be involved in my sons' activities and have an influence on their lives. I have been active as a volunteer in their school, which I find very rewarding. Some of my friends cannot understand why I stay home, but I know I'm in the place where I need to be—for them and for me.

I do intend to return to my career once Vernon and Dustin begin high school, and at times I miss the stimulation my job provided. But overall I have no regrets about our decision.

Women in Dual-Career Families

Although a career meets the needs of many women who want something more than taking care of their families, it dramatically increases their responsibilities. Unless their husbands are willing to share in the day-to-day tasks of maintaining a home and rearing children, these women often experience overload, fragmentation, and chronic fatigue. The work of homemakers is relatively invisible, frustrating, and time consuming (Matlin, 2012). Some women burden themselves with the expectation that they should perform perfectly as workers, mothers, and wives—in short, they expect they should be superwomen. Living with perfectionistic standards carries a great cost for women. Eventually, many women realize that they simply cannot continue to balance career and home responsibilities, and they finally exclaim that enough is enough! For women who are trying to do it all, Betty Friedan's advice is worth considering: Yes, women can have it all—just not all at once.

Maureen, a physician, is another woman facing the challenge of a dual career. She holds a teaching position at a hospital. In addition to practicing medicine, she must teach interns, keep current in her field, and publish.

MAUREEN'S STORY

I enjoy pretty much everything I'm doing, but I do feel a lot of pressure in doing all that needs to be done. Much of the pressure I feel is over my conviction that I have to be an outstanding practitioner, teacher, and researcher and must also be fully available as a mother and a wife. There is also pressure from my husband, Daniel, to assume the bulk of the responsibility for taking care of our son and for maintaining the household. With some difficulty Daniel could arrange his schedule to take an increased share of the responsibility, but he expects me to consider his professional career above my own. I need to leave my job early each day to pick up our son from the day care center. I fight traffic and get myself worked up as I try to get to the center before it closes. I put myself under a great deal of stress holding up all my roles. I feel the toll balancing family and work responsibilities is taking on my physical and emotional well-being.

Some women experience a lack of support or actual resistance from the men in their lives when the women step outside traditional roles and exercise their options. Although Maureen did not get much resistance from her husband about maintaining her career, she received very little active support to make balancing her multiple roles possible. The power resided with her husband, and she was expected to make decisions that would not inconvenience him greatly. Husbands who see themselves as liberated are put to the test when they are expected to assume increased responsibilities at home. They may say that they want their wives to "emerge and become fulfilled persons" but also send messages such as "Don't go too far! If you want, have a life outside of the home, but don't give up any of what you are doing at home." A woman who has to fight her husband's resistance may have an even more difficult fight with herself. Both husband and wife may need to reevaluate how realistic it is to expect that she can have a career and also assume the primary responsibility for the children, along with doing all the tasks to keep a home going. Both parties need to redefine and renegotiate what each is willing to do and what each considers essential. It is not uncommon now for a man to be the primary homemaker while the woman devotes most of her time to her work outside the home. Ideally, women and men should be free to choose which, if either, spouse stays at home.

Dual-career couples are often challenged to renegotiate the rules they grew up with and that governed the early phase of their relationship. In dual-career families, both partners must be willing to renegotiate their relationship. Belinda and Burt have tried to establish a more equal partnership. Belinda is a professional woman with a husband and three young children. Her husband, Burt, shows a great deal of interest in Belinda's personal and professional advancement. She often tells her colleagues at work how much support she gets from him. When Bert was offered a higher paying job that entailed a move to another state, he declined the offer after a full discussion with his wife and children. They decided that the move would be too disruptive for all concerned. During the times when Belinda is experiencing the most pressure at work, Bert is especially sensitive and takes on more responsibility for household chores and for taking care of their children. This is an example of a dual-career couple who have created a more equitable division of responsibilities.

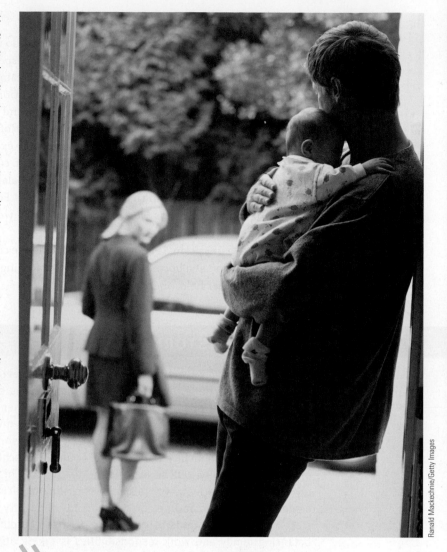

Ranald Mackechnie/Getty Images

》 Women in dual-career families can face high self-expectations.

Just as a woman can question the traditional female stereotype, she can also question the myth that a successful and independent woman doesn't need anyone and can make it entirely on her own. This trap is very much like the trap that many males fall into and may even represent an assimilation of traditional male values. Ideally, a woman will learn that she can achieve independence, exhibit strength, and succeed while at times being dependent and in need of nurturing. Real strength allows either a woman or a man to be needy and to ask for help without feeling personally inadequate.

Relationships are often challenged as one person in the relationship moves beyond restrictive role conformity. Guiza is one of the many women struggling to break out of rigid traditional roles and move toward greater choice and self-expression. She describes the nature of her struggle.

GUIZA'S STORY

In high school I was an exceptional student and had aspirations to go to college, but I was discouraged by my family. Instead, they encouraged me to marry the man I had been dating through high school, letting me know that I would risk losing David if I went off to college. My parents told me that David could provide a good future for me and that it was not necessary for me to pursue college or a career. Without much questioning of what I was told, I got married and had two children. Others thought I had a good life, that I was well provided for and that David and I were getting along well. For me, I remember first feeling restless and dissatisfied with my life when my children went to school. David was advancing in his career and was getting most of his satisfaction from his work. Around him, I felt rather dull and had a vague feeling that something was missing from my life. I had never forgotten my aspiration to attend college, and I eventually enrolled. Although David was not supportive initially, he later encouraged me to complete my education.

As I was pursuing my college education, I often had to make difficult choices among multiple and sometimes conflicting roles. Sometimes I felt guilty about how much I enjoyed being away from my family. For the first time in my life I was being known as Guiza and not as someone's daughter, wife, or mother. Although at times David felt threatened by my increasing independence from him, he did like and respect the person I was becoming.

Guiza's situation illustrates that women can successfully shed traditional roles they have followed for many years and define new roles for themselves. Some of the themes that she and many women like her struggle with are finding a livable balance between dependence and independence, dealing with fears of success, looking outside of herself for support and direction, expecting to be taken care of, and questioning the expectations of others.

TAKE TIME TO REFLECT

1. Examine your beliefs regarding the roles of women. Write the number of the response that most closely reflects your viewpoint on the line at the left of each statement. Use a 5-point scale, with 5 indicating strong agreement and 1 indicating strong disagreement.

_____ Women's socialization discourages achievement in a competitive world.

_____ Like men, women pay a price for living by narrowly defined rules of what women should be.

_____ Many women are labeled unfeminine if they strive for success, especially by men.

_____ Women are naturally more nurturing than men.

_____ Women tend to respond emotionally to a situation, and because of that they are often considered to be irrational.

_____ Women are still subject to discrimination in our society.

_____ Women have more opportunity today to attain equality with men in the workplace.

_____ Most women tend to feel more fulfilled if they work in and out of the home.

_____ Many women today reject rigid gender roles.

2. What challenges must women face in dual-career families? What challenges do men face in dual-career families?_____

_____

_____

3. What challenges do marriages face in dual-career families?_____

_____

_____

4. What are your thoughts about the price women must pay for accepting traditional roles?

_____

_____

5. What specific qualities do you most respect in women? _____

_____

_____

6. As you reflect on your life, what family scripts did you learn about gender roles? _____

_____

_____

ALTERNATIVES TO RIGID GENDER-ROLE EXPECTATIONS

We can actively define our own standards of what we want to be like as women or as men. We do not have to uncritically accept roles and expectations that have been imposed on us or remain bound to the effect of our early conditioning—or of our own self-socialization. It is possible for us to begin achieving autonomy in our gender identity by looking at how we have formed our ideals and standards and who our models have been. We can then decide whether these are the standards we want to use in defining our gender-role identity now.

We are in a transitional period in which men and women are redefining themselves and ridding themselves of old stereotypes; yet too often we needlessly fight with each other when we could be helping each other be patient as we learn new patterns of thought and behavior. We are challenged to develop gender empathy for each other. As women and men alike pay closer attention to deeply ingrained attitudes, they may find that they have not caught up emotionally with their intellectual level of awareness.

Monica McGoldrick (2011) maintains that traditional marriage and family patterns are no longer working for women and that women are increasingly refusing to accept the status quo. She contends that we need to work out new equilibriums in relationships that are not based on the patriarchal family hierarchy. She hopes that "both men and women will be able to develop their potential without regard for the constraints of gender stereotyping that have been so constricting of human experience until now" (p. 58).

Androgyny as an Alternative

One alternative to rigid gender stereotypes is the concept of **androgyny,** the blending of typical male and female personality traits and behaviors in the same person. Androgyny refers to the flexible integration of strong masculine and feminine traits in unique ways; androgynous people are able to recognize and express both feminine and masculine dimensions.

To understand androgyny, it is essential to remember that both biological characteristics and learned behavior play a part in how gender roles are actualized. We all secrete both male and female hormones, and we all have both feminine and masculine psychological characteristics, which Carl Jung labeled the *animus* and the *anima.* Taken together, the animus and the anima reflect Jung's conception of humans as androgynous beings. (See Harris [1996] for a more complete discussion of Jung's theory of personality.) Because women share some of the psychological characteristics of men (through their animus) and men possess some feminine aspects (through their anima), both can better understand the other. Jung was insistent that women and men must express both dimensions of their personality to become fully human.

Androgynous individuals are able to adjust their behavior to what the situation requires in integrated and flexible ways. They are not bound by rigid, stereotyped behavior. Androgynous people have a wider range of capacities and can give expression to a richer range of behaviors than those who are entrapped by gender-typed expectations. Thus, they may perceive themselves as being both understanding, affectionate, and considerate and self-reliant, independent, and firm. The same person has the capacity to be an empathic listener to a friend with a problem, a forceful leader when a project needs to be moved into action, and an assertive supervisor.

Crooks and Baur (2011) suggest that androgynous people tend to be flexible and comfortable with their sexuality. Such women and men have the capacity to enjoy both the physical and emotional dimensions of sexual intimacy. Crooks and Baur claim androgynous lovers tend to be comfortable in both initiating and receiving invitations for sexual sharing, and they are probably not restricted by preconceived gender-role notions pertaining to sexuality. Androgynous individuals "can choose to be independent, assertive, nurturing, or tender, based not on gender-role norms but rather what provides them and others with optimum personal satisfaction in a given situation" (p. 144).

Matlin (2012) believes contemporary psychologists are disenchanted with androgeny and argues that the concept of androgeny has several problems. For example, androgeny leads us to believe that the solution to gender bias is centered within the individual, whereas a proper focus should be on reducing institutional sexism and discrimination against women.

Masculinity and femininity continue to be regarded as distinctive and separate ways of behaving, yet such a dualistic view of human personality is not supported by evidence. Julia (2000) points out that the concept of gender is rooted in the premise that the sexes are diametrically defined as "female" and "male." Gender-role socialization reinforces distinct and often unequal sets of behaviors for each gender. But there are wide individual differences within genders as well as across genders. In reality we are multidimensional beings, and polarities of behavioral traits are rare. People do have both feminine and masculine aspects within them. To become fully human, we need to realize the rich and complex dimensions of our being.

Gender-Role Transcendence

Gender-role transcendence involves going beyond the rigid categories of masculine and feminine to achieve a personal synthesis that allows for flexible behaviors in various situations. According to Weiten et al. (2012), "the **gender-role transcendence** perspective proposes that to be fully human, people need to move beyond gender roles as a way of organizing their perceptions of themselves and others" (p. 364). Basow (1992) suggests that we need to define healthy human functioning independently of gender-related characteristics: "When gender transcendence occurs, people can be just people—individuals in their own right, accepted and evaluated on their own terms" (p. 327).

When individuals go beyond the restrictions imposed by gender roles and stereotypes, they experience a sense of uniqueness because each person has different capabilities and interests. The transcendence model separates personality traits from biological sex. Those who advocate gender-role transcendence claim that this practice will enable individuals to free themselves from linking specific behavior patterns with a gender. If there were less emphasis on gender as a means of categorizing traits, each individual's capabilities and interests would assume more prominence, and individuals would be freer to develop their own unique potentials (Weiten et al., 2012).

TAKE TIME TO REFLECT

1. The following statements may help you assess how you see yourself in relation to gender roles. Place a "T" before each statement that generally applies to you and an "F" before each one that generally does not apply to you. Be sure to respond as you are now rather than as how you would like to be.

_____ Under pressure I tend to withdraw rather than express myself.

_____ I'm more an active person than a passive person.

_____ I'm more cooperative than I am competitive.

_____ I have clear gender expectations.

_____ Under pressure I tend to be competitive.

_____ I see myself as possessing both masculine and feminine characteristics.

_____ I'm adventurous in most situations.

_____ I feel OK about expressing difficult feelings.

_____ I'm very success-oriented.

_____ I fear making mistakes.

Now look over your responses. Which characteristics, if any, would you like to change in yourself?

_____

_____

2. What are your reactions to the changes in women's views of their gender role? What impact do you think the feminist movement has had on women? On men?

_____

_____

3. Would you like to possess more of the qualities you associate with the other sex? If so, what are they? Are there any ways in which you feel limited or restricted by rigid gender-role definitions and expectations?

_____

_____

SUMMARY

The gender-role standard of our culture has encouraged a static notion of clear roles into which all biological males and females must fit. Masculinity has become associated with power, authority, and mastery; femininity has become associated with passivity, subordination, and nurturance. These concepts of masculinity and femininity are historically and socially conditioned. They are not part of a woman's or a man's basic nature.

Many men have become prisoners of a stereotypical role that they feel they must live by. Writers who address the problems of traditional male roles have focused on characteristics such as independence, aggressiveness, worldliness, directness, objectivity, activity, logic, denial of fears, self-protection, lack of emotional expressiveness, lack of bodily awareness, denial of "feminine" qualities, rigidity, obsession with work, and fear of intimacy. An increasing number of men are questioning the restrictions of these traditional roles. Books on men's issues describe the challenges men face in breaking out of rigid roles and defining themselves in new ways.

Women, too, have been restricted by their cultural conditioning and by accepting gender-role stereotypes that keep them in an inferior position. Adjectives often associated with women include gentle, tactful, neat, sensitive, talkative, emotional, unassertive, indirect, and caring. Too often women have defined their own preferences as being the same as those of their partners, and they have had to gain their identity by protecting, helping, nurturing, and comforting. Despite the staying power of these traditional female role expectations, more and more women are rejecting the limited vision of what a woman "should be." Like men, they are gaining increased intellectual awareness of alternative roles, yet they often struggle emotionally to feel and act in ways that differ from their upbringing. Many of us are faced with keeping pace on an emotional level with what we know intellectually about living more freely.

We described androgyny as one path toward uprooting gender-role stereotypes. However, it is not the only way, or even the best way, to bring about this change. One important way to change gender-role expectations is by focusing on systemic change aimed at reducing institutional sexism. Ideally, you will be able to transcend rigid categories of "femininity" and "masculinity" and achieve a personal synthesis whereby you can behave responsively as a function of the situation. It is up to you to choose the kind of woman or man you want to be rather than to uncritically accept a cultural stereotype or blindly identify with some form of rebellion. When you examine the basis of your gender-role identity and your concept of what constitutes a woman or a man, you can decide for yourself what kind of person you want to be instead of conforming to the expectations of others.

In this chapter we have encouraged you to think about your attitudes and values concerning gender roles and to take a close look at how you developed them. Even though cultural pressures are strong toward adopting given roles as a woman or a man, we are not cemented into a rigid way of being. With awareness, we can challenge role expectations that restrict us and determine whether the costs of having adopted certain roles are worth the potential gains.

Where Can I Go From Here?

1. Write down the characteristics you associate with being a woman (or feminine) and being a man (or masculine). Then think about how you acquired these views and to what degree you are satisfied with them.

2. Men and women are challenging traditional roles. Based on your own observations, to what extent do you find this to be true? Do your friends typically accept traditional roles, or do they tend to challenge society's expectations?

3. Interview some people from a cultural group different from your own. Describe some of the common gender stereotypes mentioned in this chapter and determine if such stereotypes are true of the other cultural group.

4. List your gender-role models; include those close to you as well as prominent people you do not know personally. Explain why they are your gender-role models. What traits do they have in common? In what ways do you want to be more like them? Are there ways in which you are already like them?

5. For a week or two, pay close attention to the messages you see on television, both in programs and in commercials, regarding gender roles and expectations of women and men. Record your impressions in the journal pages at the end of this chapter.

6. Suggested Readings. The full bibliographic entry for each of these sources can be found in the References and Suggested Readings at the back of the book. For books that deal with how boys are socialized into manhood, see Real (1998) and Pollack (1998). For a treatment of separate gender worlds and how to bring women and men together, see Philpot, Brooks, Lusterman, and Nutt (1997). For a discussion on psychotherapy with men, see Rabinowitz and Cochran (2002).

WEBSITE RESOURCES

Included here are some valuable websites. For access to these websites, video activities, and other supporting materials, visit Cengage Learning's Counseling CourseMate website for *I Never Knew I Had a Choice*, 10th Edition, at **www.cengagebrain.com.**

SOCIETY FOR THE PSYCHOLOGICAL STUDY OF MEN AND MASCULINITY (SPSMM)
www.apa.org/about/division/div51.html

Recommended Search Words: "APA division 51"

A division of the American Psychological Association, SPSMM promotes the "critical study of how gender shapes and constricts men's lives" and is "committed to the enhancement of men's capacity to experience their full human potential." This site presents contemporary psychological approaches to masculinity and includes extensive links to other related resources.

GENDER AND RACE IN MEDIA
www.uiowa.edu/~commstud/resources/ GenderMedia

Recommended Search Words: "University of Iowa gender and race resources"

The University of Iowa's Communication Studies program presents a number of articles and links about the ways in which gender and racial differences are expressed in various media, including advertising, cyberspace, feminist media, print media, television and film, and mixed media.

THE WELLESLEY CENTERS FOR WOMEN
www.wcwonline.org

Recommended Search Words: "Wellesley centers for women"

The Wellesley Centers for Women works with the Center for Research on Women and the Stone Center for Developmental Services and Studies by "facilitating the development of new research, increasing efficiency, and expanding the Centers' outreach." It shares with them "a joint mission to educate, inform and expand the ways we think about women in the world." Resources for research and publications for purchase are offered.

WOMEN'S STUDIES DATABASE
www.mith2.umd.edu/WomensStudies

Recommended Search Words: "University of Maryland women's studies"

This resource has links to many different areas of interest including conferences, computing, employment, government and history, film reviews, program support, and publications.

FEMINIST MAJORITY FOUNDATION ONLINE
www.feminist.org

Recommended Search Words: "feminist majority foundation"

This site offers many links to a variety of feminist issues including news and events, the National Center for Women and Policing, global feminism, and a feminist online store.

GENDER TALK
www.gendertalk.com

Recommended Search Words: "gender talk"

This site provides explanations and challenges to conventional attitudes about gender issues and gender identity.

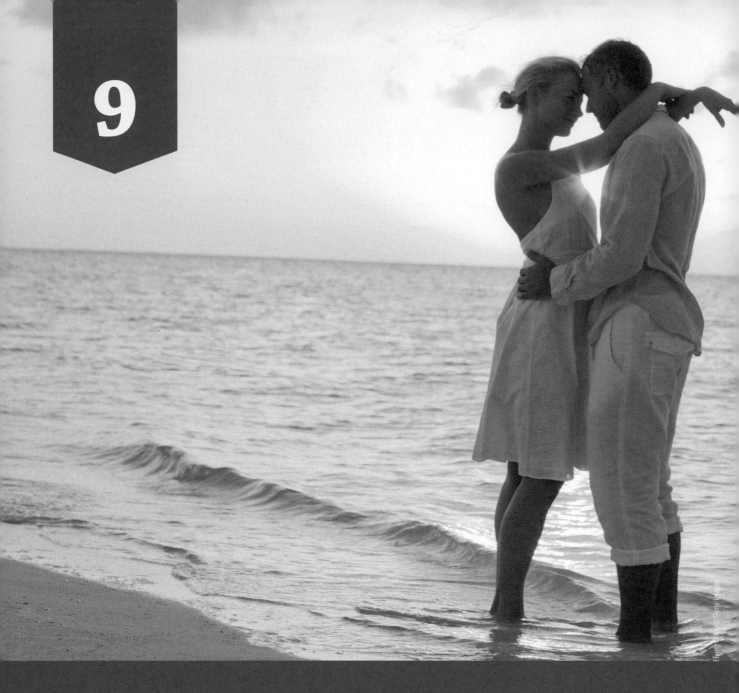

9

SEXUALITY

> Where Am I Now?

> Learning to Talk Openly About Sexual Issues

> Developing Your Sexual Values

> Guilt and Misconceptions About Sex

> Learning to Enjoy Sensuality and Sexuality

> The Healthy Dimensions of Sexuality

> Sex and Intimacy

> The Controversy Over Sexual Addiction

> The Hazards of Unprotected Sex

> Summary

> Where Can I Go From Here?

> Website Resources

Flying Colours/Getty Images

> *It is no easier to achieve sexual autonomy than it is to achieve autonomy in other areas of your life.*
>
> —C. MOORE/CORBIS

WHERE AM I NOW?

Use this scale to respond to these statements:

4 = I *strongly agree* with this statement.
3 = I *agree* with this statement.
2 = I *disagree* with this statement.
1 = I *strongly disagree* with this statement.

1. The quality of a sexual relationship usually relates to the general quality of the relationship.

2. I find it easy to talk openly and honestly about sexuality with my friends.

3. For me, sex without love is unsatisfying.

4. I experience guilt or shame over sexuality.

5. Gender-role definitions and stereotypes affect sexual relationships.

6. Sensual experiences differ from sexual experiences.

7. Performance expectations get in the way of my enjoying sensual and sexual experiences.

8. I am clear about my own values and how they affect my sexual behavior.

9. I acquired healthy attitudes about sexuality from my parents.

10. I am concerned and knowledgeable about HIV/AIDS and other sexually transmitted illnesses.

I t a paradox: we are bombarded with sexual images in advertising, yet talking about sexuality in a personal way is difficult for many of us. An important part of personal growth entails reflecting on your beliefs regarding sexuality. Open discussions with those you are intimate with, and with others whom you trust, can do a lot to help you evaluate the unexamined attitudes and values you may have about this significant area in your life. The goals for this chapter are to help you identify or clarify the beliefs, attitudes, and values you hold regarding your sexuality and to help you evaluate whether your sexual behavior is consistent with your beliefs, attitudes, and values.

Sex can be a positive or a negative force, depending on how it is expressed. At its best, sexuality can contribute to your physical and psychological well-being: it can be a source of joy and pleasure and an expression of love, and it can provide an intimate connection to others. At its worst, sex can be used to hurt others or to sabotage yourself: it can lead to guilt, shame, anxiety, and inhibition; and it can be a source of pain and disconnection from others. Sexual coercion is one way sex can be misused to exploit and harm others, and sexual addiction can cause harm to you. In addition, HIV/AIDS and other sexually transmitted infections are a real threat to anyone who practices unprotected sex. If you are a sexually active person, you owe it to yourself and to your partners to take an honest look at how you express your sexuality. These are the topics we address in this chapter.

LEARNING TO TALK OPENLY ABOUT SEXUAL ISSUES

People of all ages can experience difficulty talking openly about sexual matters, which contributes to the perpetuation of myths and misinformation about sexuality. Childhood socialization that entails a lack of communication about sexual matters can lead to later difficulties in communicating with a partner about sex. Increased media saturation of sexualized images has not resulted in more people talking more freely about their own sexual desires and concerns, nor has it reduced people's anxiety about sexuality. For many, sex remains a delicate topic, and people find it difficult to communicate their sexual wants, especially to a person close to them.

Crooks and Baur (2011) suggest that open communication contributes to the enjoyment of a sexual relationship and that the basis for effective sexual communication is **mutual empathy**—the awareness that each partner in the relationship cares for the other and knows that this care is reciprocated. Carroll (2013) stresses the role of good communication skills in developing healthy, satisfying relationships, including sexual relationships. Carroll adds that by talking in an honest and open way with your partner, you are able to share your sexual needs and desires, and you can learn what your partner's emotional and sexual needs are in turn. She acknowledges how difficult it is to talk about sexuality, yet says that talking about sex is a good way to move a relationship to a new level of intimacy and connection.

Although people may have a greater awareness of sexuality today, this knowledge does not always translate into a more satisfying sex life. Couples are often very uncomfortable communicating their sexual likes and dislikes, as well as their personal concerns about sex. Some people think that if their partner really loves them he or she should know intuitively how to respond sexually.

Students may discuss attitudes about sexual behavior in a general way, but they often show considerable hesitancy and embarrassment in speaking of their own sexual concerns, fears, and conflicts. If the topic of sexuality is discussed in the classroom, it is of the utmost importance that appropriate boundaries be established and respected. Although many students want to find out how others think about sexual issues, some have reservations about sharing such deeply personal matters. Students should never be pressured to disclose their personal experiences regarding their sexual attitudes and behavior. Many cultural differences exist about the norms pertaining to talking about sexual topics in public. Within the same culture and between different cultures, variation exists in how free people are to talk about sexual topics. The religious, cultural, and moral values of students need to be taken into consideration when facilitating discussions about sexuality in the classroom. As you can see in Marguerita's story, these values can influence how comfortable someone is in discussing sexuality outside the classroom, even among friends.

MARGUERITA'S STORY

As a Latina, I have been surprised by the openness with which my college friends talk about sexuality. In my family and culture, I am expected to remain a virgin until I get married; however, it seems that many of the young women my age in college don't share that value. A few of them have talked about hooking up with guys they hardly know. Sometimes that makes me feel awkward. If I tell them I have never had sex, they may think I am prudish. I don't think of myself that way, but I am not certain they would understand my reasons for wanting to wait until I am married. So I just listen to them as they talk about their sexual encounters and hope that they don't ask me directly about my experiences.

In the therapeutic groups that we lead, we take great care to create a safe and trusting climate that will be conducive for members to discuss whatever personal concerns (including sexuality) they bring to the group. When women and men are given the opportunity to talk about their concerns in a direct way, they often experience a sense of relief through hearing from others. Here are some of the concerns related to sexuality expressed by the participants in our therapeutic groups:

▶ I often wonder what excites my partner and what she [he] would like, yet I seldom ask. Am I responsible if my partner is dissatisfied?

▶ I am concerned about sexually transmitted infections.

▶ Sex can be fun, I suppose, but it is really difficult for me to be playful and spontaneous.

▶ I would really like to know how other women feel after a sexual experience.

▶ As a man, I frequently worry about performance expectations, and that gets in the way of my making love.

▶ When I feel stressed and tired, I am less interested in sex.

▶ When my partner and I have conflicts, it is difficult to initiate sex.

▶ There are times when I become involved in a sexual relationship because I feel lonely.

▶ There are times when I really do not want intercourse but would still like to be held and touched and caressed. I wish my partner could understand this about me and not take it as a personal rejection.

These are a few of the common concerns people express about sexuality. Knowing that others have similar concerns can help people to feel less alone with their anxieties about sexuality. As the comments show, discussions on sexual topics are not limited to the sexual act but encompass a range of personal feelings related to sexuality. Look over the list and identify the statements that seem to fit for you. Ask yourself if you are ready to reexamine your beliefs about some of these issues.

DEVELOPING YOUR SEXUAL VALUES

How you express your sexuality is influenced by your values. As adults, most of us make choices regarding our sexual behavior. However, for some adults, cultural and religious values determine acceptable sexual behavior. Whatever situation you are in, it is important that your sexual behavior be consistent with your value system. Take a few minutes to reflect on your attitudes about sexual behavior and consider these questions in exploring the pros and cons of being sexually active:

▶ How do I feel about my decision to be sexual or nonsexual?

▶ Does my choice to be sexually active conflict with my religious beliefs or cultural values? If so, how do I reconcile this?

▶ Do I feel pressured into having sex? If so, what can I say or do to feel more empowered and stand my ground?

▶ What are my reasons for choosing to have sex or choosing not to have sex at this time?

▶ Am I willing to talk openly with my partner about sex? If not, what are my reservations?

▶ What do I know about the emotional dimensions of a sexual relationship?

▶ If birth control is an issue, have my partner and I considered options and chosen a safe and effective method?

▶ Am I prepared to discuss and effectively use protection against sexually transmitted infections?

Formulating Your Sexual Values and Ethics

Designing a personal and meaningful set of sexual ethics is not easy. It can be accomplished only through a process of honest questioning. Examine the role of your family of origin and your culture as the background of your sexual ethics. Are the values you received from your family and your culture congruent with your views of yourself in other areas of your life? Which of them are important in enabling you to live responsibly and with enjoyment? Which values might you want to modify?

Developing our personal values means assuming responsibility for ourselves, which includes taking into consideration how others may be affected by our choices. For instance, some people struggle with wanting to be sexual with several partners, even though this behavior goes against their personal value system. Their struggle over giving behavioral expression to their sexual desires may be fraught with guilt because what they are doing is not congruent with their values. In an adult relationship, the parties involved are capable of taking personal responsibility for their own actions. For example, in the case of premarital or extramarital sex, each person must weigh these questions: "Do I really want to pursue a sexual relationship with this person at this time?" "What are some of the possible emotional consequences of getting sexually involved?" "What are my commitments?" "Who else is involved, and who might be affected?" "How does my decision fit in with my values?"

When developing your personal values and behavior regarding sexuality, a key component is taking responsibility for the choices you make. Sexually responsible decisions involve considering the possible consequences of sexual behavior, both for yourself and for your partner. You might ask, "Do I feel enhanced or embarrassed by my past or present experiences?" Consider Zachary's experience.

ZACHARY'S STORY

My parents divorced when I was 12 and it has influenced the way I view relationships today. My father cheated on my mother with his secretary, and I saw how devastated my mother was for years afterward. I have always considered myself to be a person with high moral convictions, and I vowed never to allow myself to follow in my father's footsteps. I have had several long-term relationships, and even though they didn't work out, I was always faithful.

Around a year ago things with my now ex-girlfriend were pretty rocky, and I immersed myself in work as a distraction. I found myself attracted to a coworker who had just gotten out of a bad relationship. We commiserated about our relationship problems over a few drinks one night after work, and one thing led to another. We had sex, and I knew I had made a big mistake almost immediately afterward. Honestly, I think my girlfriend and I were headed for a breakup, but my actions sealed the deal. I confessed to her within days, and she dumped me. I don't blame her; I would have done the same thing.

There is really no excuse for what I did, but it has given me greater insight into what my father did years ago and how he may have felt. As for my own feelings, I have felt tremendous guilt and am working on forgiving myself. I let my ex-girlfriend down, but just as important, I let myself down. If my mother knew, she would be deeply disappointed in me, which really bothers me the most. Before I move on to another relationship or even start dating again, I need to understand how I fell down that slippery slope so history will not repeat itself.

Just as Zachary had to take an honest look at the boundary he crossed, which resulted in violating his own set of sexual values, we can all benefit from examining the congruence between our behavior and the values we hold. Learning to establish your boundaries is of major importance in being true to your own values. Ask yourself, "Can I stand by my convictions and not allow others to persuade me to cross my own sexual boundaries?" If the answer is "no," consider ways to strengthen your boundaries so you can confidently engage in interpersonal relationships without fear that you may compromise your own values. It is important to respect the boundaries of others as you would want them to respect yours.

Sexual Abstinence as an Option

Some people choose **sexual abstinence,** refraining from sexual intercourse until they enter a committed, long-term, monogamous relationship. But what does abstinence really mean? Does it merely mean to abstain from sexual intercourse? The Centers for Disease Control's definition of **abstinence** includes "refraining from sexual activities which involve vaginal, anal, and oral intercourse" (Hales, 2012, p. 294). But Hales points out that abstinence means different things to different people, cultures, and religious groups. Some who decide to be abstinent refrain from all sexual activity. Others may engage in a range of sexual behaviors, such as masturbation, but choose not to engage in interpersonal sexual contact.

Celibacy may be chosen out of moral, cultural, or personal convictions. Some make this choice to prevent pregnancy. Others choose temporary celibacy after a disappointing sexual relationship in the hope of establishing a new relationship without the complication of sex (Crooks & Baur, 2011). Many people who were sexually active in the past are also choosing abstinence because the risks of medical complications associated with sexually transmitted infections increases with the number of sexual partners one has (Hales, 2013). Some decide that the only completely safe route is abstinence.

If you are choosing to be sexually abstinent, it may be important to clarify your own reasons for your choice. Answering these questions can help you understand the values that support your decision: "What meaning do I attach to celibacy?" "Is my choice to be celibate based on a full acceptance of my body?" "Do I believe I am a sexually desirable person?" "Do I fear that being celibate stands in the way of the level of intimacy I desire?"

TAKE TIME TO REFLECT

1. What influences have shaped your attitudes and values concerning sexuality? In the following list, indicate the importance of each factor using this scoring system:

> 1 = This is a *very important* influence.
> 2 = This is a *somewhat important* influence.
> 3 = This is *unimportant* as an influence.

For each item you mark 1 or 2, briefly indicate the nature of that influence.

_____ Parents _____

_____ Spouse/Partner _____

_____ Relatives _____

_____ Friends _taught me to not be sleezy_____

_____ Siblings _____

_____ Your own experiences _it's unattractive_____

_____ Religious background _____

_____ Movies _shows me romantic_____

_____ Music _____

_____ Internet/Social networking sites _____

_____ School _____

_____ Books _____

_____ Magazines _____

_____ Television _____

_____ Other influential factors _____

2. Try making a list of specific values that guide you in dealing with sexual issues. To help you get started, respond to the following questions:

a. How do you feel about sex with multiple partners versus monogamous sex? Give your reasons.

_____

_____

b. What is your view of sex outside of marriage or a committed relationship?

_____

_____

GUILT AND MISCONCEPTIONS ABOUT SEX

Guilt Over Sexual Feelings

Many people express fears as they begin to recognize and accept their sexuality. It is important to learn that we can accept the full range of our sexual feelings yet decide for ourselves what we will do behaviorally. For instance, we remember a man who said that he felt satisfied with his marriage and found his wife exciting but he was troubled because he found other women appealing and sometimes desired them. Even though he had made a decision not to have extramarital affairs, he still experienced a high level of anxiety over having sexual feelings toward other women. At some level he believed he might be more likely to act on his feelings if he fully accepted that he had them. It was important for him to learn to discriminate between having sexual feelings and deciding to take actions to express them.

In making responsible, inner-directed choices about whether to act on your sexual feelings, consider these questions:

▶ Will my actions negatively affect another person or myself?

▶ Will my actions bring me joy?

▶ Will my actions exploit another's rights?

▶ Are my actions consistent with my values and commitments?

Each of us decides our own moral guidelines, but it is unrealistic to expect that we can or should control our feelings in the same way we control our actions. By controlling our actions, we define who we are; by denying our feelings, we become alienated from ourselves.

Guilt Over Sexual Experiences

Some college students, whether single or married, young or middle-aged, report a variety of sexual experiences over which they feel guilt. Guilt may be related to masturbation, extramarital (or "extrapartner") affairs, sexual promiscuity, same-sex behavior, or sexual practices that are sometimes considered abnormal.

Crooks and Baur (2011) present some perspectives on **masturbation,** or self-stimulation of one's genitals for sexual pleasure. Masturbation has been censured throughout Judeo-Christian history, which has resulted in medical misinformation and considerable shame and guilt. In the mid-18th century, the "evils" of masturbation received considerable attention in the name of science. It was thought that those who engaged in this sexual practice would face dire consequences, such as blindness and mental illness. This negative attitude filtered down, and some of the traditional condemnation still exists. Some people avoid masturbation because their religious teachings equate masturbation with morally unacceptable behavior.

Today, this form of sexual expression generally is viewed more positively. According to Crooks and Baur (2011), most men and women, whether they are in a relationship or not, masturbate on occasion. Masturbatory practices are viewed as normal and healthy, unless such practices interfere with mutually enjoyable sexual intimacy in a relationship. It is a mistaken notion that a partner's desire to masturbate is a sign of a troubled relationship. Although masturbation is chosen by many people in various situations for various reasons, it is not something that everyone wants to do. In the attempt to help people assuage guilt over self-stimulation, it may seem that the message is that people *should* masturbate. Crooks and Baur state, "Masturbation is an option for sexual expression, not a mandate" (p. 235).

Our early sexual learning is a crucial factor in later sexual adjustment because current guilt feelings often stem from both unconscious and conscious decisions made in response to verbal and nonverbal messages about sexuality. Peers often fill the void left by parents. However, reliance on the same-sex peer group usually results in learning inaccurate sexual information, which can later lead to fears and guilt over sexual feelings and activities. Most information about sex from the peer group is imparted during the early teen years, which results in us carrying into adulthood many distorted and inaccurate notions about sex.

The media provide information that is often a source of biased learning about sexuality. Children are exposed to material that is inappropriate for their age. This negative information often produces unrealistic and unbalanced attitudes about sexuality and can foster fears and guilt that can have a powerful impact on the ability to enjoy sex as an adult.

Those who have been victimized by sexual coercion often struggle with feelings of guilt, shame, and self-blame (see Chapter 5). These negative experiences can interfere with the ability to enjoy one's sexuality or to form any kind of interpersonal relationships. Those traumatized by any form of sexual coercion should not be blamed for what happened, and they deserve to get help in the healing process.

We acquire a sense of guilt over sexual feelings and experiences as a result of a wide diversity of sources of information and misinformation. Not all guilt is neurotic, nor should it necessarily be eliminated. When we violate our value system, guilt is a consequence. This guilt can serve a useful purpose, motivating us to examine the behavior to determine whether it is congruent with our ethical standards. In freeing ourselves of undeserved guilt, the first step is to become aware of early verbal and nonverbal messages about sexuality and gender-role behavior. Once we become aware of these messages, we can explore them to determine in what ways we might want to modify them.

Misconceptions About Sexuality

Misconceptions flourish in the spaces between what we know to be true (facts based on evidence) and what we assume to be true (unsupported opinions or ideas). The following statements contain misconceptions about sex. As you read over this list, ask yourself what your attitudes are and how you developed these beliefs.

▶ If I allow myself to become sexual, I will get into trouble.

▶ Women are not as sexually desirable when they initiate sex.

▶ If my partner really loved me, I would not have to tell him or her what I liked or wanted.

▶ My partner should know what I need intuitively without my asking.

▶ It is impossible to overcome negative conditioning about sexuality learned in childhood.

▶ Acting without guilt or restrictions is what is meant by being sexually free.

▶ Being sexually attracted to a person other than my partner implies that I don't really find my partner sexually exciting.

▶ Being attracted to someone of the same gender is abnormal.

▶ The more physically attractive a person is, the more sexually exciting he or she is.

▶ With the passage of time, some, if not most, sexual relationships are bound to lose a sense of excitement.

Could any of these statements apply to you? Are your information sources credible, or is it possible you have accepted some ideas based on misinformation? How might some of these statements affect your ability to make choices concerning sexuality?

TAKE TIME TO REFLECT

1. Complete the following statements pertaining to sexuality:

a. I first learned about sex through _____
b. My earliest memory about sex is _____
c. The way this memory affects me now is _____
d. One verbal sexual message I received from my parents was _____
e. One nonverbal sexual message I received from my parents was _____
f. An expectation I have about sex is _____
g. When the topic of sexuality comes up, I usually _____
h. While I was growing up, a sexual taboo I internalized was _____

2. Are there any steps you would like to take toward learning to accept your body and your sexuality more than you do now? If so, what are they?

_____

_____

3. Do you experience guilt over sexual feelings or experiences? If so, what specific feelings or experiences lead to guilt?

_____

_____

4. How openly are you able to discuss sexuality in a personal way? Would you like to be more open in discussing your sexuality or sexual issues? If so, what is preventing this openness?

_____

_____

5. How have your cultural, spiritual, and religious background and values affected your view of sex?

_____

_____

LEARNING TO ENJOY SENSUALITY AND SEXUALITY

Sensual experiences involve all of our senses and can be enjoyed separately from sexual experiences. Although sexuality involves sensual experiences, **sensuality** does not have to include sexual activity.

Performance standards and expectations often get in the way of sensual and sexual pleasure, particularly for men. Some men measure themselves by unrealistic standards. In spite of the availability of drugs such as Viagra and Cialis, men continue to be concerned about their ability to respond sexually. Instead of enjoying sexual and sensual experiences, many men become fixated on the **orgasm,** an intense sensation during the peak of sexual arousal that results in the release of sexual tension (Carroll, 2013). For some men, the fact that they or their partner experiences an orgasm signifies that they have performed perfectly. They may expect their partner always to have an orgasm during intercourse, primarily out of their need to see themselves as good lovers. For example, Roland stated in his human sexuality class that he would not continue to date a woman who did not have an orgasm with him. Several of the other male students were in full agreement with Roland's attitude. With this type of orientation toward sex, it is not surprising that these men have problems with intimacy.

Listening to Our Bodies

Erectile dysfunction (ED) is the consistent inability to achieve and maintain an erection necessary for adequate sexual relations. Men may be unable to achieve or maintain an erection on occasion for a number of reasons, including fatigue and stress. In as many as 80% of cases of ED, there is a physical reason (Hales, 2013), and sometimes this is due to circulatory issues or to the side effects of certain prescription drugs

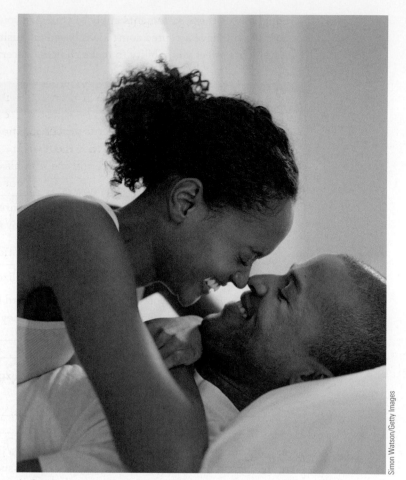

Simon Watson/Getty Images

》 Intimacy can be conceived of as a close emotional relationship and is a basic component of all loving relationships.

or alcohol. Organic causes of ED include cardiovascular disease, diabetes, kidney disease, and neurological and hormonal issues. In these cases it is important to consult with a physician about possible remedies. In addition, ED may be due to psychological factors such as feelings of guilt, prolonged depression, hostility or resentment, anxiety about personal adequacy, fear of pregnancy, or a generally low level of self-esteem. Men who experience erectile dysfunction might ask themselves, "What is my body telling me?"

Some women have difficulty responding sexually too, especially experiencing orgasm. This is often due to unrealistic expectations, which affect sexual behavior and intimacy. Stress is also a major factor that can easily interfere with being in a frame of mind that will allow a woman's body to respond. This is particularly true if the couple engages in sex late at night when they are both tired or if they have been under considerable stress. If the woman's body is not responding, it could well be a sign that stress and fatigue are making it difficult for her to relax and give in to a full psychological and physical release. Rather than interpreting her lack of responsiveness as a sign of sexual inadequacy, she would be wise to pay attention to what her body is expressing. Her body is probably saying, "I'm too tired to enjoy this." For an in-depth discussion of this subject, we recommend *For Women Only: A Revolutionary Guide to Overcoming Sexual Dysfunction and Reclaiming Your Sex Life* by Jennifer Berman and Laura Berman (2001), which addresses female sexual arousal and treatments for sexual problems.

Asking for What We Want

Paying attention to the messages of our body is a first step. We still need to learn how to express to our partner specifically what we like and enjoy sexually. Many women and men keep their sexual wishes to themselves instead of sharing them with their partner. They have accepted the misconception that their partner should know intuitively what they like, and they resist telling their partner what feels good to them out of fear that their lovemaking will become mechanical or that their partner will only be trying to please them.

Often a woman will complain that she does not derive as much enjoyment from sex as she might because the man is too concerned with his own pleasure. She may desire considerable foreplay and afterplay, but her partner may not recognize her needs. Therefore, it may be helpful for her to express to him what it feels like to be left unsatisfied. It is essential to consider the cultural context, for in some cultures there is an injunction against women asking for what they want in a sexual relationship.

It is not uncommon for a woman to ask a question such as, "Does touching always have to lead to sex?" She is probably implying that there is a significant dimension missing for her in lovemaking—namely, the sensual aspect. The case of Tiffani and Ron illustrates this common conflict in lovemaking.

TIFFANI'S STORY

Anytime I want to be affectionate with Ron, he wants to have sexual intercourse. I really resent Ron's inability to respond to my need for affection without making a sexual demand. When I sense that Ron wants to be sexual with me, I start a fight to create distance. In turn, he feels rejected, humiliated, and angry. I want to feel close to Ron both physically and emotionally, but his all-or-nothing response makes me afraid to be affectionate with him.

It is important to learn how to negotiate for what you want. Being sensual is an important part of a sexual experience. Sensuality pertains to fully experiencing all of our senses, not just sensations in our genitals. Many parts of the body are sensual and can contribute to our enjoyment of sex. Although there is great enjoyment in the orgasmic experience, many people are missing out on other sources of enjoyment by not giving pleasure to themselves and their partners with other forms of stimulation. A range of sexual behavior is open to couples if they make their expectations clear and if they talk about sexuality as part of their relationship.

THE HEALTHY DIMENSIONS OF SEXUALITY

Sexuality can bring us pleasure, and it is also a healthy dimension of our lives. Jannini, Fisher, Bitzer, and McMahon (2009) state that "sexual health correlates so much with general health that the former can be considered an efficient marker of the latter" (pp. 2641–2642). One long-term study found that "men who had fewer orgasms were twice as likely to die of any cause compared to those having two or more orgasms a week" (p. 2642). Based on a summary of research, these authors suggest that high ejaculation frequency might be associated with a lower risk of total and organ-confined prostate cancer. They also note that women's health tends to be positively influenced by endocrine events and physical and emotional reactions associated with sexual activity. Specifically, they note that oxytocin and dopamine secretions, which occur during orgasm, may change the internal neuroendocrine milieu involved in general affective states, possibly reducing the risk of depression. In a more recent study aimed at distinguishing the health benefits of different sexual activities, Brody (2010) discovered that "a wide range of better psychological and physiological health indices are associated specifically with penile-vaginal intercourse" (p. 1336). Sexuality is a fundamental aspect of being human, and as such it is vital to our mental and physical functioning.

SEX AND INTIMACY

Intimacy is a close emotional relationship characterized by a deep level of caring for another person and is a basic component of all loving relationships. Positive sexual experiences contribute to our deepest need to connect to another person. In our discussions with college students, we often hear that they are seeking to be loved by a special person, and they want to trust giving their love in return. Crooks and Baur (2011) cite studies suggesting that although there are gender differences regarding ways of viewing sex and love, people generally value love and affection in sexual relationships. The attributes that both men and women rank as being important include good communication, commitment, and a high quality of emotional and physical intimacy. Two excellent resources for a very comprehensive treatment of all aspects of human sexuality are Janell Carroll's (2013) *Sexuality Now: Embracing Diversity* and Robert Crooks and Karla Baur's (2011) *Our Sexuality*.

Some people engage in sex without being in love, and many forms of intimate relationships do not involve sex (see Chapter 7). Crooks and Baur (2011) raise the question "What is the relationship between love and sex?" and conclude that the connection is not always clear. Sex without love is a relatively common practice, and love can exist independent of any sexual expression.

Take a moment to reflect on what sex means to you and how sex can be used to either enhance or diminish you and your partner. Is sex a form of stress release? Does it make you feel secure? Loved? Accepted? Nurtured? Is it fun? Does it signify commitment? Is it abusive? Pleasurable? Is it shameful or positive? Ask yourself, "Are my intimate relationships based on a genuine desire to become intimate, to share, to experience joy and pleasure, to both give and receive?"

Asking yourself what you want in your relationships and what value sex serves for you may also help you avoid the overemphasis on technique and performance that frequently detracts from sexual experiences. Although technique and knowledge are important, they are not ends in themselves, and overemphasizing them can cause us to become oblivious to the needs of our partner. An abundance of anxiety over performance and technique can only impede sexual enjoyment and rob us of the experience of genuine intimacy and caring.

Examine where your views about sex come from and the meaning you attach to sexuality. Knowing where you stand can make it easier to make choices about what you want sexually.

Enjoying Sexual Intimacy in Later Life

One common misconception is that people no longer engage in sexual intimacy as they get older. This mistaken notion persists quite possibly because our society equates sexuality with youth (Carroll, 2013). Crooks and Baur (2011) point out that the number of people who engage in sexual activity decreases with each decade, but "many people remain sexually active well into their 80s and even later" (p. 396). Poor health is the factor that carries the most weight in influencing one's level of sexual activity in older adulthood. In long-term relationships, "the

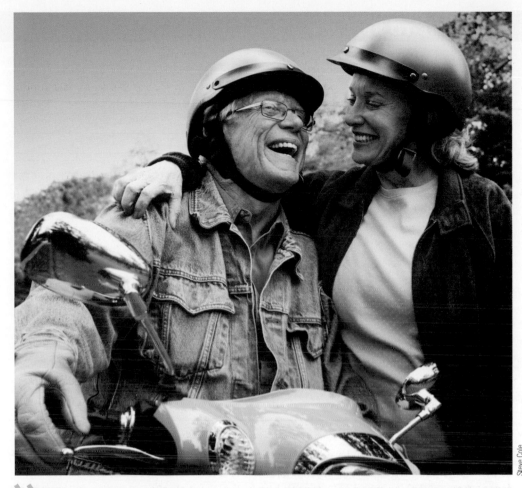

>> Enjoying intimacy and sexuality later in life can be an important part of a relationship.

Steve Cole

poor health and loss of sexual interest by one person limits the partner's sexual expression as well" (p. 397). Rosemary, in her mid-60s, shares her feelings about how difficult it has been to adjust to her husband's declining health and decreasing interest in sexual intimacy.

ROSEMARY'S STORY

I sometimes feel guilty that I am angry at Alfred for getting sick. Honestly, sometimes I resent that he didn't take better care of himself over the past couple of decades. I suppose the warning signs are easy to ignore if they are not severe enough. It's human nature; but he now suffers from a number of physical ailments that prevent him from feeling well enough to engage in the kind of activities that I enjoy. Now that the kids are grown and have their own lives, and now that Alfred and I are both retired, we could be taking trips that we always wanted to take. And although I don't ordinarily talk about these matters, I was looking forward to rekindling our intimacy now that we have more free time. But he will have nothing to do with it! He seems like a grouchy old man, not the Alfred that I fell in love with nearly 40 years ago. I am not ready to live like a nun, but Alfred seems so disconnected from his sexuality. I'm not sure what to do about that.

1. Complete the following sentences:

a. To me, being sensual means _____

b. To me, being sexual means _____

c. Sex without intimacy is _____

d. Sex can be a disappointing experience when _____

e. Sex can be most fulfilling when _____

2. Look over the following list, quickly checking the words that you associate with sex:

___ fun   ___ pressure

___ ecstasy   ___ performance

___ procreation   ___ experimentation

___ beautiful   ___ routine

___ duty   ___ closeness

___ trust   ___ release

___ shameful   ___ vulnerability

___ joy

Now look over the words you have checked and see whether there are any significant patterns in your responses. Are there any other words you associate with sex? Summarize your attitudes toward sex.

_____

_____

3. Imagine that you are an older adult. How do you think you will express your sexuality as you age? If either you or your partner becomes less interested in sexual activity for any reason, how might you communicate with him or her about that?

_____

_____

THE CONTROVERSY OVER SEXUAL ADDICTION

Inundated with seemingly countless new sex-related websites on a daily basis, the Internet generates $13 billion each year from people in search of sex (Ropelato, 2006), so it is not surprising that we are seeing an increase in problematic sexual behaviors (Carnes, 2003). The sexual escapades of high-profile married men are a hot topic on cable news shows, and the term *sexual addiction* has become a buzzword in society. However, there is no consensus among mental health professionals and sexologists as to whether this is the most appropriate way to describe the behavior of one who is obsessed with sex.

Having recurrent and intense sexual urges, fantasies, and behaviors that tend to interfere with a person's daily functioning is commonly referred to as **compulsive sexual behavior** (Carroll, 2013). However, "the official proposal of Hypersexual Disorder [has been] submitted for the new Diagnostic and Statistical Manual of Mental Disorders [DSM–V]" (Woody, 2011, p. 301). Although the debate continues regarding the terminology and definition of sexual addiction, without question this is not a problem only experienced by people in the media spotlight.

Early estimates of sexual addiction for the online population were 3 to 5%, but Weiss and Samenow (2010) state "that those numbers may now be rapidly escalating related to the increasing accessibility of online sexual content and the immediate connectivity now provided by Smartphones and social networks" (p. 241). In a recent study, Wetterneck, Burgess, Short, Smith, and Cervantes (2012) found that "the more hours per week an individual views IP [Internet pornography], the more they report sexual urges and problems with sexual compulsivity. Additionally, as use of IP increases, impulsivity and use of avoidant coping methods increase and individuals report both more perceived positive and negative effects of IP use" (p. 9). They suggest that "like substance abusers, problematic IP users who experience negative outcomes may continue to use IP due to the positive reinforcement (i.e., sexual gratification or perceived enhancement of relationships) they receive from its use" (p. 12).

Could you determine whether you, your partner, or someone you know is hypersexual (or is addicted to sex)? What would you do if you suspected your intimate partner was addicted to sex or to Internet pornography? If you do not believe sex can become an addiction, what do you think are the causes of problematic sexual behavior?

THE HAZARDS OF UNPROTECTED SEX

There are many positive aspects of sexuality, but we would be remiss if we failed to discuss the risks of participating in unprotected sex. As a responsible adult, it is imperative that you make informed choices about your sexual behavior. To safeguard your well-being, you need to be aware of the potential consequences of having unprotected sex. You are not safeguarded from HIV/AIDS and other sexually transmitted infections if you choose to participate in risky, unprotected sexual acts.

HIV/AIDS

If you have not already done so, you will inevitably come in contact with people who have tested positive for HIV, people who have AIDS, people who have had sexual contact with someone who has tested HIV-positive, and people who are close to individuals with HIV or AIDS.

AIDS affects a wide population and will continue to be a major health problem. You need to be able to differentiate between fact and fiction about the virus and about this disease. You simply cannot afford to be unaware of the personal and societal implications of this epidemic. Unless you are educated about the problem, you are more likely to engage in risky behaviors or live needlessly in fear. Accurate information is vital if you are to deal with the personal and societal implications of the AIDS epidemic. Since HIV/AIDS was first discovered, a great deal has been learned about the subject, and new information continues to expand our knowledge base.

Ignorance and fear of AIDS is fueled by misinformation about the ways in which the disease is spread, but there is no reason to remain ignorant today. The basic information you need about this disease and how to prevent it is readily available from your doctor, your state or local health department, your local chapter of the American Red Cross, and the Centers for Disease Control and Prevention (CDC) National Center for HIV/AIDS, Viral Hepatitis, STD, and TB Prevention. These sources offer free written material, updated information, and answers to your questions about what HIV/AIDS is, how it is transmitted and spread, who is most at risk for contracting HIV, what the most promising treatments are, and what you can do to protect yourself. Become informed, then make an honest inventory of your sexual practices and drug use that might put you at greater risk of contracting HIV. By examining your attitudes, values, and fears, you will be better equipped to make informed, wise choices.

Other Sexually Transmitted Infections

Unprotected sexual practices frequently result in contracting some form of sexually transmitted infection (STI) other than HIV/AIDS. Some of the more common STIs include human papillomavirus (HPV), which can lead to cervical cancer in women and genital warts and other forms of cancer in both sexes, genital herpes, chlamydia, gonorrhea, and syphilis. Some STIs can be transmitted without direct genital-to-genital contact. Effective and consistent protection is necessary to protect yourself and your partner. All STIs are treatable, but all are not curable. If you or someone you know discovers symptoms associated with STIs, seek medical treatment as soon as possible. If STIs go untreated, they can cause sterility, organ damage, and life-threatening complications. We introduce this topic in the hope that you will seek sources of more detailed information so that you can learn more about a range of STIs, what causes them, and what can be done to prevent them. Two good sources of information are the American Red Cross and the Centers for Disease Control and Prevention (CDC) National Center for HIV/AIDS, Viral Hepatitis, STD, and TB Prevention. Gaining a realistic picture of the potential dangers, and measures to prevent negative consequences, can help you make better choices.

If you choose to be sexually active, it is essential that you develop the skills to negotiate your safer sex plan with your partner. Magic Johnson (1992), who retired from the NBA in 1991 after announcing he had contracted HIV, has some useful advice for those who are considering becoming sexually active. He suggests asking yourself these questions:

▶ Am I prepared to practice safer sex each time I have sex?

▶ Am I prepared to consistently and effectively use contraception each time I have heterosexual sex?

▶ Am I prepared to deal with the consequences if my partner or I become infected with HIV or another STI or becomes pregnant?

▶ Am I prepared to say "No" when I think it is not right for me?

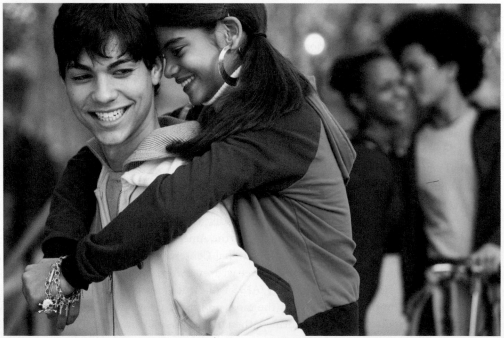

Radius Images

》 Only a small percent of young people who are sexually active use condoms with regularity.

If you cannot answer "Yes" to each of these questions, you may not be ready to take on the responsibilities that are basic to this level of intimacy.

Young adults often feel that they are immune from any harm, and thus they tend to disregard good advice or sound practices. Others may remain in a state of denial because they do not want to change their sexual lifestyle. Only a small percentage of young people who are sexually active use condoms with regularity, and fear-arousing campaigns are not effective in changing these patterns of sexual behavior. Aronson (2000) encourages young adults to persuade themselves to change dysfunctional attitudes and behavior, and his work in schools teaching self-persuasion has had results far superior to traditional external approaches. If you learn to challenge your own beliefs and make new decisions based on internal motivation, you have gained personal power over your life. By persuading yourself to act in accordance with what you know, you can lessen your chances of contracting a sexually transmitted illness.

TAKE TIME TO REFLECT

1. What are your attitudes, values, and fears pertaining to HIV/AIDS and other STIs?

_____

_____

2. What steps are you willing to take to avoid contracting HIV and other STIs? What knowledge or information do you need to obtain to feel more prepared? Visit credible websites (such as the CDC) to empower yourself with up-to-date information.

_____

_____

3. If you have had personal experience with STIs, what can you do moving forward to make healthier choices regarding your sexual practices?

_____

_____

SUMMARY

Sexuality is part of who we are, and the way we express our sexuality is influenced by our values. Although childhood and adolescent experiences do have an impact on shaping our present attitudes toward sex and our sexual behavior, we are in a position to modify our attitudes and behavior if we are not satisfied with ourselves as sexual beings.

If we are successful in dealing with barriers that prevent us from acknowledging, experiencing, and expressing our sexuality, we increase our chances of learning how to enjoy both sensuality and sexuality, which can enhance our physical and psychological well-being. Sensuality can be a significant path toward creating satisfying sexual relationships, and we can learn to become sensual beings even if we decide not to have sexual relationships with others. Sensuality encompasses full awareness of and

sensitivity to the pleasures of sight, sound, smell, taste, and touch. We can enjoy sensuality without being sexual, and sensuality does not always lead to sexual behavior. Nevertheless, sensuality is very important in enhancing sexual relationships. Intimacy, or the emotional sharing with a person we care for, is another ingredient of joyful sex.

One significant step toward evaluating your sexual attitudes is to become aware of the myths and misconceptions you may harbor. Review where and how you acquired your views about sexuality. Have the sources of your sexual knowledge and values been healthy models? Have you questioned how your attitudes affect the way you feel about yourself sexually? Is your sexuality an expression of yourself as a complete person? The place that sex occupies in your life and the attitudes you have toward it are very much a matter of your choice.

A significant step toward developing your own sexual views is to learn to be open in talking about sexual concerns, including your fears and desires, with at least one other person you trust. Guilt feelings may be based on unfounded premises, and you may be burdening yourself needlessly by feeling guilty about normal feelings and behavior. You may feel very alone when it comes to your sexual feelings, fantasies, fears, and actions. By sharing some of these concerns with others, you are likely to find out that you are not the only one with such concerns.

The AIDS crisis has had a significant impact on sexual behavior. Along with a better understanding of this disease and of other STIs, education can put you in a good position to make informed choices in expressing your sexuality.

The themes explored in the chapters on love and relationships are really impossible to separate from the themes of this chapter. Think about love, sex, and relationships as an integrated dimension of a rich and full life.

Where Can I Go From Here?

1. Write down some of your major questions or concerns regarding sexuality. Consider discussing these issues with a friend, your partner (if you are involved in an intimate relationship), or your class group.

2. In your journal trace the evolution of your sexual history. What were some important experiences for you, and what did you learn from these experiences?

3. How was sexuality modeled by your parents? What attitudes and values about sex did they convey to you, both implicitly and explicitly? What would you most want to communicate to your children about sex?

4. Reflect for a moment on the particular slang words regarding sex that are used in your culture. What attitudes about sex are conveyed by these words?

5. Go to a community family-planning agency or the campus health center. Pick up pamphlets on HIV, AIDS, STIs, and safer sex practices. As an alternative, contact any of the following sources for some updated information on HIV/AIDS. The National AIDS Clearinghouse (1-800-458-5231) provides information on HIV/AIDS. Additional sources of information on HIV/AIDS and other STIs include these agencies:

▶ HIV/AIDS Treatment Information Service, 1-800-HIV-0440

▶ National Gay and Lesbian Task Force AIDS Information Line, 1-800-221-7044

▶ AIDS National Interfaith Network, 202-546-0807

▶ Public Health Service AIDS Hotline, 1-800-342-AIDS

▶ National Institute on Drug Abuse Hotline, 1-800-662-HELP

▶ National Sexually Transmitted Diseases Hotline, 1-800-227-8922

▶ Centers for Disease Control and Prevention, 404-639-3534

▶ American Red Cross, 1-800-375-2040

▶ World Health Organization, 202-861-4354

6. Suggested Readings. The full bibliographic entry for each of these sources can be found in the References and Suggested Readings at the back of the book. Two excellent textbooks that provide a comprehensive discussion of sexuality are Crooks and Baur (2011) and Carroll (2013).

WEBSITE RESOURCES

Included here are some valuable websites. For access to these websites, video activities, and other supporting materials, visit Cengage Learning's Counseling CourseMate website for *I Never Knew I Had a Choice*, 10th Edition, at **www.cengagebrain.com.**

SEXUAL HEALTH NETWORK
www.sexualhealth.com

Recommended Search Words: "sexual health network"

This site is "dedicated to providing easy access to sexuality information, education, counseling, therapy, medical attention, and other sexuality resources," especially for people with disabilities, illness, or other health-related problems.

SEXUALITY INFORMATION AND EDUCATION COUNCIL OF THE UNITED STATES (SIECUS)
www.siecus.org

Recommended Search Words: "SIECUS"

This organization is devoted to providing information on a range of topics pertaining to sexuality. SIECUS promotes comprehensive education about sexuality and advocates the rights of all individuals to make responsible sexual choices.

HIV/AIDS AEGIS
www.aegis.com

Recommended Search Words: "AIDS aegis"

This is an important resource dealing with HIV and AIDS. This site provides an extensive collection of related links, documents, and news articles.

NATIONAL CENTER FOR HIV/AIDS, VIRAL HEPATITUS, STD, AND TB PREVENTION
www.cdc.gov/nchhstp/

Recommended Search Words: "nchhstp"

The Centers for Disease Control and Prevention (CDC) offers current information, fact sheets, conferences, publications, and information on the prevention and treatment of HIV/AIDS, viral hepatitis, sexually transmitted diseases and infections, and tuberculosis.

AMERICAN RED CROSS
www.redcross.org

Recommended Search Words: "American red cross"

Considered the nation's premier emergency response organization, the American Red Cross offers domestic disaster relief and a variety of services and programs that aim to relieve human suffering. This site offers a wealth of information about domestic and international services.

SEXUAL ADVICE ASSOCIATION
www.sda.uk.net/

Recommended Search Words: "sexual dysfunction association"

Formerly called the Sexual Dysfunction Association, this charitable organization is dedicated to helping

men and women become more aware of the extent to which sexual conditions affect the general population.

WEB MD: ERECTILE DYSFUNCTION HEALTH CENTER
www.webmd.com/erectile-dysfunction/default.htm

Recommended Search Words: "Web md"

Visit this site to get news and information about erectile dysfunction.

NATIONAL PREVENTION INTERVENTION NETWORK
www.cdcnpin.org/

Recommended Search Words: "national prevention intervention network"

The Centers for Disease Control and Prevention (CDC) house NPIN contains useful information about the prevention of sexually transmitted diseases and infections. This site includes information about at-risk populations.

U.S. DEPARTMENT OF HEALTH AND HUMAN SERVICES: OFFICE OF ADOLESCENT HEALTH
www.hhs.gov/ash/oah/

Recommended Search Words: "office of adolescent health"

This site offers information that pertains to the health and well-being of adolescents, including content on sexual relationships, teen pregnancies, and sexually transmitted diseases and infections.

U.S. DEPARTMENT OF HEALTH AND HUMAN SERVICES: OFFICE ON WOMEN'S HEALTH
www.womenshealth.gov/

Recommended Search Words: "office on women's health"

A great deal of information about sexuality, STIs, and sexual dysfunction is available on this site. It is a rich resource for women who want information about any number of health-related topics.

SEX ADDICTS ANONYMOUS
http://saa-recovery.org/

Recommended Search Words: "sex addicts anonymous"

This website offers information about a program for men and women who self-identify as having an addiction to sex.

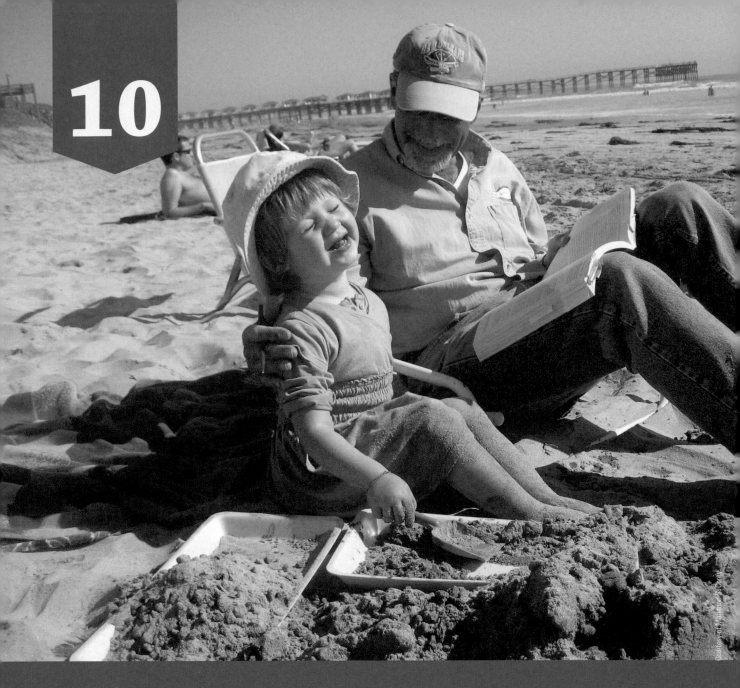

10

WORK AND RECREATION

> Where Am I Now?

> Higher Education as Your Work

> Choosing an Occupation or Career

> The Process of Deciding on a Career

> Choices at Work

> Changing Careers in Midlife

> Retirement

> The Place of Recreation in Your Life

> Summary

> Where Can I Go From Here?

> Website Resources

Courtesy of Marianne Schneider Corey

Working to live—living to work.

WHERE AM I NOW?

Use this scale to respond to these statements:

4 = I *strongly agree* with this statement.
3 = I *agree* with this statement.
2 = I *disagree* with this statement.
1 = I *strongly disagree* with this statement.

1. I am furthering my education because it is necessary for the career I have chosen.

2. My primary reasons for pursuing an education are to mature as a person and to fulfill my potential.

3. I am pursuing higher education to give me time to decide what to do with my life.

4. I would not work if I did not need the money.

5. Work is a very important means of expressing myself.

6. I expect to change jobs several times during my life.

7. A secure job is more important to me than an exciting one.

8. If I am unhappy in my job, I will need to change either the job or my attitude about my circumstances.

9. I expect my work to fulfill many of my needs and to be an important source of meaning in my life.

10. I have a good balance between my work and my recreation.

Deriving satisfaction from work and recreation are very important. Work affects many areas of our lives, and the balance we find between work and recreation can contribute to our personal vitality or to a stressful experience that ultimately results in burnout. **Recreation** is derived from "re-create," which means to restore, to refresh, to put new life into, and to create anew. Recreation involves leisure time and what we do away from work.

Work is a good deal more than an activity that takes up a certain number of hours each week. In an average day, most people spend about 8 hours sleeping, another 8 hours working, and the other 8 hours in routines such as eating, traveling to work, and leisure. If you enjoy your work, then at least half of your waking hours are spent in meaningful activities. However, if you do not look forward to going to work, those 8 hours can easily affect your relationships and your feelings about yourself. It is important to reflect on the attitudes you have toward work and recreation and to be aware of the impact of these attitudes on your life.

The fast pace of social and technological change in today's world is forcing people to adapt to a changing world of work. The changing workforce and changing workplace have implications for career decision making. In writing about these changes, Zunker (2012) emphasizes that throughout the 21st century increasing numbers of women will enter the workplace, and the workforce will become more culturally diverse. Peterson and Gonzalez (2005) pointed out that U.S. workers must take advantage of the diversity that exists within our country to remain competitive in the global marketplace, for economic reasons if not for moral ones. They see the challenge for the future as maximizing the potential of women, ethnic minorities, and immigrants so that all people can contribute to workplace productivity.

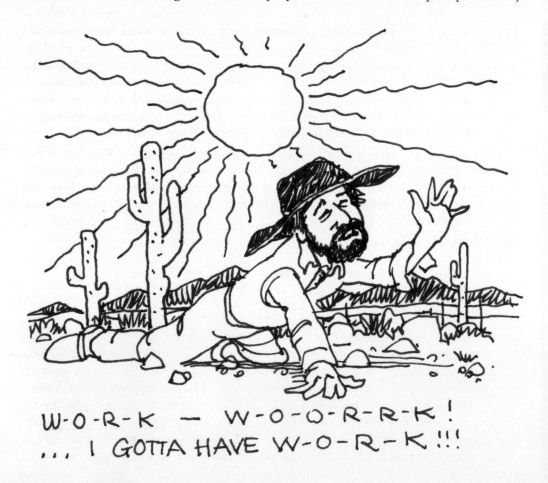

Before continuing further into the world of work, let's clarify a few terms. A **career** can be thought of as your life's work. A career spans a period of time and may involve one or several occupations; it is the sequence of a person's work experience over time. An **occupation** is your vocation, profession, business, or trade, and you may change your occupation several times during your lifetime. A **job** is your position of employment within an occupation. Over a period of time you may have several jobs within the same occupation. A job is what you do to earn money to survive and to do the things you would like to do. **Work** is a broad concept that refers to something you do because you want to, and we hope, because you enjoy it. Ideally, your job and your work involve similar activities. Work is fulfilling when you feel you are being compensated adequately, when you feel valued for your contributions, and when you like what you are doing. People entering the workforce need to have more than specific knowledge and skills; they need to be able to adapt to change. One career may pave the way to another.

In *Taking Charge of Your Career Direction,* Robert Lock (2005b) acknowledges that choosing an occupation is not easy. Externally, the working world is constantly changing; internally, your expectations, needs, motivations, values, and interests may change. Deciding on a career involves integrating the realities of these two worlds. Lock emphasizes the importance of *actively choosing* a career.

The process of actively choosing a career path involves making an assessment of your personal interests, needs, values, and abilities, and then matching your personal characteristics with occupational information and trends in the world of work. In deciding on a career, you may find it extremely valuable to make use of the resources available at your college or university. Most college counseling centers offer computer based programs to help students get occupational information and decide on a career. Online resources, some of which you will find at the end of this chapter, can help you assess your values and interests and link them to careers. Another way of taking an active role involves talking to other people about their job satisfaction. One of the major factors that might prevent you from becoming active in planning for a career is putting off doing what needs to be done to choose your work.

Career development researchers have found that most people go through a series of stages when choosing an occupation or, more typically, several occupations to pursue. As with life-span stages, different factors emerge or become influential at different times throughout this process. Therefore, it could well be a mistake to think about selecting *one* occupation that will last a lifetime. It may be more fruitful to choose a general type of work or a broad field of endeavor that appeals to you. You can consider your present job or field of study as a means of gaining experience and opening doors to new possibilities, and you can focus on what you want to learn from this experience. Your decisions about work are part of a developmental process, and your jobs may change as you change or may lead to related occupations within your chosen field.

HIGHER EDUCATION AS YOUR WORK

You already may have made several vocational decisions and held a number of different jobs, you may be changing careers, or you may be in the process of exploring career options and preparing yourself for a career. If you are in the midst of considering what occupations might best suit you, review the meaning that going to college or graduate school has for you now. How you approach your postsecondary education is a good gauge of how you will someday approach your career.

School may be your primary line of work for the present, but for those of you who are engaged in a career and have a family, school is not likely to be your main source of work. Regardless of your commitments outside of school, it can be beneficial to reflect on why you are in college or graduate school. Some people are motivated to pursue higher education because it offers opportunities for personal development and the pursuit of knowledge. Others do so primarily to attain their career objectives, and some go because they are avoiding making other choices in their lives. Ask yourself these questions: "Why am I in college or graduate school?" "Is it my choice or someone else's choice for me?" "Do I enjoy most of my time as a student?" "Is my work as a student satisfying and meaningful?" "Would I rather be somewhere else or doing something other than being a student? If so, why am I staying in school?" Clarifying your own reasons for pursuing higher education can be useful to the process of long-range career planning.

If you like the meaning your educational experience has for you as well as your part in creating this meaning, you are likely to assume responsibility for making your job satisfying. If you typically do more than is required as a student, you are likely to be willing to go beyond doing what is expected of you in your job. If you fear making mistakes and do not risk saying what you think in class, you may carry this behavior into a job. Reflect for a moment on the degree to which your attitudes and behavioral patterns as a student might show up in your work.

CHOOSING AN OCCUPATION OR CAREER

What do you expect from work? What factors do you stress in selecting a career or an occupation? What do you value the most, and to what extent can your values be attained in your chosen vocation? John Holland's (1997) theory of career decision making is based on the assumption that career choices are an expression of our values and personality. Holland believes the choice of an occupation should reflect the person's motivation, knowledge, personality, and ability. Occupations represent a way of life. Dave's personal story illustrates this search for a satisfying career. Dave chose college without knowing what he wanted. Eventually he found a direction by pursuing what interested him.

DAVE'S STORY

I went to college right out of high school because I thought I needed a college degree to get a good job and to succeed. My first year was a bit rough because of the new surroundings. In my classes I felt like a number, and it didn't seem to matter if I attended classes or not. I was the one who was responsible to show up for class, and it was hard for me to handle this freedom. Needless to say, my grades took a nosedive. I was placed on academic probation. As a result, I decided to go to a community college. But my pattern of not taking school seriously persisted. Although I wanted to eventually finish college, I knew that university life was not right for me at this time. I decided to move out of my parents' home, work full time, and attend community college on a part-time basis. I knew that if I left college completely it would be harder to return.

Eventually I accepted a job with a promotional marketing firm. I was given more responsible assignments, and I really enjoyed what I was doing. I asked myself, "How can I apply what I enjoy doing and make it a career?" This question led me to doing research on the sports entertainment field, which gave me a career path. Knowing what I wanted as a career made selecting a major relatively easy. I majored in business with a marketing emphasis and did extremely well. My journey took me from academic disqualification to graduating with honors.

Following my interests has led to an exciting career. I look forward to getting up and going to work, which is both fun and challenging. I am able to combine my sports hobbies with my profession. This work is personally rewarding, and I feel energized and motivated on the job. My work doesn't seem like "work." To me, it has become a key to a meaningful life.

The Disadvantages of Choosing an Occupation Too Soon

So much emphasis is placed on what you will do "for a living" that you may feel compelled to choose an occupation or a career before you are really ready to do so. In the United States children are encouraged to identify with some occupation at an early age. Children are often asked, "What are you going to be when you grow up?" Embedded in this question is the implication that we are not grown up until we have decided to be something. By late adolescence or young adulthood, the pressure increases to make decisions and commitments. Young adults are expected to make choices that will affect the rest of their lives, even though they may not feel ready to make these commitments. The implication is that once young people make the "right decision" they are set for life. Yet deciding on a career is not that simple.

One of the disadvantages of focusing on a particular occupation too soon is that students' interest patterns are often not sufficiently reliable or stable in high school or sometimes even in the college years to predict job success and satisfaction. Furthermore, the typical student does not have enough self-knowledge or knowledge of educational offerings and vocational opportunities to make realistic decisions. The pressure to make premature vocational decisions often results in choosing an occupation for which you do not have the interests and abilities required for success. Be cautious and resist pressures from the outside to decide too quickly on your life's vocation, but remain alert to the tendencies within yourself to expect that what you want will be yours without effort. You may remember from Chapter 2 that Erikson calls for a *psychological moratorium* during adolescence to enable young people to get some distance from the pressure of choosing a career too soon. A moratorium can reduce the pressure of having to make key life choices without sufficient data. As young people gain experience, they are likely to develop a new perspective about what they want from a career and from life.

Factors in Career Decision Making

Factors that have been shown to be important in the occupational decision-making process include motivation and achievement; attitudes about occupations; abilities and aptitudes; interests; values; self-concept; temperament and personality styles; socioeconomic level; parental influence; ethnic identity;

The fast pace of social and technological change in today's world is forcing people to adapt to a changing world of work.

gender; and physical, mental, emotional, and social disabilities. In choosing your vocation (or in evaluating the choices you have previously made), consider which factors really mean the most to you. Let's take a closer look at how some of these factors may influence your vocational choice, keeping in mind that a career choice is a developmental process, not a one-time event.

Motivation and Achievement Setting goals is at the core of the process of deciding on a vocation. If you have goals but do not have the energy and persistence to pursue them, your goals will not be met. Your need to achieve along with your achievements to date are related to your motivation to translate goals into action plans. In thinking about your career choices, identify those areas where your drive is the greatest. Also, reflect on specific achievements. What have you accomplished that you feel particularly proud of? What are you doing now that moves you in the direction of achieving what is important to you? What are some of the things you dream about doing in the future? Did you ever have a dream of what you wanted to be when you grew up? What happened to that dream? Were others encouraging or discouraging of this dream? Thinking about your goals, needs, motivations, and achievements gives you a clearer focus on your career direction.

Attitudes About Occupations We develop our attitudes toward the status of occupations by learning from the people in our environment. Typical first graders are not aware of the differential status of occupations, but through the socialization process these children quickly begin to rank occupations in a manner similar to that of adults. As students advance to higher grades, they reject more and more occupations as unacceptable. Unfortunately, they rule out some of the very jobs from which they may have to choose if they are to find employment as adults. It is difficult for people to feel positive about themselves if they have to accept an occupation they perceive as low in status. At this point ask yourself, "What did I learn about work from my parents?" "What did I learn about work from my culture?" "What did I learn about work from other sources (such as the media)?"

Abilities and Aptitudes Ability and aptitude have received a great deal of attention in the career decision-making process, and they are probably used more often than any other factors to evaluate potential for success. **Ability** refers to your competence in an activity. **Aptitude tests** are designed to measure the specific skills needed to acquire certain proficiencies. Both general and specific abilities should be considered in making career choices. (See Chapter 1 for a discussion of how multiple intelligences influence our abilities.) You can measure and compare your abilities with the skills required for various professions and academic areas of interest to you. Ask yourself, "How did I determine what abilities I have?" "What influence did my family of origin have on my perception of my abilities?" "How did others, such as teachers and friends, influence my perception?"

Interests Your interests reflect your experiences or ideas pertaining to work-related activities that you like or dislike. In career planning, primary consideration is given to assessing interests, which can be done in a three-step process: (1) discover your areas of interest, (2) identify occupations in your interest areas, and (3) determine which occupations correspond to your abilities and aptitudes.

Interest inventories are useful tools because the results can help you compare your interests with those of others who have found job satisfaction in a given area (Zunker, 2012). These inventories are not designed to predict job success but to give some indication of job satisfaction. Interest alone does not necessarily mean that you have the ability or aptitude to succeed in a particular occupation. Both abilities and interests are integral components of career decision making.

Several interest inventories are available to help you assess your vocational interests. One of these instruments is Holland's Self-Directed Search (SDS), which is probably the most widely used interest inventory. For further information about other interest inventories, contact the counseling center at your college or university.

Values Your values indicate what is important to you and what you want from life. It is important to assess, identify, and clarify your values so you will be able to choose a career that enables you to achieve what you value. An inventory of your values can help you discern patterns in your life and see how your values have emerged, taken shape, and changed over time. Work value inventories measure values associated with job success and satisfaction (Zunker, 2012).

Your **work values** pertain to what you hope to accomplish through your role in an occupation. Work values are an important aspect of your total value system, and identifying what brings meaning to your life is crucial if you hope to find a career that has personal value for you. A few examples of work values are helping others, influencing people, finding meaning, achievement, prestige, status, competition, security, friendships, creativity, stability, recognition, adventure, physical challenge, change and variety, opportunity for travel, moral fulfillment, and independence. Because specific work values are often related to particular occupations, they can be the basis of a good match between you and an occupation.

Self-Concept People with a poor self-concept are not likely to envision themselves in a meaningful or important job. They are likely to keep their aspirations low, and thus their achievements will probably be low. They may select and remain in a job they do not enjoy or derive satisfaction from because they are convinced this is all they are worthy of. Choosing a vocation can be thought of as a public declaration of the kind of person you want to be.

Personality Types and Choosing a Career

According to John Holland (1997), people are attracted to a particular career by their unique personalities. People who exhibit certain values and particular personality traits are a good match with certain career areas. Holland identified six worker personality types, and his typology is widely used as the basis for books on career development, vocational tests used in career counseling centers, and self-help approaches for making career decisions.* Holland's six personality types are realistic, investigative, artistic, social, enterprising, and conventional. Because his work has been so influential in vocational theory, it is worth going into some detail about it here.

As you read the descriptions of Holland's six personality types, take the time to think about the patterns that fit you best. Remember that most people do not fall neatly into one category but have characteristics from several types. When you come across a phrase that describes you, put a check mark in the space provided. Then look again at the six personality types and select the three types (in rank order) that best describe the way you see yourself. As you become more aware of the type of person you are, you can apply these insights in your own career decision-making process.

Realistic Types
_____ value nature, common sense, honesty, practicality

_____ are attracted to outdoor, mechanical, and physical activities, hobbies, and occupations

Our discussion is based on Holland's work as refined by Jim Morrow (retired professor of counseling, Western Carolina University, North Carolina).

_____ like to work with things, objects, and animals rather than with ideas, data, and people

_____ tend to have mechanical and athletic abilities

_____ like to construct, shape, and restructure and repair things around them

_____ like to use equipment and machinery and to see tangible results

_____ are persistent and industrious builders but seldom creative and original, preferring familiar methods and established patterns

_____ tend to think in terms of absolutes, dislike ambiguity, and prefer not to deal with abstract, theoretical, and philosophical issues

_____ are materialistic, traditional, and conservative

_____ do not have strong interpersonal and verbal skills and are often uncomfortable in situations in which attention is centered on them

_____ tend to find it difficult to express their feelings and may be regarded as shy

Investigative Types

_____ value inventiveness, accuracy, achievement, independence

_____ are naturally curious, inquisitive, precise, analytical, reserved

_____ need to understand, explain, and predict what goes on around them

_____ are scholarly and scientific and tend to be pessimistic and critical about nonscientific, simplistic, or supernatural explanations

_____ tend to become engrossed in whatever they are doing and may appear to be oblivious to everything else

_____ are independent and like to work alone

_____ prefer neither to supervise others nor to be supervised

_____ are theoretical and analytic in outlook and find abstract and ambiguous problems and situations challenging

_____ are original and creative and often find it difficult to accept traditional attitudes and values

_____ avoid highly structured situations with externally imposed rules but are themselves internally well-disciplined, precise, and systematic

_____ have confidence in their intellectual abilities but often feel inadequate in social situations

_____ tend to lack leadership and persuasive skills

_____ tend to be reserved and formal in interpersonal relationships

_____ are not typically expressive emotionally and may not be considered friendly

Artistic Types

_____ value beauty, self-expression, imagination, creativity

_____ are creative, expressive, original, intuitive, unconventional, individualistic

_____ like to be different and strive to stand out from the crowd

_____ like to express their personalities by creating new and different things with words, music, materials, and physical expression like acting and dancing

_____ want attention and praise but are sensitive to criticism

_____ tend to be uninhibited and nonconforming in dress, speech, and action

_____ prefer to work without supervision

_____ are impulsive in outlook

_____ place great value on beauty and aesthetic qualities

_____ tend to be emotional and complicated

_____ prefer abstract tasks and unstructured situations

_____ find it difficult to function well in highly ordered and systematic situations

_____ seek acceptance and approval from others but often find close interpersonal relationships so stressful that they avoid them

_____ compensate for their resulting feelings of estrangement or alienation by relating to others primarily indirectly through art

_____ tend to be introspective

_____ enjoy creative work in music, writing, performance, sculpture

Social Types

_____ value service to others, fairness, understanding, empathy

_____ are friendly, warm, trusting, generous, enthusiastic, outgoing, cooperative

_____ enjoy the company of other people

_____ like helping and facilitating roles like teacher, mediator, adviser, or counselor

_____ express themselves well and are persuasive in interpersonal relationships

_____ like attention and enjoy being at or near the center of the group

_____ are idealistic, sensitive, and conscientious about life and in dealings with others

_____ like to deal with philosophical issues such as the nature and purpose of life, religion, and morality

_____ dislike working with machines or data and at highly organized, routine, and repetitive tasks

_____ get along well with others and find it natural to express their emotions

_____ are tactful in relating to others and are considered to be kind, supportive, and caring

_____ enjoy working with others and tend to prefer team approaches

Enterprising Types

_____ value success, status, power, responsibility, initiative

_____ are outgoing, self-confident, assertive, persuasive, adventurous, ambitious, optimistic

_____ like to organize, direct, manage, and control the activities of groups toward personal or organizational goals

_____ like to feel in control and responsible for making things happen

_____ are energetic and enthusiastic in initiating and supervising activities

_____ like to influence others

_____ enjoy social gatherings and like to associate with well-known and influential people

_____ like to travel and explore and often have exciting and expensive hobbies

_____ see themselves as popular

_____ tend to dislike activities requiring scientific abilities and systematic and theoretical thinking

_____ avoid activities that require attention to detail and a set routine

_____ enjoy leading, selling, motivating, persuading others, producing a great deal of work

Conventional Types

_____ value accuracy, honesty, persistence, order

_____ are well organized and practical

_____ enjoy clerical and computational activities that follow set procedures

_____ are dependable, efficient, and conscientious

_____ enjoy the security of belonging to groups and organizations and make good team members

_____ are status-conscious but usually do not aspire to high positions of leadership

_____ are most comfortable when they know what is expected of them

_____ tend to be conservative and traditional

_____ usually conform to expected standards and follow the lead of those in positions of authority, with whom they identify

_____ like to work indoors in pleasant surroundings and place value on material comforts and possessions

_____ are self-controlled and low-key in expressing their feelings

_____ avoid intense personal relationships in favor of more casual ones

_____ are most comfortable among people they know well

_____ like for things to go as planned and prefer not to change routines

Relationships Among the Personality Types As you were reading the descriptions of the six personality types, you probably noticed that each type shares some characteristics with some other types and also is quite different from some of the others. To help you compare and contrast the six types, Holland's "hexagon" illustrates the order of the relationships among the types (see Figure 10.1).

Each type shares some characteristics with those types adjacent to it on the hexagon. Each type has only a little in common with those types two positions removed from it, and

▸ **FIGURE 10.1** Holland's Hexagon

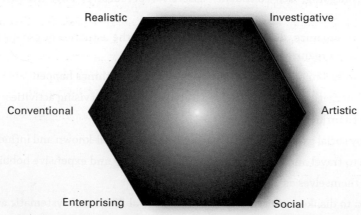

© Cengage Learning 2014

it is quite unlike the type opposite it on the hexagon. For example, the investigative type shares some characteristics with the realistic and artistic types, has little in common with the conventional and social types, and is quite different from the enterprising type. If you read the descriptions of the six types once more with the hexagon in mind, the relationships among the types will become clearer.

People who feel that they resemble two or three types that are not adjacent on the hexagon may find it difficult to reconcile the conflicting elements in those type descriptions. It is important to remember that the descriptions provided are for "pure" types and that very few people resemble a single type to the exclusion of all others. This is why we ask you to select the three types that you think best describe you.

Once you have compared your personal traits with the characteristics of each of the six types, it is possible to find a general area of work that most matches your personal qualities, interests, and values. This topic is addressed in the next section. The Take Time to Reflect exercise will help you become familiar with Holland's personality types and will assist you in assessing your personality type. It is important to have someone you know assess you as well as doing so yourself.

TAKE TIME TO REFLECT

1. Read the descriptions and other information furnished about Holland's six personality types at least two or three times.

2. Which of the six personality types best describes you? No one type will be completely "right" for you, but one of them will probably sound more like you than the others. Consider the overall descriptions of the types; do not concentrate on just one or two characteristics of a type. As soon as you are satisfied that one type describes you better than the others, write that type down on the space for number 1 at the end of this exercise.

3. Which of the six types next best describes you? Write that type down in the space for number 2. Write down the type that next best describes you in the space for number 3.

4. Next, give the descriptions of the six types to someone who knows you very well. Ask that person to read the descriptions carefully and order them in terms of their resemblance to you, just as you have done. Do not show or tell this person how you rated yourself.

5. After the other person finishes rating you, compare your own rating with his or hers. If there is not close agreement among the three types on both lists, ask the other person to give examples of your behaviors that prompted his or her ratings. The other person may not have rated you very accurately, or your behavior may not portray you to others as you see yourself. The purpose of this exercise is to familiarize you with Holland's personality types. It may have a "bonus" effect of better familiarizing you with yourself.

Your rating of yourself:

1. _____

2. _____

3. _____

Rating by someone who knows you well:

1. _____

2. _____

3. _____

THE PROCESS OF DECIDING ON A CAREER

Holland (1997) originally developed his system as a way of helping people make occupational choices. After you have identified the three personality types that most closely describe you, this information can be used in your career decision-making process.

Personality Types and Careers

It is more likely that you will be successful in your career if your own personality types match those of people who have already proven themselves in the career that you hope to pursue. Central to Holland's theory is the concept that we choose a career to satisfy our preferred person orientation. However, you will need to have at least basic skills in all areas. For example, if you are a strong investigative type, you might need to brush up on your enterprising skills to do well in the interview situation. Holland has developed elaborate materials that can help you assess your personality type and compare it with the dominant types in various occupations or fields of study. Here are examples of possible occupations or fields of interest associated with each personality type:

Realistic: carpenter, cook, electrician, industrial arts teacher, materials engineer, mechanical engineer, metal shop supervisor, paramedic

Investigative: chemical engineer, computer programmer, drafter, laboratory assistant, pharmacist, surgeon, systems analyst, veterinarian

Artistic: advertising executive, architect, author, English teacher, film editor, interior designer, musician, photographer

Social: counselor, elementary school teacher, employee relations specialist, nurse, occupational therapist, personnel manager, police officer, political scientist

Enterprising: financial planner, judge, lawyer, management trainee (any industry), operations manager, project director, sales manager, urban planner

Conventional: accountant, bookkeeper, building inspector, editorial assistant, investment analyst, mortgage processor, payroll clerk, website editor

Keep in mind that there are many career fields to choose from and that new career fields are emerging all the time. For instance, as existing technologies have become more advanced and new technologies have been developed, the very real threat of cyberattacks has necessitated the creation of jobs in cybersecurity. For links to these new career fields and their respective professional associations, visit the website of *Imagine* magazine (see Website Resources at the end of the chapter).

Some Suggestions Identify any fields of interest from the previous list that appeal to you, and make notes on why certain occupations or fields of study are attractive to you. Reflect on occupations that appeal to you as well as areas you would want to avoid. What are your reasons for picking certain fields of study or occupations and for rejecting others?

Visit the career counseling center at your college or university and inquire about standardized assessments that are available. Consider also using the Computer-Assisted Career Guidance (CACG) assessment. The use of CACG assessment has steadily increased because results are immediately available. Computer-based assessment programs interpret results by occupational fit with lists of career options (Zunker, 2012).

Steps You Can Take

The process of selecting a career is more than a simple matter of matching information about the world of work with your personality type. You will find it useful to go through some of these steps several times. For example, gathering and assessing information is a continual process rather than a step to be completed. When you gather basic information about occupations, consider the nature of the work, rewards of the job, challenges you may need to face, job entry requirements, monetary aspects, opportunities for advancement, intrinsic job satisfaction, security, and future outlook.

▶ **Begin by focusing on yourself.** Continue to identify your interests, abilities, aptitudes, values, beliefs, wants, and preferences. Keep these questions in mind: "Who am I?" "How do I want to live?" "Where do I want to live?" "What kind of work environment do I want?" "What do I want to do for a living?" This self-assessment includes taking into consideration your personality style. Ask yourself, "Do I function well in a system that is structured or unstructured?" "How much and what type of supervision do I need?" "Do I prefer to work alone or with others?"

▶ **Generate alternative solutions.** This stage is closely related to the next two. Rather than first narrowing your options, consider a number of alternatives or different potential occupations that you are drawn to. In this step it is wise to consider your work values and interests, especially as they apply to Holland's six personality types.

▶ **Gather and assess information about the alternatives generated.** In the process of expanding your list of career possibilities, recognize that you will likely devote a great deal of time to your occupation. Be willing to research the occupations that attract you. Doing so will increase your chances of being able to choose the way you want to live. Ask yourself, "Where do I best fit?" "Will the occupation I am considering be psychologically and financially satisfying to me?" "Do I have the resources to meet the challenges and responsibilities of the occupation?" "What are the typical characteristics of people who enter into this occupation?" Find an occupation that matches your interests, values, and talents, and read about the educational requirements of the occupation. Talk to as many people as you can who are involved in the occupations you are considering because they can provide valuable information and practical suggestions. Ask them how their occupation may be changing in the years to come. Examine the social, political, economic, and geographic environment as a basis for assessing factors that influence your career choice.

▶ **Weigh and prioritize your alternatives.** After you arrive at a list of alternatives, spend adequate time prioritizing them. Consider the practical aspects of your decisions. Integrate occupational information and the wishes and views of others with your knowledge of yourself.

▶ **Make the decision and formulate a plan.** It is best to think of a series of many decisions at various turning points. In formulating a plan, read about the preparation required for your chosen alternative. Ask, "How can I best get to where I want to go?"

▶ **Carry out the decision.** After deciding, take practical steps to turn your vision into reality. Realize that committing yourself to implementing your decision does not mean that you will have no fears, but do not allow these fears to stop you from taking action. You will never know if you are ready to meet a challenge unless you put your plan into action. This action plan includes knowing how to market your skills to employers. You need to learn how to identify employment sources, prepare résumés, and meet the challenges of job interviews.

▶ **Get feedback.** After taking practical steps to carry out your decision, you will need to determine whether your choices are viable for you. Both the world of work and you will change over time, and what may look appealing to you now may not seem appropriate at some future time. Remember that career development is an ongoing process, and it will be important to commit yourself to repeating at least part of the process as your needs change or as occupational opportunities open up or decline.

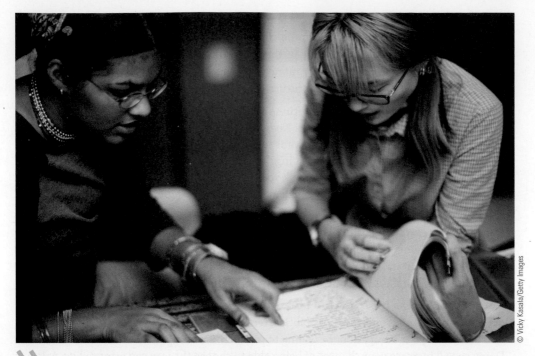

© Vicky Kasala/Getty Images

》 Choosing a career is best thought of as a process, not a one-time event.

A useful book with practical information about getting a job or changing careers is *The 2012 What Color Is Your Parachute? A Practical Manual for Job Hunters and Career-Changers* by Richard Bolles (2012).

TAKE TIME TO REFLECT

This survey is aimed at getting you to reflect on your basic attitudes, values, abilities, and interests in regard to occupational choice.

1. Rate each item, using the following code:

1 = This is a *most important* consideration.
2 = This is *important* to me, but not a top priority.
3 = This is *slightly important*.
4 = This is of *little* or *no importance* to me.

_____Financial rewards

_____Security

_____Challenge

_____Prestige and status

_____Opportunity to express my creativity

_____Autonomy—freedom to direct my project

_____Opportunity for advancement

_____Variety within the job

_____Recognition

_____Friendship and relations with coworkers

_____ Serving people

_____ Source of meaning

_____ Chance to continue learning

_____ Structure and routine

Once you have finished the assessment, review the list and write down the three most important values you associate with selecting a career or occupation.

_____

_____

2. In what area(s) do you see your strongest abilities?

_____

_____

3. What are a few of your major interests?

_____

_____

4. Which of your values have the most bearing on your choice of an occupation?

_____

_____

5. At this point, what kind of work do you see as most suitable to your interests, abilities, and values?

_____

_____

CHOICES AT WORK

Just as choosing a career is a process, so is creating meaning in our work. If we experience deadness in our job or do not find avenues of self-expression through the work we do, we eventually lose vitality. In this section we look at ways to find meaning in work and at approaches to keeping our options open.

The Dynamics of Discontent in Work

You may like your work and derive satisfaction from it, yet at times feel drained because of irritations produced by factors that are not intrinsic to the work itself such as low morale or actual conflict and disharmony among fellow workers. Chamberlain and Hodson (2010) describe three types of toxic working conditions: *occupational, organizational,* and *interpersonal.* Although it may be unrealistic to expect never to experience conflict with coworkers, chronic conflict or abuse from coworkers is not acceptable and should not be tolerated. Unfortunately, coworker abuse is part of the organizational culture in some workplaces, and it "can have devastating consequences for worker morale and job performance" (p. 457). Harris, Harvey, and Booth (2010) conducted research on personality and situational variables that contribute to coworker abuse. Their research showed that employees who view the world through a negative lens are likely to take out their frustrations on coworkers.

Abusive supervision may pose an even more challenging problem due to the power differential inherent in the relationship between an employee and his or her supervisor. Abusive supervision can have a "deleterious impact on both the attitudes (e.g., psychological distress, job dissatisfaction, work-family conflict) and behaviors (e.g., job performance, workplace deviance) of its victims" (Kiazad, Restubog, Zagenczyk, Kiewitz, & Tang, 2010, p. 512). Although some contend that abusive supervisory treatment reflects hostility aimed at convenient targets when retaliation against the original source of frustration is not feasible, Kiazad and his colleagues propose an alternative explanation. They see a link between destructive leader behaviors and *Machiavellianism*—a personality characteristic that predisposes an individual to manipulate and exploit others to maximize his or her own self-interests. Machiavellian supervisors may be more inclined to adopt an authoritarian style of leadership.

Even if you are not dealing with abusive supervisors or coworkers, countless pressures and demands can sap your energy and lead you to feel dissatisfied. These include having to meet deadlines and quotas, having to compete with others instead of simply doing your best, facing the threat of losing your job, feeling stuck in a job that offers little opportunity for growth, dealing with difficult customers or clients, or having to work long hours or perform exhausting or tedious work. Another source of dissatisfaction might be encountering people at your work who are younger and less experienced than you but who make close to your current salary or perhaps even more.

Bryce's story illustrates how abusive behavior and the negative attitude of his boss affected Bryce's overall satisfaction with work.

BRYCE'S STORY

Some people overreact and consider any behavior they don't approve of to be "abusive," especially from authority figures. Sometimes the label "abusive" isn't warranted, but at other times it might well be. I do think my boss abuses his power. He has a negative attitude about virtually everything—from the work we submit to him to the policies he is supposed to implement. There is little incentive for us to work hard and produce quality work, and he is sabotaging his own success by limiting the productivity of his staff with his negative attitude and behavior. He has screamed at certain employees for making him "look bad" in front of the company executives, yet he fails to take responsibility for his own behavior.

My boss's behavior is making my work life hell. Every morning when I hear my alarm clock go off, I hit the snooze button at least two times. Quite frankly, I dread getting up and going to work because the dynamics in the office are upsetting. Because of the dismal job market, the odds of finding a different job with a similar salary and benefits are slim. I would even consider taking a reduction in salary to escape this situation, but I haven't found a job listing that would be a good match for me. In light of this reality, I have decided to come up with a strategy to deal with the day-to-day turmoil I face until a decent job becomes available.

I am trying to remain focused on the tasks I need to accomplish while limiting my interactions with my boss. I realize that I cannot change my boss, yet I do have control over my reactions to this situation. I am also taking on freelance projects to provide myself with an outlet for my creativity. Even though I feel discouraged at times, I keep my eyes open and search for new employment opportunities.

A stress that is particularly insidious—because it can compound all the other dissatisfactions you might feel—is the threat of cutbacks or layoffs, an anxiety that becomes more acute when you think of your personal commitments and responsibilities. In today's unstable economic climate and politically divisive society, the outrage felt by many Americans is palpable. The Occupy movement—an international effort that has spread to many U.S.

cities—embodies the anger, frustration, and disgust people feel about economic and social inequality. At its core, these protestors "are hoping for the creation of more and better jobs, more equal distribution of wealth, bank reform, and a reduction of the influence of corporations on politics" (Lowenstein, 2011). An uncertain job market and global pressures make it even more important that you continually reevaluate the path you are on as you move through today's marketplace for work.

If you are fortunate and have a job that you enjoy, you may still have the daily stress of commuting to and from work. You may be tense before you even get to work, and the trip home may only increase the level of tension or anxiety you bring home with you. Relationships with others can be negatively affected by this kind of pressure. If your work is exhausting, you may have little to give your children, partner, and friends, and you may not be receptive to their efforts to give to you. There are times when you may not be able to avoid working in a less than desirable job, but you cannot afford to ignore the effects this may have on your overall life. If you are in an unsatisfying work situation, you would do well to find other ways of nourishing yourself.

All these factors contribute to a general discontent that robs your work life of whatever positive benefits it might otherwise provide. Experiencing this kind of discontentment in your work can spoil much of the rest of your life as well. The alternative is to look at the specific things that contribute to your unhappiness or tension and to ask yourself what you can do about them. You may not be able to change everything about your job that you do not like, but you might be surprised by the significant changes you can make to increase your satisfaction. It is essential to focus on those factors within your job that you can change. Even in cases where it is impractical to change jobs, you can still change your attitude and how you respond to a less than ideal situation.

Self-Esteem and Work

Making a career choice is a very personal matter. Niles, Jacob, and Nichols (2010) observe that "the substantial surge in downsizing has helped most people realize that when career situations go awry, the ripple effects are quite personal and, often, devastating" (p. 249). Self-esteem is based on feelings of worth and acceptance, which for many people are dependent on feedback from the external world (Guindon, 2002). If you have been laid off or have been unsuccessful in finding work, your self-esteem may have suffered a blow. If you do not feel valued at work or are prevented from working to your full potential, your self-esteem is likely to suffer. If you encounter difficult times in your career, be vigilant about self-care. You can help yourself by tapping into your internal resources and by seeking external supports.

Unemployment is a reality that can erode self-esteem. Nevertheless, even when job prospects are limited, you may be able to buoy your self-concept. Nina's experience with losing a job shows how this loss can affect self-esteem and lead to a sense of powerlessness. She found that shifting her attitude increased her possibilities and provided a sense of hope.

NINA'S STORY

When the company I had worked at for 21 years filed for bankruptcy, I found myself going through the stages of grief that Elisabeth Kübler-Ross wrote about. It felt like I had experienced the death of a close relative. Once my initial shock and denial wore off, I became stuck in anger for a period of time. I couldn't believe that the owners of the company, whom I held in such high regard, had mismanaged the business and drove their company—and along with it, my career—into the ground. My anger eventually turned into depression, which led me to feel lethargic and unmotivated to look for a new position. At this point, I knew I needed to seek help from a trusted friend or the professional assistance of a counselor.

In counseling, I began to realize how much my sense of identity was attached to my work. My self-esteem naturally plummeted when I lost my job. With the support of my counselor, I took steps to take charge of my life, which helped to counteract the sense of powerlessness that I had been feeling. Instead of sleeping until 11:00 A.M. every day, I started to get up early, go to the gym, and use my time more efficiently. I created tasks for myself and set deadlines so that I would be productive. For example, I assigned myself the task of researching local companies via the Internet during a 2-week period and sending out my résumé to prospective employers. Prior to that, I had contacted the career development office at my alma mater to seek advice on improving my résumé and to brush up my interviewing skills. Although technically I was not employed, I was definitely working. I was using my skills to improve myself as a job candidate, and that bolstered my self-esteem and sense of hope.

Creating Meaning in Work

Work can be a major part of your quest for meaning; it can also be a major source of distress. Work can be a way for you to be productive and to find enjoyment in daily life. Through your work you may be making a significant difference in the quality of your life or the lives of others, and this provides real satisfaction. Sometimes work is devoid of any self-expressive value. It can be merely a means to survival and a drain on your energy. Instead of giving life meaning, your work may be contributing to burnout. Ask yourself. "To what degree is my work life-giving and a source of meaning in my life?"

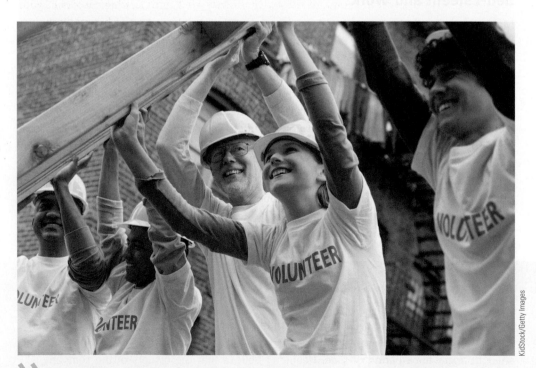

KidStock/Getty Images

» Through your work you may be making a significant difference in the quality of your life or the lives of others.

If your job is depleting you physically and emotionally instead of energizing you, what course of action can you consider? Are there some ways to constructively deal with the sources of dissatisfaction within your job? When might it be time for you to change jobs as a way of finding meaning? One strategy is to explore what you most want from your work, such as variety, a flexible schedule, and direct contact with people. If what you want is lacking in your work environment, perhaps you can discuss alternatives with your employer. Many employers will renegotiate rather than lose a quality person. Of course, if you decide to broach this topic with your boss or supervisor, be sure you do so in a respectful manner, and be careful not to make disparaging remarks about your current duties or circumstances. There are no guarantees that your employer will be receptive to your ideas or be in a position to implement them, so it is wise to handle situations like this with tact.

If you decide that you must remain in a job that allows little scope for personal effort and satisfaction, you may need to accept the fact that you will not find much meaning in the hours you spend on the job. It is important, then, to be aware of the effects that your time spent on the job has on the rest of your life. More positively, it is crucial to find something outside your job that fulfills your need for recognition, significance, productivity, and excitement.

Making changes in your present job might increase your satisfaction in the short term, but the time may come when these resources no longer work and you may decide to leave a job. Changing jobs as a way to create meaning is possible, but you have to be prepared to deal with the potential costs, both financial and psychological, of making such a change. It is up to you to weigh the cost-benefit ratio in making your decisions.

Shifting Your Attitudes About Work

It is worthwhile to consider those attitudes you hold about work that may either help or hinder you in achieving success in your career. What would help you deal with the demands of the future world of work? Some of the attitudes that are key to finding success in your work include assuming responsibility for the future, being committed to lifelong learning, viewing the future with vision and creativity, being able to tolerate uncertainty, and viewing change as both positive and necessary.

You may be enthusiastic about some type of work for years and yet eventually become dissatisfied because of the changes that occur within you. With these changes comes the possibility that a once-fulfilling job will become less than satisfying. If you outgrow your job, you can learn new skills and in other ways increase your options. Because your own attitudes are crucial, when a feeling of dissatisfaction sets in, it is wise to spend time rethinking what you want from a job and how you can most productively use your talents. Look carefully at how much the initiative rests with you—your expectations, your attitudes, your behaviors, and your sense of purpose and perspective.

CHANGING CAREERS IN MIDLIFE

Being aware of options is an important asset at midlife. Many people we know have changed their jobs several times, and they may also have experienced a career change. Does this pattern fit any people you know? Whether or not you have reached middle age, ask yourself about your own beliefs and attitudes toward changing careers. Although making large changes in our lives is rarely easy, it can be a good deal harder if our own attitudes and fears are left unquestioned and unexamined.

A common example of midlife change is the woman who decides to return to college or the job market after her children reach high school age. Women who want to develop new facets of themselves are enrolling in community colleges and state universities. This phenomenon is not unique to women. Some men quit a job they have had for years, even when they are successful, because they want new challenges. This flexibility may be less common during tough economic times, but some people will be positioned to pursue a new career path. Men often define themselves by the work they do, and work thus becomes a major source of the purpose in their lives. If they feel successful in their work, they may feel successful as persons. If they become stagnant in work, they may feel that they are ineffectual in other areas. Father Tom is a career-changer who was able to translate a dream into reality later in life.

Thomas Bonacum was drafted into the Army at age 21 and became a drill instructor. After leaving the army, Tom completed his degree in engineering, which led to a job as an industrial engineer. A few years later he was laid off and then joined the police department. During the time he was a police officer, he returned to college to get another degree in criminal justice. He became a police sergeant and eventually taught criminal justice for 4 years in the police academy during his 22 years in police work.

After the death of his wife of 35 years, Tom made a significant change of careers. With the support and encouragement of his four grown children, he entered the seminary in his late 50s and was ordained as a Catholic priest at age 60. Even after Father Tom retired, at the age of 77, he still kept active in a mountain community church and conducted services on weekends as long as his health allowed him to do so. He died at the age of 81.

When Tom graduated from high school, he tried to become a priest but discovered that he was not ready for some of the people in church, and they were not ready for him. He exemplifies a man who was willing to make career changes throughout his life and who dared to pursue what might have seemed like an impossible career choice. Many of us would not even conceive of such a drastic career change, yet Father Tom not only entertained this vision but also realized his dream.

You may believe it is extremely risky and unrealistic to give up your job, even if you hate it, because it provides a measure of financial security. This sentiment is especially strong during economically difficult times when unemployment rates are high. The costs involved in achieving optimal job satisfaction may be too high. You might choose to stay with a less-than-desirable career yet at the same time discover other avenues for satisfaction. If you feel stuck in your job, ask yourself these questions: "Does my personal dissatisfaction outweigh the financial rewards?" "Is the price of my mental anguish, which may have resulted in physical symptoms, worth the price of keeping this job?"

RETIREMENT

Many people look forward to retirement as a time for them to take up new projects. Others fear this prospect and wonder how they will spend their time if they are not working. The real challenge of this period, especially for those who retire early, is to find a way to remain active in a meaningful way. Some people consciously choose early retirement because they have found more significant and valuable pursuits. For other people, however, retirement does not turn out as expected, and it represents a major loss. For those who derive their major source of identity from work and have a strong work ethic, leaving a job may lead to a void, feelings of deprivation, and dissatisfaction in retirement (Peterson & Gonzalez, 2005). A deeply engrained Puritan work ethic may push these individuals to continue to work beyond retirement in order to feel valuable (Genevay, 2000). Other older adults want to continue working because it provides a meaningful existence. For folks like William and Jenny, however, a desired retirement may be delayed due to unanticipated financial hardships that occur later in life.

WILLIAM AND JENNY'S STORY

William and I have always had an active social life and value our leisure time. We have both worked for the same company for many years and, until recently, expected to retire when we turn 65. Some people live to work, but William and I have always worked to live. Unlike some retirees who don't know what to do with their free time, we have plenty of activities lined up and can hardly wait to retire. Unfortunately, the economy and a combination of other factors have made it impossible for us to retire at 65. Not only have our retirement accounts shrunk, our stock in the company has lost value, and we have had to agree to a 15% cut in salary in order to avoid layoffs. Also, our daughter, who has been independent for a long time, recently was laid off and is in the process of moving back home with us. We love our daughter, but this new arrangement will be an adjustment for all three of us. I guess one lesson we can all learn is that there are no guarantees in life.

Options at Retirement

It is a mistake to think of retired people as sitting around doing nothing. Many retired individuals keep themselves actively involved in community affairs, do volunteer work, pursue new ventures, engage in recreation more fully and with more enjoyment, and have a fuller life than when they were employed full time. At the age of 76 Angela finally retired. Soon after her retirement, she became deeply involved in managing a retirement community. Doing this as a volunteer did not lessen the meaning of this kind of work for Angela.

For people who were in positions of power, the adjustment to retirement can be difficult. They need to come to terms with the reality that once they retire they may no longer have the respect and admiration that they received in their professional roles. If the meaning of their lives was derived from their work position, they may be at a loss when they are without the work to fulfill these needs. Those who are retired may experience a loss of status over not having a professional role.

It is important to prepare for retirement and to find other sources of meaning so you remain engaged with life. Here are some key questions to explore: "Is there life after retirement?" "What are some options to working full time at retirement?" "If you have relied largely on your job for meaning or structure in life, can you deal with having much time and little to do?" "How can you retain your sense of purpose and value apart from your work life?"

Adjustments at Retirement

Some individuals are at a loss when they retire, and they really did not want to quit working as soon as they did. Ray worked for 32 years as a salesman for a large dairy company. Here is Ray's description of his experience with work and retirement.

RAY'S STORY

I loved my work. My job was my life. I looked forward to going to work, I liked helping people, and I thrived on the challenges of my career. I worked for 50 hours a week, and at age 57 I stopped very abruptly. Although I had made some plans for my financial retirement, I was not prepared for the emotional toll that not working would take on me. My work was my identity, and it helped me to feel worthwhile. For at least 2 years, I did not know what to do with myself. I sat around and began feeling depressed. It took me some time to adjust to this new phase in my life, but eventually I began to feel that I mattered. With the help of some friends I began to take on small jobs outside the home. I managed rentals, did repair work, and did some volunteer work at my church. Simply getting out of the house every day gave me another opportunity to contribute, which changed my attitude.

Today, at 86, I can honestly say that I like my life. Leisure is something I value now, rather than fearing it, which was the case in my younger years. There are plenty of work projects to keep me busy. Fortunately, I love fishing and golfing. Each year I go on several fishing trips, and my wife and I do a lot of traveling. By being active in the church, I've learned the value of fellowship and sharing with friends. I've found that I don't have to work 50 hours a week to be a productive human being. Just because I'm retired doesn't mean that I want to sit in a rocking chair most of the day. I retired from my career, but I have not retired from life.

Retirement is an opportunity to redesign your life and tap unused potentials, or it can be a coasting period where you simply mark time until the end. Genevay (2000) asserts that there is life after work and that most retired people need to use their talents and gifts to feel that they are valuable and are contributing to society. Many people continue some type of work after they retire from their career. The skills that people develop in the workplace over a lifetime can be transferred to retirement years in a way that results in satisfaction and high self-esteem beyond formal or paid work (Genevay, 2000). Due to the importance placed on an occupation or career, the transition to retirement can either be a period of upheaval or a positive experience with many benefits (Peterson & Gonzalez, 2005).

Leona and Marvin are a couple who did not deal well with retirement. Both had very active careers and retired relatively early. They began to spend most of their time with each other. After about 2 years they grew to dislike each other's company. They both began to have physical symptoms of illness and became overly preoccupied with their health. Leona chronically complained that Marvin did not talk to her, to which he usually retorted, "I have nothing to say, and you should leave me alone." They were referred by their physician for marital counseling. One of the outcomes of this counseling was that they both secured part-time work. They found that by spending time apart they had a greater interest in talking to each other about their experiences at work. They also began to increase their social activities and started to develop some friendships, both separately and together. Marvin and Leona recognized that it wasn't that they retired too early, but that they had retired without a plan.

Just because people no longer work at a job does not mean that they have to cease being active. Many options are open to retired people who would like to stay active in meaningful ways. It is a time for them to get involved with the projects they had so often put on the back burner due to their busy days.

Retirees do have choices and can create meaning in their lives by keeping themselves vital as physical, psychological, spiritual, and social beings. People can discover that retirement is not an end but rather a new beginning. Schlossberg (2004) points out that retirement is not simply an event in a person's life: retirement is best viewed as an evolving process that changes over time. Retirement is a major transition in a person's life that brings a unique set of choices and challenges. Transitions change our lives by altering our relationships, routines, roles, and assumptions. These shifts are characterized by leaving old patterns and moving onto new paths. Once people retire, says Schlossberg, they have different relationships with their colleagues, different daily routines, different roles, and different assumptions that affect both the structure of their lives and their interactions. Replacing these relationships, routines, roles, and assumptions is an evolutionary process that often gives rise to considerable uncertainty and anxiety.

There are many choices open to us as we embark on the path toward retirement. Indeed, a major challenge we face as we retire is deciding which path we will take to continue to find meaning in life. Schlossberg (2004) identified five retirement paths: continuers, adventurers, searchers, easy gliders, and retreaters:

Continuers do more of the same, but they package their main activities in new ways. They use their skills and maintain their interests and values associated with their previous work, but they modify them to fit retirement.

Adventurers are characterized by seeking something new. They view retirement as an opportunity to create a new path, and they look for new ways of organizing their time and space.

Searchers spend much of their time engaged in trial and error activities. Although they are separating from their past, they have not yet found their niche. They may pursue a path and discover that it is not rewarding, and then continue looking for a more satisfying path.

Easy gliders are content to go with the flow. They thrive on unscheduled time and select activities that appeal to them. In short, they value the newfound freedom that retirement provides for them to embrace life.

Retreaters are those who have given up on forging a new and rewarding life. They often feel disengaged from life.

Schlossberg reminds us that the word *retirement* is often used to imply giving up work. However, there are now many different models of retirement, and people can choose from a combination of paths. We are not locked into one path but instead may be traveling on several paths.

THE PLACE OF RECREATION IN YOUR LIFE

Work alone does not take care of all aspects of life. Even rewarding work takes energy, and most people need a life outside of work to enrich their lives, broaden their perspectives, and reenergize their work (Schwartz & Flowers, 2008). Whereas work requires a certain degree of perseverance and drive, recreation requires the ability to let go, to be spontaneous, and to avoid being obsessed with what we "should" be doing. **Recreation** involves creating new interests that become our path to vitality. Recreation implies flowing with the river rather than pushing against it and making something happen.

Leisure is "free time," the time that we control and can use for ourselves. Pursuing personal interests in our leisure time can be especially rewarding if work is not as fulfilling as it might be. Leisure can become a substitute for work and provide opportunities to try out new activities and find meaning apart from our work. Leisure gives us a respite from the responsibilities of work, helps relieve work stress, and refocuses our work perspective (Peterson & Gonzalez, 2005). In addition, leisure time activities can satisfy self-expressive needs and provide balance in our lives, leading to a healthier lifestyle regardless of age. Pursuit of leisure activities are associated with improved physical and cognitive functioning, increased happiness, and greater longevity (Menec, 2003).

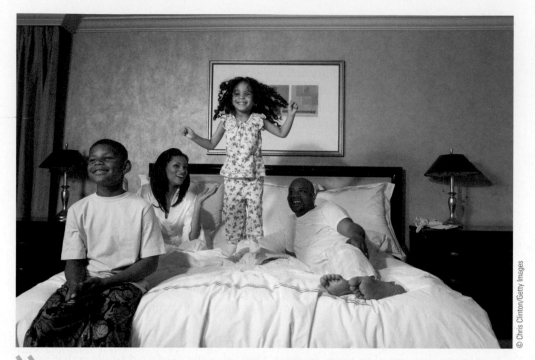

>> Recreation implies flowing with the river rather than pushing against it and making something happen.

Recreation and the Meaning of Your Life

Perhaps a major challenge you will face is balancing work, family, and leisure pursuits. We need to remind ourselves to pause long enough to really savor and enjoy experiences such as a cool breeze, a sunrise or sunset, the silence of the woods, a rainbow, and passing clouds in the sky. If we use our imagination, we can identify a range of activities that not only provide a time out from work but enhance our relationships with others and our lives. However, recreation can lose its benefits if we "work hard at having a good time." Some people schedule recreational activities in such a manner that they actually miss the point of recreation. Others become quickly bored when they are not doing something. For Bob and Jill, leisure is a way of connecting with each other. He is a laborer, she is a hairstylist, and both of them work hard all week. They say they like a weekend trip to the river, and they find that it revitalizes them to get ready for the upcoming workweek.

   As a couple, we (Marianne and Jerry) attribute different meanings to our leisure time. I (Jerry) tend to plan most of the things in my life, including my leisure time. I often combine work and leisure. Until recently, I seemed to require little leisure time because most of my satisfactions in life came from my work. Although at one point in my life I was doing everything I wanted to do professionally, I continued to feel challenged to learn the limits and find a balance in the nonwork areas of my life. A hard lesson for me to learn was to pause before too readily taking on additional professional engagements. Because I lived with an overcrowded schedule and accepted too many professional invitations, I was challenged to learn the value of carefully reflecting on the pros and cons of accepting any invitation, no matter how tempting it appeared. Although I enjoyed most of what I was doing, I eventually recognized that it left little room for anything else. I had the difficult task of learning to say "No" to some attractive and meaningful offers of work.

Many of my "hobbies" are still work-related, and although my scope tends to be somewhat narrow, this has been largely by choice. I am aware that I have had trouble with unstructured time. I am quite certain that leisure has represented a personal threat; as if any time unaccounted for is not being put to the best and most productive use. However, I am learning how to appreciate the reality that time is not simply to be used in doing, producing, accomplishing, and moving mountains.

Although it is a lesson that I am learning relatively late in life, I am increasingly appreciating times of being and experiencing, as well as time spent on accomplishing tasks. Experiencing sunsets, watching the beauty in nature, and being open to what moments can teach me are ways of using time that I am coming to cherish. Although work is still a very important part of my life, I am realizing that this is only a part of my life, not the totality of it.

In contrast, I (Marianne) want and need unstructured and spontaneous time for unwinding. I am uncomfortable when schedules are imposed on me, especially during leisure time. I do not particularly like to make detailed life plans, for this gets in the way of my relaxing. Although I plan for trips and times of recreation, I do not like to have everything I am going to do on the trip planned in advance. I like the element of surprise. It feels good to flow with moments and let things happen rather than working hard at making things happen. Also, I do not particularly like to combine work and leisure. For me, work involves considerable responsibility. It is difficult for me to relax and enjoy leisure if it is tainted with the demands of work, or if I know that I will soon have to function in a professional role. It is ironic that I am working on the revision of this chapter while sitting on a beautiful beach in Kauai, Hawaii. I guess I am balancing work and leisure today.

The objectives of planning for a career and planning for creative use of leisure time are basically the same: to help us develop feelings of self-esteem, reach our potential, and improve the quality of our lives. If we do not learn how to pursue interests apart from work, we may well face a crisis when we retire. If we do plan for creative ways to use leisure, we can experience both joy and continued personal growth.

A Couple Who Are Able to Balance Work and Recreation

Judy and Frank have found a good balance between work and recreation. Although they both enjoy their work, they have also arranged their lives to make time for leisure.

Judy and Frank were married when she was 16 and he was 20. They now have two grown sons and a couple of grandchildren. At 59 Frank works for an electrical company as a lineman, a job he has held for close to 35 years. Judy, who is now 55, delivers meals to schools.

Judy went to work when her two sons were in elementary school. She was interested in doing something away from home. Judy continues her work primarily because she likes the contact with both her coworkers and the children whom she meets daily.

Frank is satisfied with his work, and he looks forward to going to the job. Considering that he stopped his education at high school, he feels he has a good job that both pays well and offers many fringe benefits. Although he is a bright person, he expresses no ambition to increase his formal education. A few of the things Frank likes about his work are the companionship with his coworkers, the physical aspects of his job, the security it affords, and the routine.

Judy and Frank have separate interests and hobbies, yet they also spend time together. Both of them are hardworking, and they have achieved success financially and personally. They feel pleased about their success and can see the fruits of their labor. Together they enjoy their grandchildren, their friends, and each other.

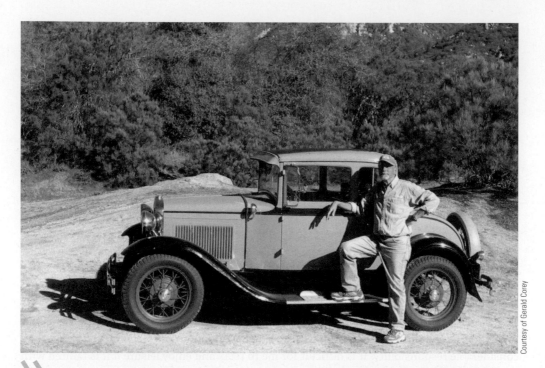

» If we do plan for creative ways to use leisure, we can experience both joy and continued personal growth.

Judy and Frank enjoy their work life and their leisure life, both as individuals and as a couple. A challenge that many of us will face is finding ways of using our leisure as well as they do. Just as our work can have either a positive or a negative influence on our life, so, too, can leisure. These Take Time to Reflect exercises will help you consolidate your thoughts on how work and leisure are integrated in your life.

TAKE TIME TO REFLECT

1. How would you describe the balance between work and recreation in your life right now? What do you envision the optimal balance between work and leisure to be for you 5 years from now? How about 10 or 20 years from now?

_____

_____

2. What was modeled by way of leisure time and recreation in your family of origin? Are there any ways that you would like to spend your leisure time differently?

_____

_____

3. How would you describe the interpersonal dynamics at your workplace (if you are currently employed)? To what extent do these dynamics seem to affect your attitudes and behaviors as an employee?

_____

_____

4. How do you think your self-esteem has been affected by your experiences as a student and, if applicable, as an employee?

_____

_____

5. What choices have you made in the past that have helped you to find meaning in your work (either as a student or an employee)? Looking forward, what choices can you make that will help you to find meaning in your career?

_____

_____

6. As you think about retirement, what are your main concerns? How would it be for you if you had to stop working prematurely? How would it be for you if you had to postpone your planned retirement?

_____

_____

SUMMARY

Choosing a career is best thought of as a process, not a one-time event. The term *career decision* is misleading because it implies that we make one choice that we stay with permanently. Most of us will probably have several occupations over our lifetimes, which is a good argument for a general education. If you prepare too narrowly for a specialization, that job may become obsolete, as will your training. In selecting a career or an occupation, it is important to first assess your attitudes, abilities, interests, and values. The next step is to explore a wide range of occupational options to see what jobs would best fit your personality. Becoming familiar with Holland's six personality types is an excellent way to consider the match between your personality style and the work alternatives you are considering. Choosing an occupation too soon can be risky because your interests may change as you move into adulthood. If you accept a job without carefully considering where you might best find meaning and satisfaction, this is likely to lead to dissatisfaction and frustration.

Retirement can be a time with new opportunities to redesign one's life, or it can be a time when one is coasting and feeling lost. Especially for those who retire early, the real challenge is to find a way to keep involved in a meaningful way.

Some people choose early retirement because they have found more significant and valuable pursuits. People who are retired do have choices, and they can create meaningful lives without employment. Many retired people have found that retirement is not an end to life but rather a new beginning.

Because we devote about half of our waking hours to our work, it behooves us to actively choose a form of work that can express who we are as a person. Much of the other half of our waking time can be used for leisure. Just as our work can profoundly affect all aspects of our lives, so, too, can leisure have a positive or negative influence on our existence. Our leisure time can leave us feeling drained, or it can be a source of replenishment that energizes us and enriches our lives.

A key idea in this chapter is that we must look to ourselves if we are dissatisfied with our work. Although work conditions may be less than optimal, especially during difficult economic times, we can choose how we want to react to these conditions. It is important to recognize what you are able to change, and what is beyond your control. Focus your attention on factors that you can control and aspects of your life that you can change.

Where Can I Go From Here?

1. Interview someone you know who dislikes his or her career or occupation. Here are some questions you might ask to get started:

▸ If you don't find your job satisfying, what has prevented you from leaving and finding a different job?

▸ What other options, if any, are you considering right now? Given the economic outlook, how much choice to you feel you have right now?

▸ What aspects of your job bother you the most? If you could change any aspects of your job to make your situation better, what would you change?

▸ How does your attitude toward your job affect the other areas of your life?

2. Interview a person you know who feels fulfilled and excited by his or her work. Begin with these questions:

▸ How does your work bring you fulfillment? What meaning does your work have for the other aspects of your life?

▸ What are the most satisfying aspects of your work?

▸ What is a typical work day like for you?

▸ What challenges or barriers did you have to deal with in getting established in your work?

▸ How do you think you would be affected if you could no longer pursue your career?

3. If your parents have not yet retired, interview them and determine what meaning their work has for them. How satisfied are they with their jobs? How much choice do they feel they have in selecting their work? In what ways do they think the other aspects of their lives are affected by their attitudes toward work? After you have talked with them, determine how your attitudes and beliefs about work have been influenced by your parents. Are you pursuing a career that your parents can understand and respect? Is their reaction to your career choice important to you? Are your attitudes and values concerning work like or unlike those of your parents?

4. If you are leaning toward a particular occupation or career, seek out a person who is actively engaged in that type of work and arrange for a time to talk with him or her. You might even see if job shadowing is a possibility. Ask questions concerning the chances of gaining employment, the experience necessary, the satisfactions and drawbacks of the position, and so on. In this way, you can make the process of deciding on a type of work more realistic and perhaps avoid disappointment if your expectations do not match reality.

5. We briefly oriented you to Holland's typology in this chapter. If you are interested in a more complete self-assessment method that also describes the relationship between your personality type and possible occupations or fields of study, we strongly recommend that you take the Self-Directed Search (SDS), which is available online (see Website Resources at the end of the chapter). The SDS takes 20 to 30 minutes to complete and costs $4.95. Your personalized report will appear on your screen.

6. Here are some steps you can take when exploring the choice of a major and a career. Place a check before each item you are willing to seriously consider. I am willing to:

_____ talk to an adviser about my intended major

_____ interview at least one instructor about potential majors

_____ interview at least one person I know in a career that I am interested in

_____ make a trip to the career development center and see what resources are offered

_____ make use of computer-assisted career guidance assessments

_____ inquire about taking a series of interest and work values tests in the career development center

_____ take an interest inventory online or at a career center on campus

_____ talk to my parents about the meaning work has for them

_____ write in my journal about my values as they pertain to work

_____ read books that deal with careers

_____ surf the Internet for sites that introduce different career fields

7. Apply the seven steps of the career-planning process to your own career planning. Set realistic goals to do one or more of the following or some other appropriate activity:

▸ Choose a major that most fully taps my interests and abilities.

▸ Take time to investigate a career by gathering further information.

▸ Develop contacts with people who can help me meet my goals.

▸ Take steps that will enable me to increase my exposure to a field of interest.

In the journal pages at the end of this chapter, write down at least a tentative plan for action. Begin by identifying some of the key factors associated with selecting a career. Write down the steps you are willing to take at this time. (Your plan will be most useful if you identify specific steps you are willing to take. Include seeking the help of others somewhere in your plan.)

8. In this chapter we emphasized the role recreation plays in maintaining your vitality. If you are experiencing an imbalance between work and recreation, consider what you need to do to restore balance in your life. If you could benefit from more recreation, do a web search to gain preliminary information about hobbies you might enjoy or skills you would like to learn. If you have always wanted to learn to play a musical instrument, learn how to oil paint, or learn Salsa dancing, use the Internet as a tool to find out about these recreational activities and class schedules.

9. Suggested Readings. The full bibliographic entry for each of these sources can be found in the References and Suggested Readings at the back of the book. A practical book that can assist you in the process of career decision making is Bolles (2012). For an interesting treatment on the subject of retirement, see Schlossberg (2004).

WEBSITE RESOURCES

Included here are some valuable websites. For access to these websites, video activities, and other supporting materials, visit Cengage Learning's Counseling CourseMate website for *I Never Knew I Had a Choice*, 10th Edition, at **www.cengagebrain.com.**

IMAGINE
http://cty.jhu.edu/imagine
Recommended Search Words: "Imagine magazine"

A five-time winner of the Parents' Choice Gold Award, *Imagine* is a resource magazine for academically talented teens, produced at the Johns Hopkins Center for Talented Youth. *Imagine's* webpage provides links to numerous opportunities and resources. Although aimed at a precollege audience, this site offers links to an impressive number of career-related sites and professional associations that will be useful for people of all ages who are exploring career opportunities.

THE OCCUPATIONAL OUTLOOK HANDBOOK
http://stats.bls.gov/oco
Recommended Search Words: "occupational outlook handbook"

The *Occupational Outlook Handbook* is a "nationally recognized source of career information, designed to provide valuable assistance to individuals making decisions about their future work lives." It "describes what workers do on the job, working conditions, the training and education needed, earnings, and expected job prospects in a wide range of occupations." Users can download pages on the careers of their choice.

THE SELF-DIRECTED SEARCH
www.self-directed-search.com
Recommended Search Words: "self-directed search"

This is a widely used career interest test, which is a very useful resource in matching your skills and interests to specific jobs and careers.

JOB CHOICES 2012
www.jobweb.org
Recommended Search Words: "jobweb"

The National Association of Colleges and Employers has created a comprehensive set of resources for job seekers and job offerings. The site includes searching employment listings, resources for career practitioners, career library resources, and professional development resources.

U.S. DEPARTMENT OF LABOR
www.dol.gov
Recommended Search Words "department of labor"

This site explores topics such as wages, worker productivity, unsafe working conditions, and the legal rights of workers, including protection from sexual harassment.

APA HELP CENTER
http://apahelpcenter.org
Recommended Search Words: "APA help center"

This American Psychological Association site disseminates information to the public about coping with various aspects of life. Work and school is one category. Information on dealing with stress in the workplace and managing your boss is available.

CAREERS.WSJ.COM
http://online.wsj.com/careers
Recommended Search Words: "career journal wsj"

This site contains daily updates of employment issues and more than 1,000 job-seeking articles.

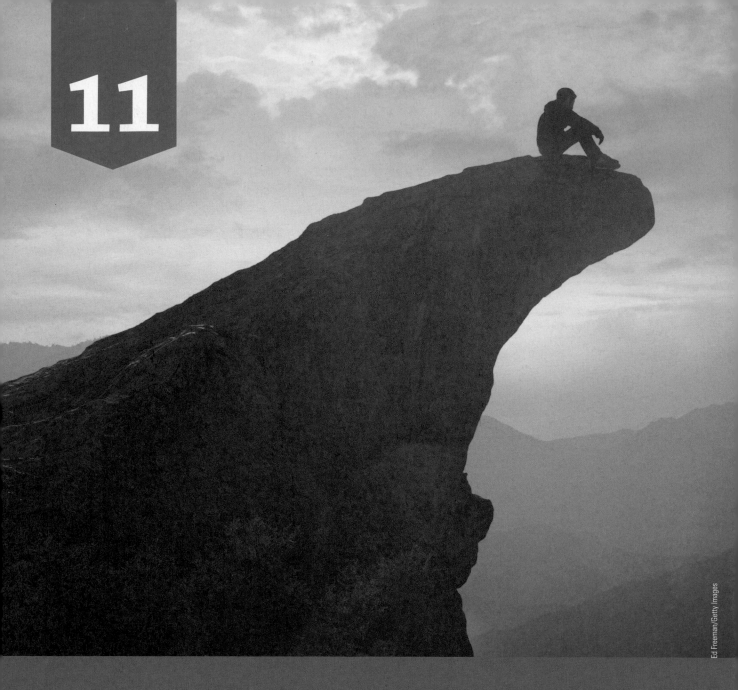

Ed Freeman/Getty Images

11

LONELINESS AND SOLITUDE

> Where Am I Now?

> The Value of Solitude

> The Experience of Loneliness

> Learning to Confront the Fear of
  Loneliness

> Creating Our Own Loneliness Through
  Shyness

> Loneliness and Our Life Stages

> Time Alone as a Source of Strength

> Summary

> Where Can I Go From Here?

> Website Resources

> *In solitude we make the time to be with ourselves, to discover who we are, and to renew ourselves.*

WHERE AM I NOW?

Use this scale to respond to these statements:

4 = I *strongly agree* with this statement.
3 = I *agree* with this statement.
2 = I *disagree* with this statement.
1 = I *strongly disagree* with this statement.

	1.	I stay in unsatisfactory relationships to avoid being lonely.
	2.	I like being alone.
	3.	I don't know what to do with my time when I am alone.
	4.	Even when I'm with people I sometimes feel lonely and shut out.
	5.	At this time in my life I like the balance between my solitude and my time with others.
	6.	I seek distractions to avoid feelings of loneliness.
	7.	My childhood was a lonely period of my life.
	8.	My adolescent years were lonely ones for me.
	9.	Currently I am satisfied with the way in which I cope with my loneliness.
	10.	I sometimes arrange for time alone so that I can reflect on my life.

We invite you to think of being alone not as something to be avoided at all costs but as a part of the human experience. If we are not able to enjoy time alone, it will be difficult to truly enjoy time with others. If we have a good relationship with ourselves and enjoy our solitude, we have a better chance of creating solid, give-and-take relationships with others. Although the presence of others can surely enhance our lives, no one else can completely share our unique world of feelings, thoughts, hopes, and memories. In some respects we are alone, even though we may have meaningful connections with others.

THE VALUE OF SOLITUDE

It is important to distinguish between being lonely and being alone. Loneliness and solitude are different experiences, and each has its own potential value. **Loneliness** is generally triggered by certain life events—the death of someone we love, the decision of another person to leave us (or we them), a move to a new city, a long stay in a hospital, or a major life decision. Unlike loneliness, solitude is something that we choose for ourselves. In **solitude,** we make time to be with ourselves, to discover who we are, and to renew ourselves. Psychotherapist and writer Thomas Moore (1995) was a monk as a young man, and he views loneliness as a way for us to understand solitude: "Loneliness is sometimes a sign that we need to learn what it takes for us to be constructively alone, grounded in our own natures, willing to take responsibility

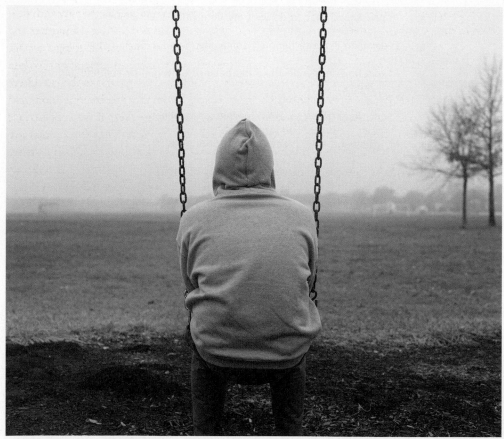

Rod Morata/Getty Images

>> In solitude, we make time to be with ourselves, to discover who we are, and to renew ourselves.

for making our own decisions and shaping our own lives" (p. 29). Moore encourages us to reflect on our need for connection with others and on our need for solitude.

If we do not take time for ourselves but instead fill our lives with activities and projects, we run the risk of losing a sense of centeredness. Solitude provides us with the opportunity for examining our life, assessing what we are doing, and gaining a sense of perspective. Solitude gives us time to ask significant questions such as, "Have I become a stranger to myself?" and "Have I been listening to myself, or have I been distracted and overstimulated by my busyness?" We can use times of solitude to look within ourselves, to come to know ourselves better, to renew our sense of ourselves as the center of choice and direction in our lives, and to learn to trust our inner resources instead of allowing circumstances or the expectations of others to determine the path we travel. Some people believe that when they are alone they are lonely. However, if we accept our aloneness, we can give ourselves to our projects and our relationships out of our freedom instead of running to them out of our fear. The Dalai Lama (2001) stresses that to make changes in our lives we need solitude, by which he means "a mental state free of distractions, not simply time alone in a quiet place" (p. 78).

We may miss the valuable experience of solitude if we allow our life to become too frantic and complicated. We may fear that others will think we are odd if we express a desire for solitude. Others may sometimes fail to understand our desire to be alone and may try to persuade us to be with them. Some people who are close to you may feel vaguely threatened, as if your need for time alone means that you have less affection for them. Indeed, their own fears of being left alone may lead them to try to keep you from taking time away from them.

We need to remind ourselves that most of us can tolerate only so much intensity with others and that ignoring our need for distance can breed resentment. For instance, a mother and father who are constantly with each other and with their children may not be doing a service either to their children or to themselves. Eventually they might resent their "obligations." When they take time out, they may be able to be more fully present to each other and to their children.

Many of us fail to experience solitude because we allow our lives to become more and more frantic and complicated. We may fear that we will alienate others if we seek private time, so we alienate ourselves instead. Society provides us with many distractions that are often hard to resist. The constant intrusion of 24-hours-a day electronic media and smart phones can rob us of the opportunity to be alone with our thoughts. It seems that solitude is neither valued nor encouraged in our world today. The message that it is better to be constantly busy rather than inactive begins early in childhood. An abundance of activities are planned for children, which allows for little quiet time. Counselors see children who suffer from stress and an already overscheduled life. These children learn early on to become impatient with lack of stimulation, and they are quick to point out that they are bored with the absence of activity.

BECKY'S STORY

As a counselor who serves bright middle school and high school students, I am constantly reminded that today's youth have very little down time. Students lead busy lives, and much of their daily life is structured with little time for rest. Once, a student who held very high standards for herself told me that she wanted to talk on the phone about college options, and she asked if I could call her between 2 and 4 o'clock in the morning! I asked her when she found time to sleep, and she mentioned that she is in the habit of taking catnaps during the day. Students like this often graduate from high school with exemplary credentials, yet at what cost?

We may feel uneasy about wanting and taking time alone for ourselves. We might even make up excuses if we want to have some time alone. Claiming what we need and want for ourselves can involve a certain risk; failing to do so also involves a risk—a loss of a sense of self-direction and being centered, which does require a certain amount of solitude. One way to use solitude to our advantage is to develop a practice of daily meditation, which is an ideal way to quiet the mind and body. Jack Canfield (1995) tells us that in times of solitude we can rekindle the fires of our soul. He reminds us that our soul nourishes us, if we allow it to happen: "Our challenge as human beings is to open ourselves to receive this nourishment—to rekindle our connection with our spirit, the spirit that is always there waiting to nurture, heal, and direct our lives" (p. 87). Canfield asserts that we will be more creative, productive, and peaceful if we make some time each day for quiet reflection and meditation.

THE EXPERIENCE OF LONELINESS

We often experience loneliness when our network of social relationships is lacking, when there are strains on these relationships, or when these relationships are not satisfying to us. Loneliness can occur when we feel set apart in some way from everyone, which can have its roots in the lack of attachment in early childhood. Sometimes feelings of loneliness are simply an indication of the extent to which we may have failed to listen to ourselves. However it occurs, loneliness generally happens to us rather than being chosen by us. If we acknowledge these feelings, loneliness can inspire us to become the person we want to be. By experiencing our loneliness, even if it is painful or unsettling, we can discover sources of strength and creativity within ourselves. Some loneliness is a natural dimension of the human condition, and we can choose to avoid pathologizing the experience.

There are different kinds of loneliness. Weiten, Dunn, and Hammer (2012) distinguish between transient loneliness and chronic loneliness. **Transient loneliness** involves brief feelings of loneliness that occur when people have had satisfactory social relationships in the past but experience some disruption in their social network, such as a breakup of a relationship or moving to a new place. A common form of transient loneliness that many new college students experience is homesickness; much attention has been given to this topic in the scholarly literature (see Beck, Taylor, & Robbins, 2003; Scopelliti & Tiberio, 2010; Tognoli, 2003). **Chronic loneliness** exists when people are unable to establish meaningful interpersonal relationships over a relatively long period of time. Although most of us experience loneliness at different times in our lives for short periods of time, chronic loneliness presents more of a problem in living. People who are particularly vulnerable to loneliness include those who are divorced, separated, or widowed; those who live alone or solely with children; gay and lesbian adolescents; and, as briefly noted, beginning college students.

Yalom (2008) writes about two kinds of loneliness: everyday and existential loneliness. **Everyday loneliness** involves the pain of being isolated from other people. This is an interpersonal loneliness often associated with the fear of intimacy and feelings of shame, rejection, or of being unlovable. **Existential loneliness** (or *existential isolation*) is associated with a profound sense of an unbridgeable gap that separates us from others. This gap is due to our awareness that each of us inhabits a world fully known only to ourselves. According to Yalom, existential loneliness refers not only to our physical death, but to the loss of our "own rich, miraculously detailed world, which does not exist in the same manner in the mind of anyone else" (p. 121). Existential loneliness takes on special meaning as we get older and move closer to death, a time when we become increasingly aware that our world will disappear and that others cannot accompany us to our final destiny.

LEARNING TO CONFRONT THE FEAR OF LONELINESS

There is good reason to have some fear of loneliness because evidence suggests that loneliness influences both our physical health and our psychological well-being. We may think of loneliness in a negative light if we associate the lonely periods in our lives with pain and struggle. Furthermore, we may identify being alone with being lonely and either actively avoid having time by ourselves or fill such time with distractions and diversions. We sometimes associate being alone with rejection of self and being cut off from others. Paradoxically, out of fear of rejection and loneliness, we may even make ourselves needlessly lonely by refusing to reach out to others or by holding back in our intimate relationships. At other times, because of our fear of loneliness, we may deceive ourselves into thinking that we can overcome loneliness only by anchoring our life to another's life. The search for relationships, especially ones in which we think we will be taken care of, is often motivated by the fear of being isolated.

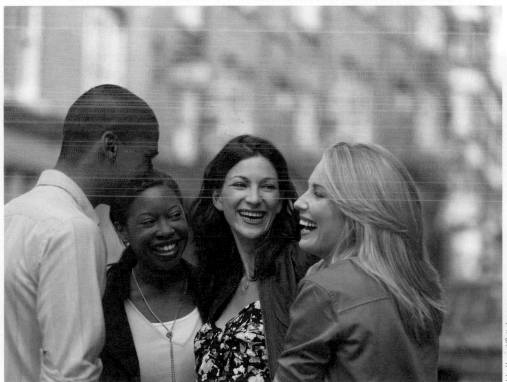

John Howard/Getty Images

» We can sometimes cope with the fear of loneliness by surrounding ourselves with people and social functions.

Silence forces us to reflect and touch deep parts of ourselves. We may attempt to escape from facing ourselves by keeping so busy that we leave little or no time to reflect. Here are some ways we do this:

▶ We schedule every moment and overstructure our lives, so we have no opportunity to think about ourselves and what we are doing with our lives.

▶ We strive for control of our environment, so we will not have to cope with unexpected happenings.

▶ We surround ourselves with people and become absorbed in social functions in the hope that we will not have to feel alone.

▶ We sometimes use relationships to avoid being alone.

▶ We numb ourselves with alcohol or drugs.

▶ We use antidepressant medications.

▶ We immerse ourselves in our responsibilities.

▶ We eat for emotional reasons, hoping that doing so will fill our inner emptiness and protect us from the pain of being lonely.

▶ We spend many hours with the computer, video games, and television.

▶ We use technology as an escape instead of as a way to make connections with others.

▶ We go to centers of activity, trying to lose ourselves in a crowd. By escaping into crowds, we avoid coming to terms with deeper layers of our inner world.

The world we live in surrounds us with entertainment and escapes, which makes it difficult to hear the voice within us. Paradoxically, in the midst of our congested cities and with all the activities available to us, we are often lonely because we are alienated from ourselves. To better understand this paradox, listen to Dianne talk about her life and her fears.

DIANNE'S STORY

I'm always wanting to surround myself with people. I don't just *dislike* being alone, I *hate* it. This realization struck me after I graduated from college and moved into an apartment on my own. In college, I never had any down time, and I liked it that way. There was always an activity of some sort going on to keep me busy, to keep me from thinking too deeply about things. And I always had at least one roommate. My friends regarded me as an outgoing and confident person because I was involved in so many things and knew so many people.

Now (a year out of college), I spend much of my free time on Facebook and texting friends from college. Technology is wonderful in that it helps me stay connected with my friends, but in a way it is also a curse—a curse that I cannot resist. Technology lets me avoid having to deal with myself. The moment I start to feel lonely, I just log onto Facebook, which makes me feel less empty for a while. But the feelings return, and I look for something else to distract me from my thoughts and feelings. If I don't face the underlying reasons why I need to fill every single moment of my time doing something, I am worried that it is going to catch up with me one of these days. Lately, I have not been feeling like the confident person my friends admired so much. If they only knew how I felt inside, I think they would be surprised.

Dianne is a young woman who often fears separateness from others, even though she immerses herself in many relationships and activities. Outsiders tend to envy her "fun-filled" life and wish they were in her place. In a moment of candor, however, she admits that she feels her life to be empty and that she is in a desperate search for substance. In some ways Dianne illustrates the quiet desperation that is captured in Edward Arlington Robinson's poem "Richard Cory" (1897/1943):

Whenever Richard Cory went down town,
We people on the pavement looked at him:
He was a gentleman from sole to crown,
Clean favored, and imperially slim.
And he was always quietly arrayed,
And he was always human when he talked;
But still he fluttered pulses when he said,
"Good morning," and he glittered when he walked.
And he was rich—yes, richer than a king—
And admirably schooled in every grace:
In fine, we thought that he was everything
To make us wish that we were in his place.
So on we worked and waited for the light,
And went without the meat, and cursed the bread;
And Richard Cory, one calm summer night,
Went home and put a bullet through his head.

The way we present ourselves to the world oftentimes belies the loneliness we feel. Many of us have known someone who appeared to have everything in life who suddenly committed suicide. The loneliness that some individuals experience is often not apparent to others. Pretending to others to be what we are not, as well as anchoring our lives to others as a way of avoiding facing ourselves, results in losing our sense of self and leads to alienation.

We often surround ourselves with people, trying to convince ourselves that we are not lonely. From our perspective, if we want to get back into contact with ourselves, we must begin by looking at the ways we have learned to escape from our loneliness. We can examine our relationships to see if we at times use others to fill that void. We can ask whether the activities that fill our time actually satisfy us or whether they leave us empty and discontented. For some of us, being alone may be less lonely than being in a relationship.

CREATING OUR OWN LONELINESS THROUGH SHYNESS

Shyness is expressed in discomfort, anxiety, inhibition, and excessive caution in interpersonal relationships.* Some specific characteristics that identify shy individuals are timidity in expressing themselves; being overly sensitive to how they are perceived and reacted to; being embarrassed easily; and experiencing bodily symptoms such as blushing, upset stomach, anxiety, and racing pulse (Carducci, 2000a; 2008). Shyness exists on a continuum. That is, some people see themselves as chronically shy, whereas others are shy with certain people or in certain situations. Shyness may be perceived and evaluated differently across cultural contexts. For instance, researchers have identified three distinct forms of shyness in Chinese children: shyness toward strangers; anxious shyness; and regulated shyness (nonassertive and

*We appreciate the contributions of Dr. Bernardo J. Carducci, Director, Shyness Research Institute, Indiana University Southeast, in updating this section on shyness.

unassuming shyness), which is an asset in Confucian cultures (Xu, Farver, Yu, & Zhang, 2009). Shyness is multifaceted, so it is important to define "shyness" for yourself. You may be shy in some situations, yet in many situations shyness may not be a part of your personality.

Shy people are generally uncomfortable in social situations, especially if they become the center of attention, are in the presence of authority figures, are interacting with someone with whom they find attractive, or if they are expected to speak up. Shyness does not necessarily have to be a problem for you. In fact, you might decide you like this quality in yourself—and so might many others who know you. Shyness becomes a problem only when you hold back from expressing yourself in ways you would like. You can learn to say and do what you would like when you are with others and still retain your shy nature. To determine how shyness may be affecting you, complete the Take Time to Reflect exercise that follows.

TAKE TIME TO REFLECT

How shy are you? Take the *Shyness Quiz** to find out.

A. How often do you experience feelings of shyness?

1. Once a month or less
2. Nearly every other day
3. Constantly, several times a day

B. Compared with your peers, how shy are you?

1. Much less shy
2. About as shy
3. Much more shy

C. "Shyness makes me feel symptoms such as a racing heart and sweaty palms." This description is . . .

1. Not like me
2. Somewhat like me
3. A lot like me

D. "Shyness makes me think others are reacting negatively to what I do and say." This description is . . .

1. Not like me
2. Somewhat like me
3. A lot like me

E. "Shyness keeps me from behaving appropriately in social settings: for example, introducing myself or making conversation." This description is . . .

1. Not like me
2. Somewhat like me
3. A lot like me

F. "Shyness appears when I'm interacting with someone to whom I'm attracted." This description is . . .

1. Not like me
2. Somewhat like me
3. A lot like me

G. "Shyness appears when I'm interacting with someone in a position of authority; for example, supervisors at work, professors, experts in their field." This description is . . .

1. Not like me
2. Somewhat like me
3. A lot like me

Scoring: Add together the numbers that correspond to your responses to each of the seven items:

7–11: *Not at all to slightly shy*: Shyness does not seem to be much of a problem for you.
12–16: *Moderately shy*: Shyness seems to be a frequent barrier in your life.
17–21: *Very Shy*: Shyness is preventing you from reaching your full potential in life.

*Reproduced with permission from Bernardo J. Carducci, Director, Shyness Research Institute, Indiana University Southeast.

If you are shy, you are not alone, for shyness is an almost universal experience. In one study 80% of those questioned reported that they had been shy at some point in their lives (Zimbardo, 1994). Additional research on shyness over the last few decades indicates that approximately 40% of people who were surveyed considered themselves to be shy (Carducci, 2000a; Carducci, Stubbins, & Bryant, 2008; Carducci & Zimbardo, 1995; Zimbardo, 1994), including 46% of adolescents (Burstein, Ameli-Grillon, & Merikangas, 2011).

Shyness can lead directly to feelings of loneliness. Zimbardo (1994) believes shyness can be a social and psychological handicap as crippling as many physical handicaps. Here are some of the negative consequences of shyness that have been identified (Carducci, 2000a, 2000b; Zimbardo, 1994):

▶ Shyness prevents people from expressing their views and speaking up for their rights.

▶ Shyness may make it difficult to think clearly and to communicate effectively.

▶ Shyness holds people back from meeting new people, making friends, and getting involved in many social activities.

▶ Shyness can hold people back in the progression of their careers.

▶ Shyness can prevent students from speaking up in class and seeking the assistance of their professors outside of class.

▶ Shyness often results in feelings such as depression, anxiety, and loneliness.

▶ Shyness can lead some individuals to develop a dependency on alcohol as a way to feel more relaxed and sociable.

According to Henderson (2011), normal shyness can be helpful in some circumstances; however, this pattern can lead to chronic shyness because of negative self-talk, avoidance, and withdrawal. Shyness becomes problematic when it interferes with your life goals, evolves into social anxiety disorder, or leads to "learned pessimism." Severe shyness is referred to as "social anxiety disorder."

You may be aware that shyness is a problem for you and that you are creating much of your own loneliness in your life because you are shy. You may ask, "What can I do about it?" You can begin by challenging those personal fears that keep you from expressing the way you truly think and feel. Put yourself in situations where you will be forced to make contact with people and engage in social activities, even if you find doing this is scary and uncomfortable.

Lynne Henderson (2011), of the Shyness Institute, describes the social fitness model as a way to help shy individuals develop their capacities. We need to achieve and maintain fitness if we hope to function optimally. Social fitness in demanding social situations is achieved through practice. With effort and practice, most of us can achieve an adaptive state of social fitness in the same way that we can attain an adaptive state of physical fitness.

It helps to understand the context of your shyness, especially to identify those social situations that stimulate your shy behavior as well as to pinpoint the reasons or combination of factors underlying your shyness (Carducci, 2005; Carducci & Fields, 2007). According to Zimbardo (1994), a constellation of factors explain shyness: being overly sensitive to negative feedback from others, fearing rejection, lacking self-confidence and specific social skills, being frightened of intimacy, and personal handicaps.

A good way to identify those factors that contribute to your shyness is to keep track in your journal of those situations that elicit your shy behavior. It helps to write down what you are truly experiencing and then what you actually do in such situations. Pay attention to your self-talk in these difficult situations because negative self-talk may be setting you up to fail. For example, do you recognize some of these thoughts? "I'm unattractive, so who would want anything to do with me?" "I'd better not try something new because I might look ridiculous." "I'm afraid of being rejected, so I won't even approach a person I'd like to get to know." "People are not really interested in what I am thinking and feeling." "Others are evaluating and judging me, and I'm sure I won't measure up to what they expect." These are the kinds of statements that are likely to keep you a prisoner of your shyness and prevent you from making real contact with others. You can do a lot yourself to control how your shyness affects you by learning to challenge your self-defeating beliefs and by substituting constructive statements. Coping with shyness involves becoming aware of, examining, and changing your thinking about shyness and yourself (Zimbardo, 1994). Carducci, director of the Shyness Research Institute, has said, "We'd rather understand shy people than change them" (personal communication, January 10, 2012). Increasing your understanding of your shyness is a good first step in deciding what, if anything, you may want to change about how you behave in social situations. Learning new ways of thinking about yourself involves pushing yourself to test out your new beliefs by acting in new ways.

In addition to thinking about yourself in new ways, you need to be willing to get out of your comfort zone (Carducci, 2000a, 2009). According to Carducci, shy individuals tend to operate in a limited comfort zone—doing the same things at the same places with the same small group of people again and again because such familiar places and people are comfortable. Carducci notes that shy people tell him that their biggest social barrier to stepping out of their comfort zone is approaching individuals in social situations and initiating and maintaining a conversation.

People who have difficulty dealing with shyness often withdraw socially, and social withdrawal generally exacerbates matters and can lead to loneliness. Tracy's experience in coping with shyness illustrates how she overcame her inhibitions and came out of her shell of shyness.

TRACY'S STORY

When I first began college, I was really shy. I would not ask questions in class, I studied by myself, and I did not pursue friendships with my peers. My shyness developed out of a belief that I would look stupid if I asked questions and that my peers would think I was not really smart if they studied with me. I was convinced that people would eventually realize I was not fun or outgoing. Needless to say, I had set myself up to feel like a failure. I eventually decided to transfer to a different college to get a fresh start. Although I don't usually run from my problems, I considered this change a good decision.

After transferring, I made a commitment to myself that I would do what it took to succeed. I was determined to reinvent myself at my new school. Part of this commitment was to speak up in class, ask questions, form study groups, and make friends. This was really scary for me, but I knew giving in to my shyness would lead to the same negative outcome as before. That was not an option.

I did not want to live that way anymore. I made contact with my teachers and became invested in my learning process. As I became involved with my studies and my peers, my self-confidence increased and my grades improved. I began to believe that I was smart, that I did ask good questions, that others were not judging me, and that others liked who I was, and most important, I liked who I was.

If you are shy, the best first step to take is to accept this as part of who you are. Then challenge yourself to get involved in activities and to make contact with others. Even though you are shy, you can monitor your thoughts, feelings, and actions as a way of becoming more aware of the process you are going through. Like Tracy, you can take steps to make contact with others and challenge negative self-talk that is keeping you in your shell. If you are interested in learning more about shyness, we recommend *Shyness: A Bold New Approach* (Carducci, 2000a), *The Shyness Workbook: 30 Ways to Dealing Effectively With Shyness* (Carducci, 2005), and *Shyness* (Zimbardo, 1994).

TAKE TIME TO REFLECT

1. In what ways do you try to escape from your loneliness?

_____

_____

2. Does this avoidance work for you? If not, how might you change it?

_____

_____

3. If shyness is a problem for you, in what ways does it affect your relationships?

_____

_____

4. To what extent do you enjoy time alone?

_____

_____

5. List a few of the major decisions you have made in your life. Did you make these decisions when you were alone or when you were with others?

_____

_____

Journal suggestion: If you find it difficult to be alone, try being alone for a little longer than you are generally comfortable with. You might simply let your thoughts wander freely, without hanging on to one line of thinking. In the journal pages at the end of this chapter describe what this experience is like for you.

LONELINESS AND OUR LIFE STAGES

How we deal with feelings of loneliness depends to a great extent on our experiences of loneliness in childhood and adolescence. Later in life we may feel that loneliness has no place or that we can and should be able to avoid it. It is important to reflect on our past experiences because they are often the basis of our present feelings about loneliness. We may fear loneliness less when we recognize that it is an inevitable part of living in every stage of life. There are many areas in which we may experience loneliness. Our differences, such as gender, race, sexual orientation, cultural background, language, or being a foreigner in a foreign land can trigger feelings of loneliness.

Loneliness and Childhood

Reliving childhood experiences of loneliness can help us come to grips with our present fears about being alone or lonely. Here are some typical memories of lonely periods that people have worked on in their personal therapy:

▶ A woman recalls the time her parents were fighting in the bedroom and she heard them screaming and yelling. She was sure that they would divorce, and in many ways she felt responsible. She remembers living in continual fear that she would be deserted.

▶ A man recalls attempting to give a speech in the sixth grade. He stuttered over certain words, and children in the class began to laugh at him. Afterward he developed extreme self-consciousness in regard to his speech, and he long remembered the hurt and loneliness he had experienced.

▶ An African American man recalls how excluded he felt in his all-White elementary school and how the other children would talk to him in derogatory ways. As an adult, he can still, at times, experience the pain associated with these memories.

▶ A woman recalls the fright she felt as a small child when her uncle made sexual advances toward her. Although she did not really understand what was happening, she remembers the terrible loneliness of feeling that she could not tell her parents for fear of what they would do.

▶ A man recalls the boyhood loneliness of feeling that he was continually failing at everything he tried. To this day, he resists undertaking a task unless he is sure he can handle it for fear of rekindling those old feelings of loneliness.

▶ A woman vividly remembers being in the hospital as a small child for an operation. She remembers the loneliness of not knowing what was going on or whether she would be able to leave the hospital. No one talked with her, and she was all alone with her fears.

Our childhood fears may have been greatly exaggerated, but the feeling of fright may remain with us even though we may now think of it as excessive. Being told by adults that we were foolish for having such fears may only have increased our loneliness while doing nothing to lessen the fears themselves.

It is important to understand how some of the pain we felt as children may still be affecting us now. We can also look at some of the decisions we might have made during these times of extreme loneliness and question whether these decisions are still appropriate. Frequently, strategies we adopted as children remain with us into adulthood even though they are no longer appropriate. For instance, suppose that your family moved to a strange city when you were 7 years old and that you had to go to a new school. Children at the new school laughed at you, and you lived through several months of anguish. You felt desperately alone in the world. During this time you decided to keep your feelings to yourself and build a wall around yourself so others could not hurt you. Although this experience is now long past, you still defend yourself in the same way because it is now a reflex response. In this way old fears of loneliness might contribute to a real loneliness in the present. If you allow yourself to experience your grief and work it through, emotionally as well as intellectually, you can overcome past pain and create new experiences for yourself.

TAKE TIME TO REFLECT

Take some time to decide whether you are willing to recall and relive a childhood experience of loneliness. If so, try to recapture the experience in as much detail as you can, reliving it in fantasy. Then reflect on the experience, using the following questions as a starting point.

1. Describe the most intense experience of loneliness you recall having as a child.

_____

_____

2. How do you think the experience affected you then?

_____

_____

3. How do you think the experience may still be affecting you now?

_____

_____

Journal suggestion: Consider elaborating on this exercise in the journal pages at the end of this chapter. If you could go back and put a new ending on your most intense childhood experience of loneliness, what would it be? You might also think about times in your childhood when you enjoyed being alone. Write some notes to yourself about what these experiences were like for you. Where did you like to spend time alone? What did you enjoy doing by yourself? What positive aspects of these times do you recall?

Loneliness and Adolescence

For many people loneliness and adolescence are practically synonymous. Adolescents often feel that they are all alone in their world, that they are the only ones to have had the feelings they do, and that they are separated from others by some abnormality. Bodily changes and impulses alone are sufficient to bring about a sense of perplexity and loneliness, but there are other stresses to be undergone as well. As you remember from Chapter 2, adolescents are developing a sense of identity. They want to be accepted and liked, but they fear rejection, ridicule, or exclusion by their peers. Conformity can bring acceptance, and the price of nonconformity can be steep. Many adolescents know the feeling of being lonely in a crowd or among friends.

As you recall your adolescent years—and, in particular, times in your life that were marked by loneliness—reflect on these questions:

▶ Did you feel included in a social group? Or did you sit on the sidelines, afraid of being included and wishing for it at the same time?

▶ Was there at least one person you felt you could talk to—one who really heard and understood you, so that you didn't feel alone?

▶ What was one of your loneliest experiences during these years? How did you cope with your loneliness?

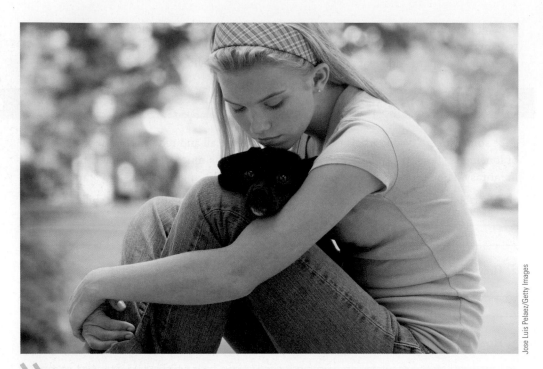

Jose Luis Pelaez/Getty Images

>> Adolescents often feel that they are all alone in the world.

▶ Did you experience a sense of confusion concerning who you were and what you wanted to be as a person? How did you deal with your confusion? Who or what helped you during this time?

▶ How did you feel about your own worth and value? Did you believe you had anything of value to offer anyone or that anyone would find you worth being with?

▶ If you were living between two cultures, in what ways did that contribute to your loneliness?

▶ Did you hear the message that loneliness is something to be avoided?

Ethnic minority adolescents often face cultural isolation. Tatum (1999) believes adolescents from the same ethnic background congregate with their own group as a way to avoid social isolation and loneliness. Young people of color face unique challenges in terms of feeling connected to others, knowing who they are, and believing in their abilities. They may buy into the stereotypes of racism that contribute to feeling alone and different. Natalie's story shows how a person can find an identity and begin to trust herself.

NATALIE'S STORY

In high school I was told that I was not college material and that "Mexicans are good with their hands." I've had to deal with the stereotype of Mexican women being submissive and unable to stand up for themselves—which I've heard all my life from many teachers.

During my senior year in high school, I met Sal, who invited me to a Chicano Youth Leadership Conference. This conference made my outlook about myself change. Up to that point I was a stranger in my own land. I had no cultural identity and no strength to speak up. People there believed in me and told me that I could go to college and be successful. It was the first time that others had more faith in my abilities than I did. Sal became my mentor and challenged me to never underestimate the power I have. He made me feel so proud as a young Latina and proud of my people. This was my spark to stand up and help the Latino community. I have continued my education and am now enrolled in a doctoral program.

Can you identify in any way with Natalie's story? Have you ever had difficulty believing in yourself? If so, did this affect your ability to feel connected to others? As you reflect on your adolescence, try to discover some of the ways in which the person you are now is a result of your experiences of loneliness as an adolescent. Do you shrink from competition for fear of failure? In social situations are you afraid of being left out? Do you feel some of the isolation you did then? If so, how do you deal with it? How might you have changed the way you deal with loneliness?

Loneliness and Young Adulthood

In our young adult years we experiment with ways of being, and we establish lifestyles that may remain with us for many years. You may be struggling with the question of what to do with your life, what intimate relationships you want to establish, and how you will chart your future. Dealing with all the choices that face us at this time of life can be a lonely process. Loneliness can be a result of not having any validation from others.

How you come to terms with your own aloneness can have significant effects on the choices you make—choices that, in turn, may determine the course of your life for years to come. For instance, if you have not learned to listen to yourself and to depend on your own inner resources, you might succumb to the pressure to choose a relationship or a career before you are really prepared to do so, or you might look to your projects or partners for the sense of identity that you ultimately can find only in yourself. Alternatively, you may feel lonely and establish patterns that only increase your loneliness. This last possibility is well illustrated by the case of Saul.

Saul was in his early 20s when he attended college. He claimed that his chief problem was his isolation, yet he rarely reached out to others. His general manner seemed to say "Keep away." It is likely that Saul's negative self-talk made it difficult for him to make contact with others, which increased the chances that others would want to stay away from him. His social withdrawal resulted in him feeling lonely.

One day, as I (Jerry) was walking across the campus, I saw Saul sitting alone in a secluded spot, while many students were congregated on the lawn, enjoying the beautiful spring weather. Here was a chance for him to do something about his separation from others; instead, he chose to seclude himself. He continually told himself that others didn't like him and, sadly, made his prophecy self-fulfilling by his own behavior. He made himself unapproachable and, in many ways, the kind of person people would avoid.

In this time of life we have the chance to decide on ways of being toward ourselves and others as well as on our vocation and future plans. We can work on our responsibility for our own loneliness and create new choices for ourselves. If you feel lonely on the campus, ask yourself what you are doing and can do about your own loneliness. Do you decide in advance that the others want to keep to themselves? Do you assume that there already are well-established cliques to which you cannot belong? Do you expect others to reach out to you, even though you do not initiate contacts yourself? What fears might be holding you back? Where do they seem to come from? Are past experiences of loneliness or rejection determining the choices you now make?

Life circumstances and cultural factors also pave the way to a lonely existence. Many young adults make the journey from their country to the United States, and for some this new life can be a very frightening and lonely experience. This is especially true of the loneliness many undocumented immigrants experience who live with the anxiety of possibly being separated from family members and the uncertainty of their future. The loneliness immigrants feel also may have a lot to do with not knowing how to be a part of a new culture. They may want to hold onto ways that are familiar to them, yet they are generally expected to give up many of their customs. They may find it difficult to connect with people in the mainstream culture and often feel isolated. Language barriers or accents may make it difficult for them to understand others or to make themselves understood to others. Depending on the country immigrants come from, they may experience discrimination. Even if they want to take on the ways of their new culture, they often miss their country of origin and struggle with retaining their original values and adopting new values. These ideas are well illustrated in Jean Kwok's (2010) novel, *Girl in Translation*, and also in Lisa See's (2010) book, *Shanghai Girls*.

We know of some young people who came from Africa to the United States to get a college education. Some of these immigrants experience guilt over leaving significant people behind, especially if their new life is better than the one at home where people are often struggling to meet their most basic needs. In one case, a young man lost the financial aid targeted for his education when it was discovered that he was sending some of this money to family members at home. He experienced a major dilemma when he was expected to help those at home who were in desperate living situations, especially when he was using money to better himself by getting an education. Although he wanted to take advantage of getting a college education, he also felt a loyalty to his family and his community at home. Not only did he experience guilt over having so much personally, but he felt the loneliness of making decisions that affected so many others.

I (Marianne) came to the United States from Germany as a young adult. Although there were many exciting aspects of moving here, I did experience the loneliness of missing my family and my country. There were times when I did not know how to fit into the mainstream of society and felt that I was not truly understood. I learned to balance embracing the American way of life with retaining my identity as a German. At times I felt disloyal and was conflicted when I was expected to make changes that were unacceptable because of the way I was brought up. I remember the loneliness I felt over conflicts of being expected to fully accept all American values, and at the same time to reject some of the values of my childhood. In speaking with other immigrants I have found a shared struggle over retaining our continued appreciation of our original culture without being seen as being disloyal to the country that many of us have chosen to live in.

Loneliness and Middle Age

Many changes occur during middle age that can result in new feelings of loneliness. Although we may not be free to choose some of the things that occur at this time in our lives, we are free to choose how we relate to these events. Here are some possible changes and crises of middle age:

▸ Our life may not turn out the way we had planned, which can pave the way to a lonely existence. We may not enjoy the success we had hoped for, we may feel disenchanted with our work, or we may feel that we passed up many fine opportunities earlier. The key point is what choices will we make in light of this reality? Will we remain stuck in loneliness and hopelessness and berate ourselves endlessly about what we could have done and should have done? Will we allow ourselves to stay trapped in meaningless work and empty relationships, or will we look for positive options for change?

▸ Our children may leave home, and with this change we may experience emptiness and a sense of loss. If so, what will we do about this transition? Can we let go and create a new life with new meaning? When our children leave, will we lose our purpose in life? Will we look back with regret at all that we could have done differently, or will we choose to look ahead to the kind of life we want to create for ourselves now that we do not have the responsibilities of parenthood?

These are just a few of the changes that many of us confront during midlife.

Although we may feel that events are not in our control, we can still choose how we respond to these life situations. Brad feels like a passive recipient of what life has in store for him and does little to change his situation, whereas Dennis decides to take responsibility for his life and make positive choices despite adversity. How do you respond to events that seem out of your control?

BRAD'S STORY

When I got married to Lauren in my mid-20s, I thought we'd be together forever. She was everything I could hope to have in a partner—beautiful, smart, funny, and nice. When we had our twin boys, our lives changed. Lauren channeled all of her energy into raising the boys, and I took on a second job to pay the bills and to start a college fund for Jake and John. Our lives have been growing apart ever since the kids were born. I feel guilty admitting that, but it is true. When I come home from work, I feel like an outsider, and I resent it. It is hard to describe the feelings I have when I am around Lauren. I still think she is beautiful and smart, but I feel distant from her and alone, and I feel angry about that. She must pick up on how I feel, but she never says anything. Does she feel the same way? If things don't improve, I fear we are headed for a divorce.

DENNIS'S STORY

I have suffered many losses over the years and have battled feelings of loneliness as a result of these losses, but I believe these struggles have made me stronger. As a result of the way I have chosen to handle them, I feel more connected to myself than ever. I was a principal dancer for a major dance company until I was injured a few years ago during a performance. My identity at the time was solely based on who I was professionally, and after being forced to retire from the company, my world was shattered. Later that year, a couple of my friends died of AIDS, and the loneliness I experienced was profound. I felt alone in this world, and the one thing that had always given me solace (dance) was something I could no longer rely on. I fell into a slump for around 8 months and started to drink heavily. But one of my best friends, Gloria, would not tolerate my whining and self-pity. She told me to stop whining and to get on with my life. Gloria was right—a bit harsh, but right! As I took steps to take charge of my life, I felt less alone. I have gotten back on track professionally (I am now a choreographer), and I have become an AIDS activist in honor of my friends. I have come to believe that the worst kind of loneliness is to feel disconnected or alienated from yourself, and that is something that we do have some measure of control over.

Loneliness and the Later Years

Our society emphasizes productivity, youth, beauty, power, and vitality. As we age, we may lose some of our vitality and sense of power or attractiveness. Many people face a real crisis when they reach retirement, for they feel that they are being put out to pasture—that they are not needed anymore and that their lives are really over. Loneliness and hopelessness are experienced by anyone who feels that there is little to look forward to or that he or she has no vital place in society, and such feelings are particularly common among older adults.

The loneliness of the later years can be accentuated by the losses that come with age—loss of sight, hearing, memory, and strength. Older people may lose their jobs, hobbies, friends, and loved ones. A particularly difficult loss is the death of a spouse with whom they have been close for many years. In the face of such losses, a person may ultimately ask what reason remains for living. It may be no coincidence that many old people die soon after their spouses have died or shortly after their retirement.

Charles, 65, lost his wife, Betsy, to cancer after a year's battle. During the last few months of Betsy's life, members of the local hospice organization helped Charles care for her at home. Here is an account of Charles's attempt to deal with her death.

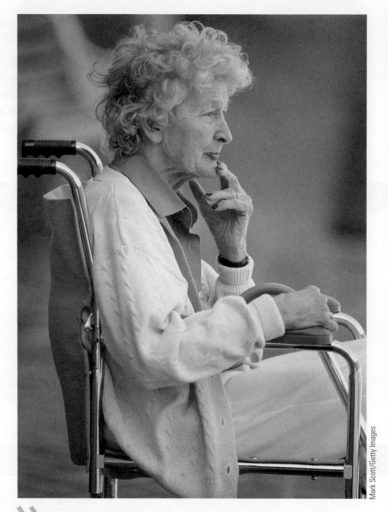

» The later years are a time for reflection and integration of life experiences.

CHARLES'S STORY

Before Betsy's death she expressed a desire to talk to me about her impending death. I could not tolerate the reality of her illness and her dying, so I never talked with her. Even though Betsy has been dead for some time, I still feel guilty for not listening to her and talking. When I look at her chair where she sat, I feel an overwhelming sense of loneliness. At times I feel as though my heart is going to explode. I rarely sleep through the night, and I get up early in the morning and look for tasks to keep me busy. I feel lost and lonely, and it is difficult for me to be in the house where she and I lived together for more than 45 years. Her memories are everywhere. My friends continue to encourage me to talk about my feelings. Although my friends and neighbors are supportive, I'm worried that I'll be a burden for them. I wish that I had died instead of Betsy, for she would have been better able to deal with my being gone than I'm able to cope with her passing.

The pangs of aloneness or the feeling that life is futile reflect a drastic loss of meaning rather than an essential part of growing old. Viktor Frankl (1969) has written about the "will to meaning" as a key determinant of a person's desire to live. He notes that many of

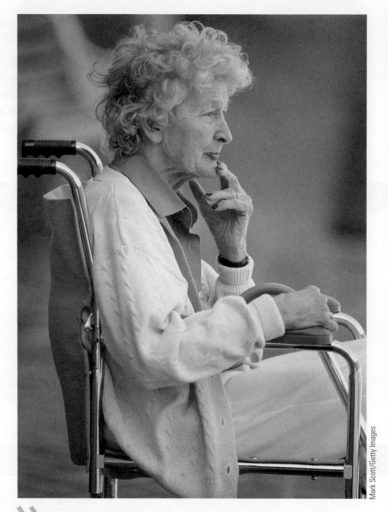

the inmates in the Nazi concentration camp where he was imprisoned kept themselves alive by looking forward to the prospect of being released and reunited with their families. Many of those who lost hope simply gave up and died, regardless of their age.

At least until recently our society has compounded the older person's loss of meaning by grossly neglecting the aged population. Although many older adults are well taken care of in convalescent homes and are visited by their family members, many others are left alone or in an institution with only minimal human contact.

TIME ALONE AS A SOURCE OF STRENGTH

You have seen that both loneliness and solitude can be positive aspects of living. Loneliness does not have to be overcome, and solitude is not something to avoid. Take a moment to reflect on the value of discovering your inner resources as a result of experiencing loneliness and consider at least one way that you might want to deal with both loneliness and solitude differently.

This chapter began with a discussion of the value of solitude and we end the chapter with the hope that you will welcome your time alone. Once you fully accept the value of time alone, this can become the source of your strength and the foundation of your relatedness to others. Maya Angelou, a poet and an extraordinarily vital person, schedules time for herself so she can retain her center. She lives a very full life, and she finds ways to retain her vitality. She schedules one day a month for herself; nothing is scheduled and her friends know not to call her. Reflecting on Maya Angelou's practice, can you see yourself as actively creating alone time? Sometimes we get so busy attending to day-to-day routines that we forget to reflect and provide ourselves with spiritual and emotional nourishment. Making time for yourself is a basic part of self-care. Taking time to be alone provides the opportunity to think, plan, imagine, and dream. It allows you to listen to yourself and to become sensitive to what you are experiencing. In solitude you can come to appreciate anew both your separateness from and your relatedness to the important people and projects in your life. If you are not a good friend to yourself, it will be difficult to find true friendship in the company of others.

SUMMARY

An essential dimension of the human experience is to be able to creatively function alone. Experiencing loneliness is part of being human, for ultimately we are alone. We can grow from such experiences if we understand them and use them to renew our sense of ourselves. We do not have to remain victimized by early decisions made as a result of past loneliness. We do have choices. It is possible to face loneliness and deal with it creatively, or another possibility is to escape from loneliness. We have some choice concerning whether we will feel lonely or whether we will make connections with others.

Some people fail to reach out to others and make significant contact because they are timid in social situations. Shyness can lead to feelings of loneliness, yet shy people can challenge the fears that keep them unassertive. Shyness is not a disorder that needs to be "cured," nor are all aspects of being shy negative. It is important to recognize that certain attitudes and behaviors can create much of the loneliness we sometimes experience.

Each period of life presents unique tasks to be mastered, and loneliness can be best understood from a developmental perspective. Particular circumstances often result in loneliness as we pass through childhood, adolescence, young adulthood, middle age, and the later years. Most of us have experienced loneliness during our childhood and adolescent years, and these experiences can have a significant influence on our present attitudes, behavior, and relationships. It helps to be able to recognize our feelings about events that are associated with each of these turning points.

Where Can I Go From Here?

1. Reflect on some of the ways you may keep yourself busy to avoid being alone. Consider writing about this in your journal. As a way of reaching out to others, consider talking about this with at least one person.

2. If you have feelings of loneliness when you think about a certain person who has been or is now significant to you, write a letter to that person expressing all the things you are feeling (you do not have to mail the letter). For instance, tell that person how you miss him or her or write about your sadness, your resentment, or your desire for more closeness.

3. Imagine that you are the person you have written your letter to, and write a reply to yourself. What do you imagine that person would say to you if he or she received your letter? What do you fear (and what do you wish) he or she would say?

4. If you feel lonely and left out, try some specific experiments for a week or so. For example, if you feel isolated in most of your classes, make it a point to get to class early and initiate some kind of contact with a fellow student. If you feel anxious about taking such a step, try doing it in fantasy. What are your fears? What is the worst thing you can imagine might happen? Record your impressions in the journal pages at the end of this chapter. If you try reaching out to other people, record in your journal what the experience is like for you.

5. Few people schedule time exclusively for themselves. If you would like to have time to yourself but have not done so, consider going to a place that might bring you solitude or that would be relaxing and spend a day completely alone. The important thing is to remove yourself from your everyday routine and experience being alone without external distractions.

6. Suggested Readings. The full bibliographic entry for each of these sources can be found in the References and Suggested Readings at the back of the book. For books dealing with shyness, we recommend Carducci (2000a), Carducci (2005), and Zimbardo (1994). A classic book on the topic of loneliness is Moustakas (1961). A highly recommended book is Cacioppo and Patrick (2008), *Loneliness: Human Nature and the Need for Social Connection*. For information on the creative use of solitude to evaluate the relationships in one's life, see Anderson (2000, 2004). To help both shy and lonely individuals of any age meet and connect more effectively with others, Carducci's (1999) *The Pocket Guide to Making Successful Small Talk: How to Talk to Anyone Anytime Anywhere About Anything* provides an easy-to-use summary of the techniques for mastering the art of conversation.

WEBSITE RESOURCES

Included here are some valuable websites. For access to these websites, video activities, and other supporting materials, visit Cengage Learning's Counseling CourseMate website for *I Never Knew I Had a Choice*, 10th Edition, at **www.cengagebrain.com.**

SHYNESS HOME PAGE
www.shyness.com

Recommended Search Words: "shyness homepage"

The Shyness Institute offers this website as "a gathering of network resources for people seeking information and services for shyness." It is an index of links to articles, associations, and agencies that work with shyness.

INDIANA UNIVERSITY SOUTHEAST SHYNESS RESEARCH INSTITUTE
http://homepages.ius.edu/Special/Shyness

Recommended Search Words: "Indiana University shyness research institute"

The Shyness Research Institute (SRI) is devoted to helping shy individuals understand the nature and underlying dynamics of shyness. It offers a variety of strategies to help shy people to become "successfully shy"—learning to control their shyness rather than allowing their shyness to control them.

SOCIAL PHOBIA/SOCIAL ANXIETY ASSOCIATION
www.socialphobia.org/

Recommended Search Words: "association for social anxiety"

This nonprofit organization offers information about social anxiety disorder. It provides news and links as well as access to a moderated mailing list.

12

DEATH AND LOSS

> Where Am I Now?

> Our Fears of Death

> Death and the Meaning of Life

> Suicide: Ultimate Choice, Ultimate Surrender, or Ultimate Tragedy?

> Freedom in Dying

> The Hospice Movement

> The Stages of Death and Loss

> Grieving Over Death, Separation, and Other Losses

> Summary

> Where Can I Go From Here?

> Website Resources

Contemplate death if you would learn how to live.

WHERE AM I NOW?

Use this scale to respond to these statements:

4 = I *strongly agree* with this statement.
3 = I *agree* with this statement.
2 = I *disagree* with this statement.
1 = I *strongly disagree* with this statement.

1. The fact that I will die makes me take life seriously.

2. I find funerals depressing.

3. If I had a terminal illness, I would want to know how much time I had left to live so I could decide how to spend it.

4. Because of the possibility of losing those I love, I do not allow very many people to get close to me.

5. If I live with integrity, I am unlikely to have regrets at the end of my life.

6. My greatest fear of death is the fear of the unknown.

7. I have had losses in my life that seemed in some ways like the experience of dying.

8. When I experience loss, I allow myself to grieve fully.

9. I am not especially afraid of dying.

10. I fear the deaths of those I love more than I do my own.

In this chapter we look at your attitudes and beliefs about death, your thoughts and feelings about your own mortality, your feelings about the eventual death of those you love, and other forms of significant loss. Like many people, you may feel overwhelmed and be preoccupied with the fear that your life will someday end. Instead of focusing on death, over which you have limited or no control, we invite you to reflect on how well you are living your life. An awareness, understanding, and acceptance of death can lay the groundwork for a meaningful life. If we accept that we have only a limited time in which to live, we can make the most of the time we do have by striving to live each day as fully as possible. It prompts us to look at our priorities and to ask what we value most. In this way our willingness to come to terms with death teaches us how to live.

The Dalai Lama (Dalai Lama & Cutler, 1998) speaks of the importance of learning to face the realities of old age, illness, and death. According to the Dalai Lama, many of us have an intense aversion to facing our pain and suffering. If we accept that suffering is a part of life, we are in a better position to deal with the problems that we will inevitably experience. The attitude we assume toward suffering is extremely important because it influences our ability to cope with suffering when it arises. We may not be able to change events or things that happen, but we have the power to choose our attitude toward these events. The late Albert Ellis, a pioneer in the development of cognitive behavior therapy, often gave the following advice in workshops about facing suffering and coping with it:

> Life has inevitable suffering as well as pleasure. By realistically thinking, feeling, and acting to enjoy what you can, and unangrily and unwhiningly accepting painful aspects that cannot be changed—you open yourself to much joy.

This discussion of death and loss has an important connection with the themes of the previous chapter, loneliness and solitude. When we accept the reality of our eventual death, we get in touch with our ultimate aloneness. This awareness of our mortality and aloneness helps us realize that our actions do count, that we do have choices concerning how we live, and that we must accept the final responsibility for the way we are living.

In their book, *Death and Dying, Life and Living*, Corr and Corr (2013) develop the theme that life and death, living and dying, are inexorably intertwined. They state "… studying death, dying, and bereavement soon reminds us that we humans are finite, limited beings. This realization clearly impacts how we live our lives, for we learn that although there are many things in life we can control, there are many others that we cannot" (p. 13). Corr and Corr believe that we cannot magically make death, loss, and grief disappear from our lives, yet by reflecting on these realities and sharing insights with other people, we can achieve a richer and fuller life. They suggest that the reality of death can serve as a catalyst in finding meaning in life. "Thus, *quality in living* and the *search for meaning* are significant issues for those who are coping with death as well as for those who are simply living their day-to-day lives" (p. 14).

This chapter is also a bridge to the next chapter, which deals with meaning and values. Our knowledge that we are mortal beings goads us to ask ourselves whether we are living by values that create a meaningful existence; if not, we have the time and opportunity to change our way of being. Steve Jobs, the late CEO of Apple Inc. and Pixar Animation Studios, truly revolutionized the world through advances in technology in his short 56 years of life. He lived each day fully and encouraged others to follow that path, as Jobs's 2005 commencement address at Stanford University*—6 years before his untimely death—clearly shows.

*To view the full transcript of Jobs's 2005 commencement speech, visit http://news.stanford.edu/news/2005/june15/jobs-061505.html

From our perspective, the theme of Jobs's commencement speech is an invitation to reflect on how we are living. Because life is precious and we are here for a limited time, we do well to think about what changes we are willing to make in the way we are living, especially if we are not satisfied with our present existence. To ensure that we will have few regrets at the end of our life, it is critical that we not put off doing what is truly significant to a later date. It is important that we have a vision and then make choices that will make this vision become a reality. The message given by Steve Jobs will be familiar as you read the different sections in this chapter. We think the following lines from Jobs's address captures a central message worth reflecting on frequently:

"Your time is limited, so don't waste it living someone else's life. Don't be trapped by dogma—which is living with the results of other people's thinking. Don't let the noise of others' opinions drown out your own inner voice. And most important, have the courage to follow your heart and intuition."

As you reflect on this profound message, contemplate whether you are living the kind of life you want. What do you most want to accomplish before you die? How much progress are you making in achieving this goal? If you are not living the life you want, what is getting in your way? To what extent do you have control over removing these barriers to living authentically and fully? Are certain barriers beyond your control?

OUR FEARS OF DEATH

There are many aspects of death, including leaving behind those we love, losing ourselves, encountering the unknown, and coping with the difficulties involved in a painful or long dying. For many people it is not so much death itself they fear as the process of dying. They may ask, "What will my process of dying be like?" Yalom (2008) describes how death anxiety is always lurking in the background with his clients in psychotherapy: The wish to survive and the dread of annihilation are always present. This is a pervasive fear to live with, yet it can teach us as much about living as about dying.

Morrie Schwartz, an elderly professor who was dying, met each Tuesday with one of his former students, Mitch Albom, to share his insights about living and dying. Morrie said: "The truth is, once you learn how to die, you learn how to live" (Albom, 1997, p. 82). For Morrie, wasting life is even sadder than dying. Morrie talked about his fears of dying, which included losing more and more of his faculties and becoming increasingly dependent. However, he chose to face his fears and deal with them rather than let his fears consume him. Even though he knew he was dying, Morrie realized that he had a choice regarding how he would deal with the end of this life: "Am I going to withdraw from the world, like most people do, or am I going to live? I decided I'm going to live—or at least try to live—the way I want, with dignity, with courage, with humor, with composure" (p. 21). One of the lessons we can learn from reading *Tuesdays With Morrie* is that we do not have to stay away from someone who is dying. Some people want to discuss what they are going through when they are dying, but their loved ones may be reluctant to engage in such conversations. There is much that we can learn by sharing in the last days of someone we love.

A close friend of ours was diagnosed with pancreatic cancer at age 82. During one of our visits with Rosemary, we asked her if she was afraid of dying and her reply was: "I have been on many journeys in my life traveling all over the world. I am now going on a new journey, and I am looking forward to where it will take me." Some may say that Rosemary was in denial, yet during her short illness she never expressed a sense of fear or panic. She was sad over leaving her friends and family behind, but she was at peace in going on this new journey. In an almost party-like atmosphere, Rosemary invited numerous family members and friends to her home to say good-bye.

Some people are reluctant to talk about dying with those close to them. For example, our daughter Heidi wrote to a friend's mother who was diagnosed with cancer. The mother did not want those close to her to talk about her condition. It was Heidi's hope that her friend's mother would recognize that she could give those who love her a gift by letting them share her struggle and allowing them to take care of her. Heidi had this kind of open relationship with her grandmother, as can be seen in Heidi's letter.

HEIDI'S LETTER

One of my greatest memories with my Gram is sitting at the foot of her big queen chair and me on the little wooden stool. My face lay in her lap and her rose soft hand stroked my cheek. We both cried over the news of her being diagnosed with bladder cancer. We cried and cried and cried, then we laughed and then cried some more. As she would say, we bared our souls and left nothing unsaid. I value that experience and others like it and see its true power. The tears washed over us, and it bathed a fear and helped us both let go and embrace. In the beginning, Gram wanted to hide her diagnosis from others. She didn't want them to worry. But I encouraged her to tell all, which she finally did. What I saw happening was those who were always taken care of by her were given the gift to nurture and take care of such a strong and powerful woman. It is a gift I personally treasure. I still carry the glow of that power.

At this point reflect on your fears about dying. Have you had the experience of being with a dying person? If so, what was this like for you? Do you tend to avoid talking with people who are dying? What seems to be your greatest fear? How might your fears influence the way you are choosing to live now?

DEATH AND THE MEANING OF LIFE

Existentialists view the acceptance of death as vital to the discovery of meaning and purpose in life. One of our distinguishing characteristics as human beings is our ability to grasp the concept of the future and, thus, the inevitability of death. This ability gives meaning to our existence, for it makes our every act and moment count. Rather than living in the fear of death, we can view life as an opportunity.

From the Stoics of ancient Greece—who proclaimed "Contemplate death if you would learn how to live"—until modern times, we have been challenged to face our future. Seneca commented that "no man enjoys the true taste of life but he who is willing and ready to quit it." And Saint Augustine said, "It is only in the face of death that man's self is born." Those who are terminally ill provide a sharply defined example of facing the reality of death and of giving meaning to life. Their confrontation with death causes them to do much living in a relatively brief period of time. The pressure of time forces them to choose how they will spend their remaining days. Irvin Yalom (1980) found that cancer patients in group therapy had the capacity to view their crisis as an opportunity to instigate change in their lives. Once they discovered that they had cancer, many experienced these inner changes that enabled them to find a powerful focus on life:

▸ A rearrangement of life's priorities, paying little attention to trivial matters

▸ A sense of liberation; the ability to choose to do those things they really wanted to do

- An increased sense of living in the moment; no postponement of living until some future time

- A vivid appreciation of the basic facts of life; for example, noticing changes in the seasons and other aspects of nature

- A deeper communication with loved ones than before the crisis

- Fewer interpersonal fears, less concern over security, and more willingness to take risks (p. 35)

We can decide to fully affirm life, or we can passively let life slip by us. We can settle for letting events happen to us, or we can actively create the kind of life we want. Our time is invaluable precisely because it is limited. In *Staring at the Sun: Overcoming the Terror of Death*, Yalom (2008) develops the thesis that confronting death allows us to reenter life in a richer and more compassionate way. He captures the essence of our death anxiety with these words:

> It's not easy to live every moment wholly aware of death. It's like trying to stare at the sun in the face: you can stand only so much of it. Because we cannot live frozen in fear, we generate methods to soften death's terror. (p. 5)

Death awareness serves as an awakening experience, which can be a profoundly useful catalyst for making significant life changes. Yalom (2008) writes about life milestones that can lead to awakening experiences such as school and college reunions, estate planning and making a will, and significant birthdays and anniversaries. These milestones can evoke a range of feelings in us about how fast life is going by and can encourage us to reflect on the choices we want to make for the rest of our life.

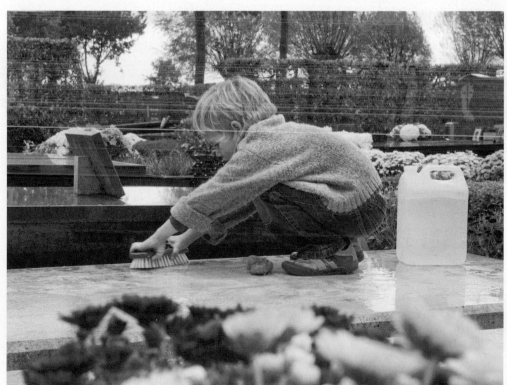

>> Cultural and religious beliefs affect the way people view death.

Choices in the Face of Death

Cultural and religious beliefs affect the way people view death. Some belief systems emphasize making the most of this life, for it is viewed as the only existence. Other belief systems focus on the natural continuity and progression of this temporal life into an afterlife. Just as our beliefs and values affect our fear of death, so do they affect the meaning we attribute to death. Regardless of our philosophical or spiritual views on the meaning of life and death, a wide range of choices is still open to us to maximize the quality of our present life.

Going through a crisis that involves facing death can be a very lonely time, and it can be difficult to find hope in continuing with life as opposed to surrendering to overpowering odds. People confronted with some forms of physical illness may find that their choices are limited. Saundra's story illustrates the challenges of coping with loneliness, isolation, physical illness, and the chance of life being cut short.

SAUNDRA'S STORY

Two months after having my second child, I became very ill, and a gall bladder condition required immediate surgery. As a result of a medical mistake that occurred during my surgery, I faced major internal damage and a life-threatening condition. Every day was a struggle to stay alive. The reality was undeniable; my health was in critical condition. My body was failing me, and I felt myself dying. Despite the circumstances, I maintained a strong desire to live. I knew that I hadn't lived my life to its completion, and I felt it was unfair that my life was being cut short.

While in the hospital, I felt isolated from the world. My family relations became distant. My husband had to visit me around his work schedule, and due to hospital policies my children weren't allowed to visit. I was totally dependent on the hospital staff who performed their jobs with minimal interaction, leaving me feeling invisible most of the time. This impersonal treatment affected my dignity and self-worth. I wanted to hold on and stay connected, but the time came when I started to let go of hope. During this very lonely time, I started to anticipate my death.

I was finally able to have reconstructive surgery, yet the months that followed were even more challenging than before. I felt tortured by the pain, constant procedures, and isolation. The recovery process was slow, but eventually I was released from the hospital. The most difficult part for me was returning home and realizing that life would never be the same. I couldn't pick up where I had left off. Everything as I knew it had changed, even the people I loved. The emotional pain associated with the experience was more intense than the physical pain.

It has been 9 years since the ordeal, but I often recall this time in my life. The experience keeps me grounded. I realize that some of the issues that arise in my daily life are insignificant, and I try not to put time and energy into matters that consume me in a negative way. With a second chance at life, I try to remain appreciative and focused on what is important to me. I try to not get discouraged and to stay positive. Being so close to death has helped me place more value on my existence and my relationships with others.

Saundra's story illustrates the isolation of facing death and the struggle to maintain a sense of hope when things seem hopeless. For Saundra, coming close to death shed a new light on what is important in living. Her illness was a catalyst for reordering her priorities and deciding how she wanted to spend her time. Indeed, she learned some lessons about the meaning of life from facing the prospects of death. What lessons can you learn when you reflect on the reality that you do not have forever to accomplish what is important to you?

Lessons About Living From Those Who Are Dying

Both of our daughters, Heidi and Cindy, were very much a part of their grandmother's final few weeks. Although this was a difficult time for them, they both learned many invaluable lessons about living from their grandmother, not only at this time when she was dying but also during the many years of her life. Cindy wrote down some of these "lessons my Gram taught me."

▶ Look the ones you love deeply in the eyes and without words let them know you love them and that they mean the world to you. Look at them so intensely and with such mindfulness that they feel as if you are the only person in the room with them.

▶ Say thank you and be grateful. Recognize your blessings, even in the face of despair.

▶ Say you are sorry when you have hurt or offended someone.

▶ Touch the ones you love and invite them to touch you. Touch heals and touch penetrates the soul and fills you up with joy.

▶ Laugh, smile, and be playful. Let laughter enter every relationship you have with every person you know.

▶ Tell people how much you care about them. If you have a compliment or a kind thought about someone, speak it in the moment.

▶ Do not judge others without trying to understand them. Even if they have done you harm or wronged you, find a way to let it go and to forgive.

▶ If you live a life of compassion and love and concern for others, you too will receive these gifts at the end of your days.

▶ Be open and share your fears and pain with each other

▶ Sit patiently with other people's pain. If you share your sorrows, they become less heavy and can easily be transformed into love and peacefulness.

▶ Take an interest in what other people do. Be genuine and curious in who they are. Ask about the welfare of others.

▶ Share your wisdom and life lessons without giving advice. Tell stories about your own struggles and accomplishments without being arrogant or self-centered.

▶ Pray and put faith in God. Always know that you are not alone and that you are connected to something beyond yourself. Trust this, ask for strength when you need to, and remember to give thanks as well.

How Well Are You Living?

We submerge ourselves in the activities of daily living, and rarely stop to evaluate how well we are living. Are you willing to take time to assess the quality of your living? Imagine that you are told that you have only a limited time to live. Would you begin to look at what you have missed and how you wish things had been different? Do you have any regrets over opportunities that you let slip away? As you review the significant turning points in your life, reflect on Norma's story to see if her experience has personal meaning for you.

I'm 53 years old, and I have accomplished more in my life than I ever thought possible. So far, my life has been rich and gratifying. I have a husband and four children with whom I generally have a good relationship. Although I know they have a need for me in their lives, they could function well without me. I am not afraid of death, but I would consider death at this time in my life terribly unfair. There is so much more I want to do. Within me are many untapped talents that I haven't had time to express. Many of my present projects take an enormous amount of time, and although they are mostly satisfying, I've put on hold many other personal and professional aspirations.

At times I feel an overwhelming sense of sadness and disappointment over the possibility of running out of time to do those things I was meant to do. Time goes by so fast, and I often wish I could stop the clock. It is my hope to live to an old age, yet I do confront myself with the reality that I may not be that fortunate, which provides me with the impetus to want to make changes in my life. The reality of mortality drives me to reflect on what I would regret not having done if I were to die soon. This reality helps me not to postpone my plans to later, because there may not be a later. The greatest tragedy for me would be, if, on my dying day, I would say that I didn't live my life, rather I lived someone else's life.

As you respond to the questions in the Take Time to Reflect section, consider whether you may benefit from making any changes in your own perspective on time and the life you are living today.

TAKE TIME TO REFLECT

1. Do you like the way you are living your life? List some specific things you are not doing now that you would like to be doing.

_____

_____

2. If you had only 6 months left to live, what would you do differently, if anything?

_____

_____

3. Does the reality of death provide you with the impetus to find meaning in your life? If so, how?

_____

_____

4. What are some ways you are living your life to the fullest at this time? _____

_____

_____

SUICIDE: ULTIMATE CHOICE, ULTIMATE SURRENDER, OR ULTIMATE TRAGEDY?

Many of you may have been personally affected by the suicide of a friend or a family member. In the United States in 2008, "36,035 persons died as a result of suicide, and approximately 666,000 persons visited hospital emergency departments for nonfatal, self-inflicted injuries" (Crosby, Han, Ortega, Parks, & Gfroerer, 2011, p. 1).What's even more alarming is that "56.8% of persons who engage in suicidal behavior never seek health services" (p. 2). As you can see, this is a public health issue in dire need of attention. Our aim, however, is to focus on the topic of suicide from a more personal perspective.

Those considering suicide often feel that they are trapped in a dead-end existence and that life is unbearable. They simply do not want to go on and feel that the chances of change are slim. Although there are undoubtedly options for living differently, they are unable to see any. Suicidal thoughts can be overwhelming during this time of emotional blindness. Some common myths about suicide include the following:

▶ Suicide often takes place with little or no warning.

▶ People who talk about committing suicide will not do it.

▶ Young people are more likely than old people to kill themselves.

▶ People who are suicidal remain so forever.

▶ People who attempt suicide are intent on dying. (Weiten et al., 2012)

Although it is true that some people do not give any signs that they intend to take their lives, generally warning signs give some indication that a person is suicidal. Here are some signs that an individual may be at risk for suicide:

▶ Suicidal thoughts and threats

▶ Absence of a sense of purpose in life

▶ Previous suicidal threats or comments

▶ Preoccupation with death, including talk of feeling hopeless and helpless

▶ Giving away prized possessions

▶ Discussing specific methods and a time for killing oneself

▶ Anxiety, agitation, and depression

▶ Increased substance use

▶ Isolation and withdrawal from friends and family

▶ Extreme changes of behavior and sudden personality changes

▶ A sudden need to get one's life in order

▶ A sudden appearance of calm or peace after a period during which some of these above-listed characteristics were evident

These signs should be taken seriously, and interventions should be made to help bring about a change in the suicidal person.

It is not possible to prevent all suicides, but preventive measures can reduce the number of suicides. When a person talks about suicide, even in vague generalities, take the matter seriously. Ask whether he or she has contemplated or is contemplating suicide. When someone displays suicidal signs or talks about suicide, it is crucial to provide empathy and support, which can be done by being present for the person in his or her struggle. In addition, a good course to follow is to encourage the person to seek professional help. Suicide prevention centers with 24-hour-a-day telephone support are available in most cities.

Is suicide an ultimate choice, an ultimate surrender, or an ultimate tragedy? This question is complex and has no easy answer. We each make conscious choices about how we are living and to some extent how we might die. Some people believe suicide to be the ultimate surrender, the result of not being willing to struggle or of being too quick to give up without exploring other possibilities. At times you may have felt a deep sense of hopelessness, and you may have questioned whether it was worth it to continue living. Often a person contemplating suicide does not wish to end his or her life but cannot see another way of ending the suffering or a dead-end existence. If any strand of hope can be found, it may provide a reason to continue living. Have you ever contemplated suicide? If so, what was going on in your life that contributed to your desire to end it? What factor or factors kept you from following through with taking your life? What hidden meanings does suicide have for you?

Taking one's life is a powerful act, and the underlying emotional messages and symbolic meanings can be equally powerful:

▶ A cry for help: "I cried out, but nobody cared!"

▶ A form of self-punishment: "I don't deserve to live."

▶ An act of hostility: "See what you made me do."

▶ An attempt to control and exert power over people: "I will make others suffer for what they did to me."

▶ An attempt to be noticed: "Maybe now people will talk about me and feel sorry for the way they treated me."

▶ A relief from a terrible state of mind: "Life is too stressful, and I see no hope."

▶ An escape from a difficult or impossible situation: "I am a burden to everybody. It will be a relief to them when I am gone."

▶ A relief from hopelessness: "I see no way out of the despair I feel. Ending my life will be better than hating to wake up every morning."

▶ An end to pain: "I suffer extreme physical pain, and there is no end to it. My suicide will end it."

▶ An expression of shame or failure: "I cannot face everyone after what I have done."

Reactions to Suicide

Often death is associated with the ending of pain. Those who commit suicide may resort to this final and deliberate act as a way to put an end to either physical or emotional suffering. Yet for survivors, the death of someone they were close to often marks the beginning of a long period of suffering. Surviving family members typical endure emotional turmoil, unanswered questions, and have a variety of thoughts and feelings that are difficult to resolve. The unexpected death of a loved one, especially due to suicide, often results in a grief-stricken process that calls for professional help for those who are left behind.

When a family member commits suicide, the immediate reaction is generally shock and distress. Soon afterward those left behind experience a range of feelings such as denial, shock, anger, shame, guilt, grief, depression, sadness, fear, blame, rejection, and abandonment. When family members are in denial, they may invent reasons that will contribute to their refusal to accept the death as a suicide. Anger is quite common and is often directed toward the deceased. Anger may also be aimed at oneself, friends, family members, health care providers, insurance companies, and others in the community (Kaslow & Aronson,

2004). There may be a sense of shame because of religious teachings about suicide. Survivors often experience guilt over what they could and should have done to prevent the tragedy— "Maybe if I had been more sensitive and caring, this terrible thing wouldn't have happened." Survivors also may experience fear over the possibility that this act will be repeated by another family member or, perhaps, even by themselves.

Survivors generally need considerable time and opportunity to process feelings such as anger, self-blame, and guilt before they can begin to accept the loss. Survivors frequently cannot understand or even feel their own numbed pain. It is extremely important that they find a person they can talk to about their loss, or their emptiness may never be filled. Eventually they face the task of reconstructing their lives without the person they lost, but this is unlikely to happen until they have dealt with their reactions to the suicide (Pehrsson & Boylan, 2004).

The nature of the unfinished business, how it is handled, and how the survivor is affected by it all have an impact on the grief process. Typically, those who are left behind experience a deep sense of abandonment, rejection, loneliness, and isolation. For those who are mourning a suicide, a good support system and communication with a nonjudgmental person can be most useful (Corr & Corr, 2013). Counseling can help survivors deal with their reactions to the suicide of a friend or family member and help them learn how to express feelings that they might otherwise keep to themselves. Additional benefits from participating in counseling include the following:

▶ Survivors are encouraged to talk about the things they may be rehearsing over and over in their heads, and it can help them to talk about their thoughts and feelings with one another.

▶ People can correct distortions they may hold, prepare for their future, learn to let go of regrets and blame, and give expression to their anger. Because of their deep sadness, without professional help it may be difficult for family members to become aware of, much less express to one another, the anger that they feel.

▶ Survivors can be helped to remember aspects of a person's life that were not defined by the way the person died. Because the intense trauma of suicide can be overwhelming, counseling that focuses on remembering conversations can help restore a balance and bring about healing (Hedtke & Winslade, 2004).

William Blau teaches a course on death and dying and finds that his students are concerned with the ethical question of whether one should interfere with a person's "right to die." He points out the difference between the physically healthy person with subjectively "unbearable" emotional pain and the terminal patient with permanent loss of quality of life. He tells his students that extreme emotional pain and hopelessness are usually subject to change and that most therapy clients hospitalized for suicidal behavior were grateful later on that they were kept from self-directed violence (personal communication, February 9, 2012). We can confirm that view. I (Marianne) recently spoke with a former client who let me know that she remembered our work together years ago when she felt desperate and wondered about ending her own life. I asked her if she was glad she had decided not to end her life, and she answered in the affirmative and told me that she is now a practicing clinical social worker.

Ending Life as an Act of Mercy

Can suicide be an act of mercy? Can suicide be rational? Some victims of painful and terminal illnesses have decided when and how to end their lives. **Rational suicide** means that a person has decided—after going through a decision-making process and without coercion from others—to end his or her life because of extreme suffering involved with a terminal illness. Many people are opposed to active measures to end life, yet they also oppose interventions that unnecessarily prolong life by artificial and unusual means. Certainly there is a difference between suicide and allowing nature to take its course in cases of extreme illness. **Assisted suicide** involves providing lethal means to cause a person's death, with the individual performing the act that ends his or her own life. **Hastened death** involves speeding up the dying process, which can entail withholding or withdrawing life support. This form of rational suicide is sometimes argued to be morally and ethically appropriate in circumstances involving terminal illness and unendurable suffering.

In *Life and Death Decisions: Psychological and Ethical Considerations in End-of-Life Care*, Kleespies (2004) writes about the importance of advance care planning. **Advance directives** are designed to protect the self-determination of people who have reached a point in their illness when they are not able to make decisions on their own about their care. The fear of being kept alive when they are in a vegetative state has resulted in directives for people at any age. Through the use of advance directives, people can go on record with their preferences for medical treatment while they are mentally capable of making decisions, with the anticipation that the time may come when they will no longer have the capacity to make these choices. Generally, there are two forms of advance directives. One form involves completing a **living will** by which the person specifies his or her preferences for end-of-life care. Another form involves identifying a person to make decisions on one's behalf when one can no longer do so. According to Kleespies, advance directives have been viewed as a means of exercising mercy and protecting the autonomy of individuals by giving them the right to make their wishes clear to both family members and treatment staff pertaining to their own end-of-life care.

FREEDOM IN DYING

The process of dying involves a gradual diminishing of the range of choices available to us. But even in dying, we can choose how we handle what is happening to us. The following account deals with the dying of Jim Morelock, a student who became a close friend of both Marianne and Jerry.*

Jim is 25 years old. He is full of life—witty, bright, honest, and actively questioning. He had just graduated from college as a human services major and seemed to have a bright future when his illness was discovered.

About a year and a half ago, Jim developed a growth on his forehead and underwent surgery to have it removed. At that time, his doctors believed the growth was a rare disorder that was not malignant. Later, more tumors erupted, and more surgery followed. Several months ago, Jim found out that the tumors had spread throughout his body and that, even with cobalt treatment, he would have a short life. Since that time he has steadily grown weaker and has been able to do less and less, yet he has shown remarkable courage in the way he has faced this loss and his dying.

Some time ago Jim came to Idyllwild, California, and took part in the weekend seminar that we had with the reviewers of this book. On this chapter, he commented that although we may not have a choice concerning the losses we suffer in dying, we do retain the ability to choose our attitude toward our death and the way we relate to it.

This account, presented by Jerry, is being repeated as it appeared in this book's first edition. Many readers have commented to us about how affected they were as they read about Jim's life and his death, and in this way he seems to have lived on in one important respect.

Jim has taught me (Jerry) many things during these past few months about this enduring capacity for choice, even in extreme circumstances. Jim has made many critical choices since being told of his illness. He chose to continue taking a course at the university because he liked the contact with the people there. He worked hard at a boat dock to support himself, until he could no longer manage the physical exertion. He decided to undergo chemotherapy, even though he knew that it most likely would not result in his cure, because he hoped that it would reduce his pain. It did not, and Jim has suffered much agony during the past few months. He decided not to undergo any further chemotherapy, primarily because he did not want to prolong his life if he could not really live fully. He made a choice to accept God in his life, which gave him a sense of peace and serenity. Before he became bedridden, he decided to go to Hawaii and enjoy his time in first-class style.

Jim has always had an aversion to hospitals—to most institutions, for that matter—so he chose to remain at home, in more personal surroundings. As long as he was able, he read widely and continued to write in his journal about his thoughts and feelings on living and dying. With his friends, he played his guitar and sang songs that he had written. He maintained an active interest in life and in the things around him, without denying the fact that he was dying.

More than anyone I (Jerry) have known or heard about, Jim has taken care of unfinished business. He made it a point to gather his family and tell them his wishes, he made contact with all his friends and said everything he wanted to say to them, and he asked Marianne to deliver the eulogy at his funeral services. He clearly stated his desire for cremation; he wants to burn those tumors and then have his ashes scattered over the sea—a wish that reflects his love of freedom and movement.

Jim has very little freedom and movement now, for he can do little except lie in his bed and wait for his death to come. To this day he is choosing to die with dignity, and although his body is deteriorating, his spirit is still very much alive. He retains his mental sharpness, his ability to say a lot in a very few words, and his sense of humor. He has allowed himself to grieve over his losses. As he puts it, "I'd sure like to hang around to enjoy all those people that love me!" Realizing that this isn't possible, Jim is saying good-bye to all those who are close to him.

Throughout this ordeal, Jim's mother has been truly exceptional. When she told me (Jerry) how remarkable Jim has been in complaining so rarely despite his constant pain, I reminded her that I'd never heard her complain during her months on duty. I have been continually amazed by her strength and courage, and I have admired her willingness to honor Jim's wishes and accept his beliefs, even though at times they have differed from her own. She has

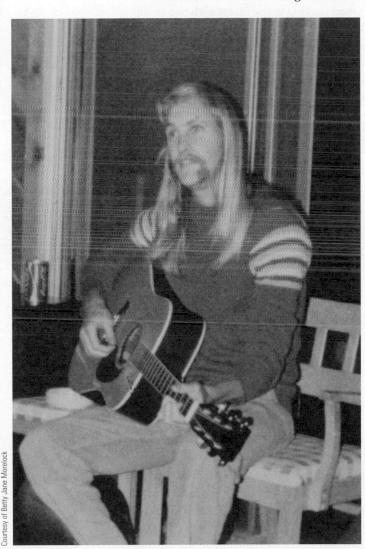

Jim Morelock enjoying playing his guitar.

demonstrated her care without smothering him or depriving him of his free spirit and independence. Her acceptance of Jim's dying and her willingness to be fully present to him have given him the opportunity to express openly whatever he feels. Jim has been able to grieve and mourn because she has not cut off this process.

This experience has taught me (Jerry) much about dying and about living. Through Jim, I have learned that I do not have to do that much for a person who is dying other than to be with him or her by being myself. So often I have felt a sense of helplessness, of not knowing what to say or how much to say, of not knowing what to ask or not to ask, of feeling stuck for words. Jim's imminent death seems such a loss, and it is very difficult for me to accept it. Gradually, however, I have learned not to be so concerned about what to say or to refrain from saying. In fact, in my last visit I said very little, but I feel that we made significant contact with each other. I have also learned to share with him the sadness I feel, but there is simply no easy way to say good-bye to a friend.

Jim is showing me (Jerry) that his style of dying will be no different from his style of living. By his example and by his words, Jim has been a catalyst for me to think about the things I say and do and to evaluate my own life.

Before he died, Jim gave me a poster showing a man walking in the forest with two small girls. At the top of the poster were the words "TAKE TIME." Jim knew me well enough to know how I tend to get caught up in so many activities that I sometimes forget to simply take time to really experience and enjoy the simple things in life. Reflect on what you can do to keep your priorities in mind and not have regrets over your life. What can you do today to ensure that you will live the life you want?

TAKE TIME TO REFLECT

1. If you were close to someone during his or her dying, how did the experience affect your feelings about your life and about your own dying?

_____

_____

2. How would you like to be able to respond if a person who is close to you were dying?

_____

_____

3. If you were dying, what would you most want from the people who are closest to you?

_____

_____

THE HOSPICE MOVEMENT

There is a trend toward more direct involvement of family members in caring for a dying person. An example of this is the **hospice program**. The term *hospice* was originally used to describe a resting place for weary travelers during the Middle Ages. Later, hospices were established for children without parents, for the incurably ill, and for the elderly. In recent years hospice programs have spread rapidly through Europe, North America, and many other parts of the world. They offer care for those who are in the final stages of the journey of life. Generally, hospice services are provided in the dying

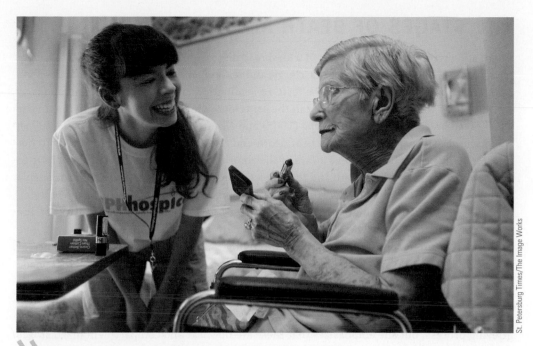

St. Petersburg Times/The Image Works

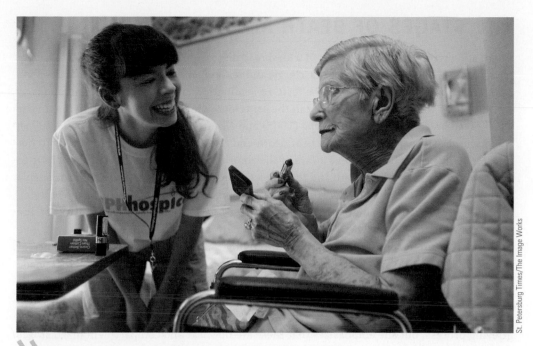
The hospice movement evolved in response to what many people perceived as inadequate care for those dying in hospitals.

person's home. Much hospice home care replaces more expensive and impersonal treatment options including multiple hospitalizations. The hospice movement also gives permission to those who are losing a significant person to feel the full range of emotions during the bereavement process.

Both volunteers and a trained staff provide health care aid, including helping the patient and the family members deal with psychological and social stresses. Hospice workers provide useful information to the patient and to family members of what to expect. Hospices are based on a holistic philosophy and aim to provide services that help dying persons experience a sense of self-worth and dignity. In addition, they provide support for the family members so that they can prepare for the eventual separation.

Sometimes the purpose of hospice is misunderstood, especially in light of the controversy surrounding physician-assisted suicide. As a family, we were confronted with one of the misconceptions regarding the aims of hospice. During the last few weeks of Josephine Corey's (Jerry's mother) life, several family members had decided to request the services of hospice. However, one family member was extremely opposed to this decision because of his mistaken belief that hospice would withhold treatment and by doing so would accelerate her death. He was willing to go to a hospice agency to talk about his concerns, which resulted in a different way of thinking about what hospice could offer. As an entire family, we felt a tremendous amount of support from the hospice staff and also came to realize how much more difficult this situation would have been had we not asked for their help. The various hospice workers were a genuine source of comfort to each of the family members. They also provided the opportunity for Josephine Corey to live out her last few weeks in her own home, which was one of her wishes.

For more information about hospice care, visit the website of the National Hospice and Palliative Care Organization (see Website Resources at the end of the chapter).

THE STAGES OF DEATH AND LOSS

Death and dying have become topics of widespread discussion among psychologists, psychiatrists, nurses, physicians, sociologists, clergy, and researchers. These topics were once taboo for many people, but they are now the focus of seminars, courses, workshops, and books.

Elisabeth Kübler-Ross is a pioneer in the contemporary study of death and dying. In her widely read books, *On Death and Dying* (1969) and *Death: The Final Stage of Growth* (1975), she discusses the psychosocial aspects of death and the experience of dying. Thanks to her efforts, many people have become aware of the almost universal need dying persons have to talk about their impending death and to complete their business with the important people in their lives. She has shown how ignorance of the dying process and of the needs of dying people—as well as the fears of those around them—can rob those who are dying of the opportunity to fully experience their feelings and arrive at a resolution of them.

A greater understanding of the process of dying can help us come to an acceptance of death, as well as be more helpful and present to those who are dying. Kübler-Ross made many people aware of the needs of the dying, and she shed light on the notion that bereavement involves some predictable stages of grief over a period of time. The **five stages of dying** that Kübler-Ross has delineated provide a starting point for understanding the grieving process, but she emphasizes that these are not neat and compartmentalized stages that every person passes through in a linear and orderly fashion. Too often people have misunderstood and misinterpreted her work because they have viewed her stages as a linear process, which is not what she intended. At times a person may experience a combination of these stages, perhaps skip one or more stages, or go back to an earlier stage he or she has already experienced. In general, however, Kübler-Ross found this sequence: denial, anger, bargaining, depression, and acceptance.

Denial

After the initial shock of learning that death will happen soon, denial is a normal first reaction. Most people move on and deal with their impending death in other ways after some time, but denial may recur at a later time. During the stage of denial, the attitudes of a dying person's family and friends are critical. If these people cannot face the fact that their loved one is dying, they cannot help him or her move toward an acceptance of death. Their own fear will blind them to signs that the dying person wants to talk about his or her death and needs support.

Anger

It is important that people recognize the need of those who are dying to express their anger, whether they direct it toward their doctors, the hospital staff, their friends, their children, or God. If this displaced anger is taken personally, any meaningful dialogue with the dying will be cut off. Moreover, people have reason to be enraged over having to suffer in this way when they have so much to live for. Rather than withdrawing support or taking offense, the people who surround a dying person can help most by allowing the person to fully express whatever he or she is feeling. In this way they help the person to ultimately come to terms with death.

Bargaining

Kübler-Ross (1969) sums up the essence of the bargaining stage as follows: "If God has decided to take us from this earth and he did not respond to any angry pleas, he may be more favorable if I ask nicely" (p. 72). Bargaining typically involves a change in behavior or a specific promise in exchange for more time to live. Such bargains are generally made in secret, often with God. Basically, the stage of bargaining is an attempt to postpone the inevitable end.

Depression

Depression occurs when a dying person faces the losses that dying brings and begins to mourn what is already lost and what is still to be lost. In *Tuesdays With Morrie* (Albom, 1997), Morrie was asked if he felt sorry for himself. He replied that in the mornings he often cries as he watches his body wilt away to nothing. "I feel around my body, I move my finger and my hands—whatever I can still move—and I mourn what I've lost. I mourn the slow, insidious way in which I'm dying" (pp. 56–57). He added that he then stops mourning and concentrates on all the good things still in his life.

Just as it had been important to allow dying people to fully vent their anger, it is important to let them express their sadness and to make their final plans. Dying people are about to lose everyone they love, and only the freedom to grieve over these losses will enable them to find some peace and accept the reality of their death.

Acceptance

Kübler-Ross (1969) found that if patients have had enough time and support to work through the previous stages, most of them reach a stage at which they are neither depressed nor angry. Acceptance of death can be reached if they work through the many conflicts and feelings that dying brings.

At this stage, the dying person is often tired and weak. Acceptance does not imply submission, defeat, or doing nothing. Instead, acceptance is a form of dealing with reality. It involves a gradual separation from people, life, ties, and roles. Of course, some people never achieve an acceptance of their death, and some have no desire to. Brenner (2002) captures this notion when he writes: "Not all people who are dying have a beautiful, blissful, insightful, forgiving, loving experience. Many are downright angry and resentful" (p. 90).

The Significance of the Stages of Dying

The value of Kübler-Ross's description of the dying process is that the stages describe and summarize in a general way what patients may experience and therefore add to our understanding of dying. But these stages should not be interpreted as a natural progression that is expected in most cases, and it is a mistake to use these stages as the standard by which to judge whether a dying person's behavior is normal or right. Just as people are unique in the way they live, they are unique in the way they die. Sometimes people who work with the terminally ill forget that the stages of dying do not progress neatly, even though they cognitively know this reality. One practitioner told us, "Although I had read Kübler-Ross's book and knew the stages that a dying person was supposed to go through, many of my terminal patients had not read the same book!"

Patients who do not make it to the acceptance stage are sometimes viewed as failures by some in the helping professions. For example, some nurses get angry at patients who take "backward" steps by going from depression to anger, or they question patients about why they have "stayed so long in the anger stage." People have a range of feelings during this process: hope, anger, depression, fear, envy, relief, and anticipation. Those who are dying have great mood fluctuations. Therefore, these stages should not be used as a method of categorizing, and thus dehumanizing, the dying; they are best used as a frame of reference for helping them. People facing death cope with this reality in a variety of ways. Some cope by becoming angry, others by withdrawing, and others by examining some meaning in their lives that would make death more acceptable. The key point is that different people cope with their death in different ways at different times and in different contexts (Corr & Corr, 2013).

A Task-Based Model for Coping With Dying

Kübler-Ross's stage-based model is one approach to understanding ways of coping with dying. Other researchers have proposed alternative approaches to understanding death and dying. One of these is Corr's (1992) **task-based model** for coping with dying. Corr believes that any useful account of coping must address the whole human being, take into account the differences among individuals, and consider all who are involved. His model identifies four main areas of task work in dealing with dying: the physical, psychological, social, and spiritual.

▸ **Physical tasks** pertain to bodily needs and physical conditions such as coping with pain and nausea, and other physical conditions. These basic bodily needs must be attended to in order to meet other needs (psychological, social, and spiritual). The aim is often to minimize physical distress.

▸ **Psychological tasks** are associated with autonomy, security, and richness in living. Personal dignity is especially important for those who are dying.

▸ **Social tasks** have to do with sustaining and enhancing the interpersonal attachments valued by the dying person. For many who are dying, their social interests narrow and their priorities shift.

▸ **Spiritual tasks** pertain to common themes such as meaningfulness, connectedness, transcendence, and fostering hope. People who are coping with dying often are concerned with the meaning of their lives, the meaning of suffering, and the impact of the reality of death on their remaining time.

These four tasks correspond to the four dimensions of human life, and they are approached differently by different individuals. Some of these tasks may not be undertaken, and some may be more or less important for different individuals. The task-based model is aimed at fostering empowerment and participation in coping with dying by focusing on choices. People have choices in the ways in which they will cope with life-threatening illness and dying. Certain tasks may be dealt with for a time and then set aside as the person works on other tasks. People can choose to work on one, all, or none of these series of tasks. According to Corr (1992), it is never possible to finish all of the tasks facing an individual. Finishing even one particular task is important. Generally, work on these tasks ends with death. For those who live on, certain tasks may be addressed in coping with bereavement.

A Relational Model of Death and Grieving

The **relational model** is an alternative way of thinking about death, dying, and the grieving process. It moves away from the idea that we are born alone and die alone as individuals, instead emphasizing that people are born into networks of relationships and remain woven into those networks long after they die. The relational perspective does not focus on individually working through emotional stages or completing tasks that lead to acceptance. Instead, those who experience the loss of someone they love can find comfort in developing a new relationship with the person who died.

Death does not end everything, for those who are dead continue to live on in the way that people remember them. In this sense, their lives continue on in the stories that are told about them long after their physical bodies perish. A focus on remembering conversations has been developed in narrative therapy by Michael White (1989, 2007) and Lorraine Hedtke and John Winslade (2004). Hedtke and Winslade claim that it is a mistaken notion that death cancels our membership (relationships) with our loved ones. By remembering loved ones in our conversations, we create new relationships, which Hedtke and Winslade refer to as "continuing membership. . . . It is about relationship going on and it is about what might continue rather than what might be lost" (p. 5). **Re-membering** is about continuing to foster the memory of a person's life even after he or she dies by involving the person in our daily lives, in our conversations, in the choices we make, and in our resources for living. This new and different relationship now requires us to remember the stories and imagine the voice of the loved one. By keeping this person's voice and thoughts alive, we have gained an ongoing resource that helps us move forward in life. We can consistently renew a dead person's presence in our "club of life," and we might even continue to introduce our dead loved one to new people who enter our life. For example, our son-in-law Brian often talks to his young daughters about his father, who died several years ago. The children never met this grandfather, but Brian has introduced his father to his children in a very caring way. The kids know a lot about who grandpa Mike was and often repeat to others the stories about their grandfather they learned from their father.

This relational view described by Hedtke and Winslade is in contrast to other models that emphasize the end goal of grief work as to "let go" of the deceased loved ones, to accept a life without them, and to complete "unfinished business" associated with death. The goal of the relational model is maintaining ongoing membership rather than detaching and moving on. The following questions are examples of conversation starters drawn from this perspective on grief counseling:

▸ What is important for you to remember about your dead loved one? What stories would you like to remember about this person?

▸ What did this person mean to you when he or she was alive?

▸ How have you continued to remember this person since his or her death? On what occasions? In what contexts? What purposes do these memories continue to serve for you?

▸ What advice would your dead loved one give you about how to deal with life's demands? How do you continue to draw upon this person's experience or wisdom?

▸ What would it mean to your loved one to know that you were continuing to honor his or her contributions to your life in the ways that you remember him or her?

▸ What difference does this way of thinking about your dead loved one make in your own life?

Many who are dying find comfort in the idea that they will not be forgotten and can be invited to actively bequeath their stories to be remembered and retold after they die. Many who are coping with the death of a person they loved find more comfort in holding their memories of a loved one close than in saying good-bye and letting go of the relationship. Hedtke and Winslade (2004) put this notion of creating a new relationship with deceased loved ones thusly:

> To remember is to include them in our daily lives, in our conversations, in our celebrations, in our decision making, and in our resources for living. To remember is to refuse to allow our loved one's memory to go by unnoticed. (p. 10)

We highly recommend *Re-membering Lives: Conversations With the Dying and the Bereaved*, by Lorraine Hedtke and John Winslade (2004), for an in-depth discussion of the relational model of grieving.

GRIEVING OVER DEATH, SEPARATION, AND OTHER LOSSES

In a way that is similar to the stages of dying, people go through stages of grief in working through death and various other losses. **Grief work**, or **bereavement**, refers to the exploration of feelings generated by a significant loss. The loss of family members, friends, and intimate relationships brings out the deepest of human wounds. After a loss, people often speak of being devastated and wonder if they will ever be able to get their lives in order. Some common feelings include sadness, sorrow, fear, hurt, confusion, depression, resentment, relief, loneliness, anger, despair, shame, and guilt. Wolfert's (2003) model of understanding grief includes 10 "touchstones," or trail markers, that can be used to navigate through the process of grief and bereavement. The touchstones are (1) opening to the presence of loss, (2) dispelling misconceptions about grief, (3) embracing the uniqueness of grief, (4) exploring the feelings of loss, (5) recognizing one is not crazy, (6) understanding the needs of mourning, (7) nurturing oneself, (8) reaching out to others, (9) seeking reconciliation, and (10) coming to appreciate one's process of transformation. These "wisdom teachings" can assist people to better understand what they are experiencing in the grief process.

In recent years, natural disasters such as earthquakes, tsunamis, hurricanes, and tornadoes have resulted in widespread loss and damage. For survivors of these catastrophes, the losses are staggering; some lost everything they owned and everyone they loved within a matter of minutes. Before they could comprehend what was happening around them, their lives were robbed of all that mattered to them. It seems unfathomable that people have the resilience to survive tragedies of such magnitude, but people do carry on with living. Their grief is profound and complex, and it will be with them for the rest of their lives.

Grief work is not a simple process. Some people refuse to accept the reality of the death of a child or a life partner. They may deny their feelings or be unable to face their pain. At some point in the grief process, people may feel numb or that they are functioning in an automatic mode. Once this numbness wears off, the pain seems to intensify. For example, my (Marianne) mother lost her first child during World War II because she was unable to get the medical help needed to save his life. My mother rarely spoke about her first-born, and most people did not even know of his brief existence. She blamed herself for her child's death, and she was never able to forgive herself for "allowing" her son to die. She had several children after losing her son, but it was difficult for her to get close to her other children, perhaps because the possibility of losing them would be more painful than she could stand.

When we deny sadness and the pain associated with loss, we inevitably suffer more in the long run and are less able to express a range of feelings. This unexpressed pain can immobilize people both physically and psychologically and can prevent them from accepting the reality of the death of a loved one. We are reminded of Verna who reported that she was overcome with emotions and could not stop crying at the funeral of an acquaintance. What surprised her was the way her reaction contrasted with her "strength and composure" over the death of her husband. What she did not realize was that she had not allowed herself to grieve over the loss of her husband and that years later she was having a delayed grief reaction. Verna's husband had died very unexpectedly after going into early retirement. She was struggling not only with his physical absence but also with the loss of all the hopes, plans, and dreams they had shared. It was difficult for her to discuss constructing a new life for herself because her future plans were so intertwined with those of her husband.

A variety of resources are available to assist people in their grieving process. A grief support group provides many benefits, especially in finding out that we are not alone in our pain and in the healing that occurs by reaching out to others and forming bonds. Those who participate in a grief group have opportunities to talk about the reality of the death of someone close to them, share the pain of this death, explore the personal meaning of the loss, adjust to loss, and eventually consider new purpose and meaning. In addition, group members comfort each other. A grief group does not necessarily resolve the issues surrounding a loss, but the group experience can teach people ways of putting their loss into perspective.

At times, professionals in the medical and psychological fields are guilty of pathologizing normal aspects of grieving. When our niece lost her father, with whom she was very close, and told her physician that she cries frequently and is very sad about her loss, his response was to prescribe antidepressants rather than to have a conversation about normalizing her loss. Psychiatric professionals are currently debating how complicated grief and bereavement issues should be classified in the upcoming fifth edition of the *Diagnostic and Statistical Manual of Mental Disorders*. Shear and her colleagues (2011) state that "[n]ormally, grief does not need clinical intervention. However, sometimes acute grief can gain a foothold and become a chronic debilitating condition called complicated grief . . . some bereaved people need to be diagnosed and treated" (pp. 103–104). As this is being sorted out among helping professionals, it is useful to remember that grieving is a part of the human condition. Some treatments may involve the use of psychopharmacological medication, but medicines alone cannot fill the void of a loss.

Allowing Yourself to Grieve

Grief is a psychologically necessary and natural process after a significant loss. However, the norms in some cultures make it very difficult for people to experience grief after they have suffered a loss. For example, in our society there appears to be a cultural norm that fosters an expectation of "moving on" and a focus on how long it is taking some people to "get back to normal" and to "get on with living." As is the case with any unexpressed emotion, unresolved grief lingers in the background and prevents people from processing their losses and sometimes from forming new relationships. Also, unresolved grief is considered a key factor in the onset of a variety of somatic complaints and physical illnesses. They may experience psychological and behavioral difficulties, yet seldom recognize the connection between these symptoms and a loss (Freeman, 2005). Most writers on the psychological aspects of death and loss agree that grieving is necessary.

Mourning pertains to the rituals and practices of an individual or community in response to a death. There is therapeutic value in the process of mourning, which entails dealing with grief on both emotional and intellectual levels. People deal with loss in different ways; there is no one correct way to grieve. Although people may successfully experience their feelings pertaining to loss differently with time, the loss will always be with them in some way. In healthy grieving, people are not immobilized by the loss, nor are they being constantly triggered by it.

Many cultures have a formal mourning period (usually a year), and in these cultures the mourners are directly involved in the funeral process. In the United States those who suffer from a loss are typically "protected" from any direct involvement in the burial, and people are often praised for not displaying overt signs of grief. Many of our rituals encourage us to deny our feelings of loss and therefore keep us from coming to terms with the reality of that loss. It has become clear that practices that include denial are not genuinely helpful. Today, increasing emphasis is being placed on providing ways for people to participate more directly in the dying process of their loved ones (such as the hospice movement) and in the funeral process as well.

Earlier we described the task-model of coping with dying and the relational model of death and grieving, and in a like manner, a task-model can be applied to processing intense grieving. Many researchers have begun to pay attention to the various *tasks* associated with bereavement, some of which include being able to verbalize what happened to their loved one, visiting the grave site, and being able to reminisce about past memories (Abeles, Victor, & Delano-Wood, 2004). Worden (2002) proposes thinking of mourning in terms of four tasks to be accomplished:

1. *Accept the reality of the loss.* Before mourning can begin, the death of a person needs to be faced. Accepting this loss needs to be done both intellectually and emotionally. For many there will be a time lag before they are able to experience the emotional impact of the reality of a loss.

2. *Work through the pain of grief.* When the bereaved accept the reality of their loss, pain usually follows. Those in mourning need to experience and express the emotional pain of a loss, and at the same time learn to nurture themselves both physically and emotionally.

3. *Adjust to an environment in which the deceased is missing.* Learning to develop a new relationship with the deceased is a gradual and unfolding process. Although the bereaved do not have to let go of all ties to the person who has died, it is important to say good-bye and to grieve the loss.

4. *Emotionally relocate the deceased and move on with life.* The phrase "moving on with life" entails finding a meaningful way to live without the person who has died. Mourners eventually need to develop a new sense of identity based on a life without the deceased. This task involves restructuring the relationship with the deceased in a way that is satisfying, but that also reflects the life circumstances that have changed after the loss.

Worden (2002) maintains that those who are mourning must accomplish these tasks before their mourning can be completed. These tasks in mourning reflect a proactive stance in managing one's loss and grief. In writing about bereavement associated with the death of one's spouse, Kaslow (2004) identifies several tasks associated with the healing process: relinquishing roles, forming a new identity, assuming control and responsibility for one's life, forgiving the loved one for dying, finding new meaning in life, and renewing hope. Although all of these tasks require effort, this effort on the part of the grieving person can be instrumental in gaining increased control over his or her life.

A chronic state of depression and a restricted range of feelings suffered by some people can be attributed to some unresolved reaction to a significant loss, as was seen in the case of Marianne's mother whose first child died during infancy. Such individuals seem to fear that the pain will consume them and that it is better to repress their feelings. They fail to realize that there is a consequence for this denial in the long run. This consequence can lead to the inability to feel closeness and joy. These people can go on for years without ever expressing emotions over their loss, being convinced that they have adequately dealt with it. Yet they might find themselves being flooded with emotions for which they have no explanation. They may discover that another's loss opens up old wounds for them, wounds they thought they had successfully healed.

My (Marianne's) father died many years ago. Although I grieved his death and found support from my friends and family, I find that even years later there are times when I am flooded with emotions of sadness over his loss. Sometimes these emotions take me by surprise, and I do not always know what triggered them. On several occasions when I felt the sadness, I realized afterward that it was a particular anniversary date that had to do with his life and death. My unconscious was more in tune than was my conscious mind. Sometimes people who have lost a loved one expect to complete their grieving in a set time, such as one year. It is important to realize that grief does not follow a linear timeline and a predictable schedule. Instead, people who are grieving need to experience their sadness and not tell themselves that they should be over this by now; they need to embrace the journey. Freeman (2005) puts this matter well when he writes:

> Grief and mourning are uniquely individual processes, and no one has the correct timetable for their completion. The process of healing might take a year, or it might take a lifetime. Whatever the time, the bereaved should not travel alone. (p. 74)

Cultural Perspectives on Grieving

There are considerable variations both within a culture and among cultures when it comes to the grieving process. Most cultures have rituals designed to help people with the grieving process. Examples are the funeral practices of the Irish, the Jewish, the Russians, and others, whereby painful feelings are actually triggered and released. In the Asian, African, and Hispanic cultures bereaved individuals are encouraged to maintain emotional connections to their dead loved ones. In these cultures, physical death does not imply the death of a relationship. Regardless of the specific form of mourning, all of the rituals have the purpose of bringing about healing and assisting the bereaved in dealing with the pain of a loss. Hannah describes how her cultural traditions provided comfort to her family at a time of great grief.

HANNAH'S STORY

Most people who are not familiar with Judaism find my family's customs and rituals very complicated. It used to bother me, but now that I am older I can understand how our traditions seem complex to those outside of our faith. Instead of feeling irritated when people look perplexed, now I try to educate them about these traditions. For instance, when my father died suddenly of a heart attack a few years ago, we sat Shiva for 7 days after he was buried. We covered the mirrors in our house and tore our shirts, which is common in Jewish culture after a family member's death. During this time, my aunt and uncle brought over meals, and my cousins were very supportive and helped to clean our house and look after us. Customs like Shiva have historical and cultural significance and are comforting. I appreciate the traditions of Judaism that helped my family navigate this most difficult time.

In my (Marianne's) culture in Germany, going to the cemetery to visit the gravesites is a standard practice and helps people in the grieving process. Our daughters were a part of this ritual when they visited their relatives in Germany. Recently, one of Jerry's American relatives called us expressing serious concerns about Heidi's psychological health because she discovered that Heidi was visiting her grandmother's grave with her young son on a regular basis. Not only did Heidi see nothing wrong with visiting her grandmother's place of rest, but she looked forward to these visits as it gave her an opportunity to introduce her son to stories about his great-grandmother.

If you are experiencing bereavement and are able to express the full range of your thoughts and feelings, you stand a better chance of adjusting to a new environment. Indeed, part of the grief process involves making basic life changes and experiencing new growth. If you have allowed yourself to grieve, you are better equipped to become reinvested with a new purpose and a new reason for living. This *post-traumatic growth* has the potential to transform you in profound ways. It can lead to a greater appreciation of life, strengthen relationships, and remind you of the human capacity of resilience (Ben-Shahar, 2011). What major losses have you had, and how have you coped with them? Have you lost a family member, a close friendship, a job that you valued, a partner through divorce, a material object that had special meaning, a place where you once lived, a pet, or your faith in some person or group? Are there any similarities in how you responded to these different types of loss? Did you allow yourself to express your feelings about your loss to someone close to you?

The stages of dying and the tasks of dying can also be applied in understanding significant losses other than the death of a loved one, such as separation from one's parents, seeing children leave home, the breakup of a relationship, miscarriages, unfulfilled dreams or life goals, retirement, and many times the loss of a pet. If people allow themselves to mourn their losses, the process of grief work usually leads to a sense of acceptance. For example, in the case of divorce, once the two persons have experienced the grief over the loss and expressed their feelings about it, new possibilities begin to open up. They can begin to accept that they must make a life for themselves without the other person and that they cannot cling to resentments that will keep them from beginning to establish that life. They may be able to let go of their resentments and experience forgiveness. They can then learn from their experience and apply that knowledge to future relationships.

TAKE TIME TO REFLECT

1. How well do you cope with loss? What do you do to help yourself grieve when you have experienced a loss?

_____

_____

2. When your life is over, how would you like to be remembered? Based on the way you are living your life now, how likely is it that you will be remembered in this way?

_____

_____

3. What stories would you like people to tell about you after your death?

_____

_____

SUMMARY

In this chapter we have encouraged you to devote some time to reflecting on your death. Doing so can help you examine the quality and direction of your life and help you find your own meaning in life. The acceptance of death is closely related to the acceptance of life. When we avoid reflecting on our finite nature, it is likely to affect the way we are living. Acceptance of death does not have to be a morbid topic, for it can lead to post-traumatic growth, revitalize our goals, and assist us in finding a deeper purpose for living. Recognizing and accepting the fact of death gives us the impetus to search for our own answers to questions like these: "What is the meaning of my life?" "What do I most want from life?" "How can I create the life I want to live?"

Although terminally ill people show great variability in how they deal with their dying, a general pattern of stages has been identified: denial, anger, bargaining, depression, and acceptance. Other models explaining how people cope with dying place emphasis on tasks to be accomplished. Both the stage and task models of coping with dying can also be applied to people who are working through grief over a significant loss. The relational model of grieving encourages people to think of ways of continuing a new and different kind of relationship with a deceased loved one. Instead of death ending a relationship, the emphasis is on keeping the person alive through our conversations and memories. In dealing with losses, grieving is necessary. If we are able to express and explore a mixture of feelings associated with a loss, we make it possible to accept the reality of loss and continue to find meaning in life.

If we are able to confront the reality of death, we can change the quality of our lives and make real changes in our relationships with others and with ourselves. We often live as though we had forever to accomplish what we want. Regardless of how much time we have left, our time is still limited. The realization that there is an end to life can motivate us to get the most from the time we have.

Where Can I Go From Here?

1. Let yourself reflect on how the loss of those you love might affect you. Consider each person separately, and try to imagine how your life today would be different if that person were not in it. What would you regret not having said to each person? Write these impressions in the journal pages at the end of this chapter.

2. One way to take stock of your life is to imagine your own death, including the details of the funeral and the things people might say about you. Try writing your own eulogy or obituary. This can be a powerful way of summing up how you see your life and how you would like it to be different. Write three eulogies for yourself. First, write your actual eulogy—the one you would give at your own funeral, if that were possible. Second, write the eulogy that you fear—one that expresses some of the negative things someone could say of you. Third, write the eulogy that you would hope for— one that expresses the most positive aspects of your life so far. After you have written your three eulogies, write down in your journal what the experience was like for you and what you learned from it. Are there any specific steps you would like to take now to begin living more fully? Reflect on how you might live your life today to bring about your hoped-for eulogy. As an additional step, consider sealing your eulogies in an envelope and putting them away for a year or so. Then, at this later date, do the exercise again and compare the two sets of eulogies to see what changes have occurred in your view of your life.

3. Write a grief letter. Think of a significant loss and express in writing your feelings about a person or thing that you have lost. In your letter, consider including how you felt about the loss and how you dealt with it when it happened; how you now feel about your loss and how you are dealing with it now; feelings that you may still have pertaining to the loss; and the perspective you would like to be able to adopt concerning how this loss is affecting you today.

4. Investigate what type of hospice program, if any, your community has. Who is on the staff? What services does it offer? If you are interested in learning more about hospice services, or to identify a local hospice program, visit the website of the National Hospice and Palliative Care Organization.

5. Suggested Readings. The full bibliographic entry for each of these sources can be found in the References and Suggested Readings at the back of the book. For a personal account of the meaning of living and dying, see Albom (1997). For a scholarly, yet personal treatment of how the reality of death can enhance living, see Yalom (2008). For a textbook that offers an in-depth treatment of death and dying, see Corr and Corr (2013). See Hedtke and Winslade (2004) for a comprehensive discussion of the process of grieving.

WEBSITE RESOURCES

Included here are some valuable websites. For access to these websites, video activities, and other supporting materials, visit Cengage Learning's Counseling CourseMate website for *I Never Knew I Had a Choice,* 10th Edition, at **www.cengagebrain.com.**

END OF LIFE, EXPLORING DEATH IN AMERICA
www.npr.org/programs/death

Recommended Search Words: "NPR end of life"

National Public Radio (NPR) has aired programs about death and dying in American culture. This website offers both printed and audio transcripts of the programs and many bibliographical and organizational resources as well.

SUICIDE . . . READ THIS FIRST
www.metanoia.org/suicide

Recommended Search Words: "metanoia suicide"

This site is for those who are dealing with suicidal issues in themselves or others. It speaks straight to the issue and guides readers through a thoughtful series of steps to resolve their issues. Suicide and suicidal feelings are dealt with, including helpful resources and links for more information.

NATIONAL HOSPICE AND PALLIATIVE CARE ORGANIZATION
www.nhpco.org

Recommended Search Words: "national hospice and palliative care organization"

For news briefs about hospice care, information about advocacy, and access to a database of service providers and programs, visit this website or call the NHPCO HelpLine at (800) 658-8898.

SUICIDE HOTLINES
http://suicidehotlines.com/

Recommended Search Words: "suicide hotlines"

This extremely valuable site offers links to suicide hotlines and crisis centers across the United States. It also contains links to other resources on suicide.

ELISABETH KÜBLER-ROSS FOUNDATION
www.ekrfoundation.org/

Recommended Search Words: "Kübler-Ross foundation"

This foundation is aimed at furthering the legacy and work of pioneering legend Elisabeth Kübler-Ross. It provides links to resources for those wanting information about advanced directives, end-of-life care, grief support, and much more.

STEVE JOBS: 2005 STANFORD UNIVERSITY COMMENCEMENT ADDRESS
http://news.stanford.edu/news/2005/ june15/jobs-061505.html

Recommended Search Words: "Steve Jobs Stanford commencement speech"

Visit this site to read the full transcript or watch the video of this remarkable commencement address.

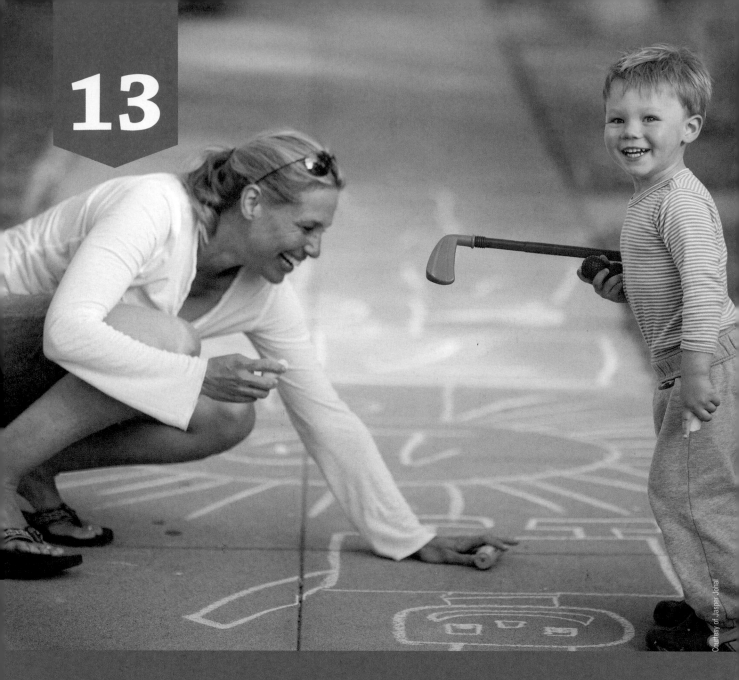

Courtesy of Jasper Johal

MEANING AND VALUES

> Where Am I Now?

> Our Quest for Identity

> People Who Live With Passion and Purpose

> When Good People Do Bad Things: The Lucifer Effect

> When Ordinary People Do Extraordinary Things

> Our Search for Meaning and Purpose

> Religion/Spirituality and Meaning

> Our Values in Action

> Embracing Diversity

> Making a Difference

> Summary

> Where Can I Go From Here?

> Website Resources

> *We need to develop the ability to listen to our inner selves and trust what we hear.*

WHERE AM I NOW?

Use this scale to respond to these statements:

4 = I strongly *agree* with this statement.
3 = I *agree* with this statement.
2 = I *disagree* with this statement.
1 = I *strongly disagree* with this statement.

1. At this time in my life I have a sense of meaning and purpose.

2. Most of my values are similar to those of my parents.

3. I have challenged and questioned most of the values I now hold.

4. Religion/spirituality is an important source of meaning for me.

5. I'm generally faithful to my values.

6. My values and my views about life's meaning have undergone much change over the years.

7. The meaning of my life is based in large part on my ability to have a significant impact on others.

8. I let others influence my values more than I would like to admit.

9. I am willing to reflect on my own biases and prejudices, and to challenge them.

10. I welcome the opportunity to learn about value systems that differ from mine.

We are the only creatures who can reflect on our existence and exercise individual choice in defining our lives. As we saw in Chapter 12, the confrontation with death is a pathway to finding meaning in life. Awareness of our mortality can create anxiety, but it also can be a catalyst for making major life decisions. Our quest for meaning involves asking three key existential questions, none of which have easy or absolute answers: "Who am I?" "Where am I going?" "Why?"

"Who am I?" is a question that will have a different answer at various times in our lives. When old values no longer seem to supply meaning or give us direction, we have the opportunity to create a different way of life.

"Where am I going?" questions our plans for a lifetime. What process do we expect to use to attain our goals? The answer to this question involves a periodic review of our life goals, which are rarely set once and for all.

Asking "Why?" and searching for understanding is a human characteristic. We face a rapidly changing world in which old values give way to new ones or to none at all. Part of the quest for meaning requires an active search to make sense of the world in which we find ourselves.

OUR QUEST FOR IDENTITY

Achieving personal identity does not necessarily mean clinging to a certain way of thinking or behaving. Instead, it may involve trusting ourselves enough to become open to new possibilities. We are challenged to reexamine our patterns and our priorities, our habits and our relationships. Above all, we must develop the ability to listen to our inner selves and trust what we hear. In this way we can come to define the core values that shape us.

Values are core beliefs that influence how we act. Our values support the choices we make in life. If we have questioned our values and found they fit us, we are more likely to live in harmony with these values.

Sometimes we may decide to go against our cultural upbringing to create an identity that is congruent with our own newly adopted values. This was true for Jenny, a Vietnamese woman who developed a different set of values from her mother.

JENNY'S STORY

There were many instances when I wanted to be alone or to take time off from work to relax. There would be an attack of accusatory statements indicating that I was selfish, that I was wasting too much time on myself, and that I wasn't devoting enough time to my family obligations. Even the way I spent my money was met with criticism, because I did not save it for a better cause like my family. I spent many hours explaining to my mother about how much it meant to me to buy myself nice things and to spend some of my time enjoying life. In the eyes of my mother and her culture, I was the selfish one. I had to understand this perspective and edit it to fit my own values.

How do you experience your identity at this time in your life? The Take Time to Reflect exercise may help you answer this question.

1. What are your core values? To identify some of your values, rate the importance of each of these items using this scale:

3 = This is *extremely important* to me.
2 = This is *somewhat important* to me.
1 = This is *not important* to me.

_____ Appreciating nature
_____ Loving others and being loved
_____ Enjoying an intimate relationship
_____ Engaging in recreation
_____ Family life
_____ Preserving and protecting the planet
_____ Security
_____ Courage
_____ Work and career
_____ Laughter and a sense of humor
_____ Intelligence and curiosity
_____ Being open to different cultures and experiences
_____ Taking risks in order to change
_____ Being of service to others
_____ Making a difference in the lives of others
_____ A relationship with God or a higher power
_____ Independence and self-determination
_____ Interdependence and cooperation
_____ Having control of my life
_____ Being financially successful
_____ Having solitude and time to reflect
_____ Being productive and achieving
_____ Being approved of by others
_____ Facing challenges
_____ Compassion and caring
_____ Engaging in competition

Look over the items you rated as "3" (extremely important). If you had to select the top three values in your life, which would they be? _____

_____

_____

2. How are these three values a part of your everyday life?

_____

_____

3. How often do you experience each of the things you have just listed? What prevents you from doing the things you value as frequently as you would like?

_____

_____

4. What are some specific actions you can take to add meaning to your life?

_____

_____

5. Who are you? Try completing the sentence "I am . . ." six different ways by writing down the words or phrases that immediately occur to you.

I am _____

I am _____

I am _____

I am _____

I am _____

I am _____

PEOPLE WHO LIVE WITH PASSION AND PURPOSE

History is replete with the stories of people who strived for a meaningful existence through their devotion to a particular cause. Consider, for instance, the extraordinary life of Dr. Martin Luther King Jr. One of the greatest nonviolent leaders in world history, King was inspired by his Christian faith and by the teachings of Mahatma Gandhi. King derived meaning from his role as an advocate for freedom, justice, equality, and peace. "During the less than 13 years of Dr. Martin Luther King, Jr.'s leadership of the modern American Civil Rights Movement, from December, 1955 until April 4, 1968, African Americans achieved more genuine progress toward racial equality than the previous 350 years had produced" ("About Dr. King," 2012).). Regardless of the resistance King encountered, he maintained fidelity to the principle that people everywhere, regardless of color or creed, were equal members of the human family. (See the King Center website, listed at the end of this chapter, for more information on this remarkable man and his work.)

Viktor Frankl (1963), a European psychiatrist, dedicated his professional life to the study of meaning in life. The approach to therapy that he developed is known as **logotherapy**, which means "therapy through meaning" or "healing through meaning." According to Frankl (1963, 1965, 1969, 1978), what distinguishes us as humans is our search for purpose. The striving to find meaning in our lives is a primary motivational force. Humans choose to live and even to die for the sake of their ideals and values. Frankl (1963) notes that "everything can be taken from a man but one thing: the last of the human freedoms—to choose one's attitude in any given set of circumstances, to choose one's own way" (p. 104). Frankl points to the wisdom of Nietzsche's words: "He who has a why to live for can bear with almost any how" (as cited in Frankl, 1963, p. 164). Drawing on his experiences in the death camp at Auschwitz, Frankl asserts that inmates who had a vision of some goal, purpose, or task in life had a much greater chance of surviving than those who had no such sense of hope. We have many opportunities to make choices, and the decisions we make or fail to make shape the meaning of our lives.

This relationship between choice and meaning is dramatically illustrated by Holocaust survivors who report that although they did not choose their circumstances they could at least choose their attitude toward their plight. Consider the example of Dr. Edith Eva Eger, a clinical psychologist, who was interviewed about her experiences as a survivor of a Nazi concentration camp (see Glionna, 1992). At one point, Eger weighed only 40 pounds, yet she refused to engage in the cannibalism that was taking place. She said, "I chose to eat grass. And I sat on the ground, selecting one blade over the other, telling myself that even under those conditions I still had a choice—which blade of grass I would eat." Although Eger lost her family to the camps and had her back broken by one of the guards, she eventually chose to let go of her hatred. She finally came to the realization that it was her captors who were the imprisoned ones. As she put it: "If I still hated today, I would still be in prison. I would be giving Hitler and Mengele their posthumous victories. If I hated, they would still be in charge, not me." Her example supports the notion that even in the most dire situations it is possible to give a new meaning to such circumstances by our choice of attitudes, and in her case, the choice to forgive.

Sometimes our choices are stripped from us, as in the extreme cases illustrated by Viktor Frankl and Edith Eger. In a like manner, Francis Bok (2003), in his very moving book, *Escape From Slavery*, tells the story of his village in the Sudan being pillaged and his being taken as a slave for many years. He reports his horrifying childhood experiences with near death and his attempts to escape, only to be recaptured. His father told Bok that he was special and that he would always do something important in life. His father's faith in him inspired him to never give up hope and to continue to struggle even in extreme circumstances. Bok found ways to avoid totally surrendering, even though almost all of his freedoms were taken from him. With his attitude and constant thoughts of escaping from slavery, Bok was able to retain some degree of control over his life. Although a couple of his attempts at escaping almost resulted in his death, he finally did escape his bondage because of his hope and the risks he took. Since that time he has devoted his life to doing whatever he could to inform people in the United States about the trials of the Sudanese people. In 2000 he became the first escaped slave to testify before the Senate Committee on Foreign Relations in hearings on Sudan. He speaks throughout the United States, has been featured in magazines and television, and met with President George W. Bush at the White House. Bok was driven by passion and purpose in extreme circumstances, and his story illustrates how he was able to find meaning at a very desperate time in his life and how his work today is motivated by giving meaning to his earlier experiences.

WHEN GOOD PEOPLE DO BAD THINGS: THE LUCIFER EFFECT

When we focus on the survivors of atrocities—torture, slavery, and genocide—we are reminded of the human capacity for resilience. But when we contemplate the behavior of the perpetrators of these atrocities, we are forced to confront the human capacity to engage in acts of evil. Stanford University Professor Emeritus Philip Zimbardo, who conducted the now classic Stanford Prison Experiment in 1971, addresses the perplexing issue of how average, decent people become perpetrators of evil. Zimbardo (2007) suggests that when we try to comprehend unusual or aberrant behavior we tend to focus solely on the inner determinants of genes, personality, and character. In doing so, we overlook two potential critical catalysts for behavior change—the external *situation* and the *system* that creates and maintains the situation. Situational forces, such as those operating during the abuses at Abu Ghraib, can seduce people into evil. As an expert witness in the trial of a military policeman involved in the Abu Ghraib prisoner abuse, Zimbardo describes how situational forces transformed a good guard into a bad guard. Zimbardo then adopts the perspective of "prosecutor" to critically examine the role of the system and its complicity in establishing and maintaining torture-interrogation centers across many military prisons.

The officer was sentenced to 8 years of hard time in military prison, dishonorably discharged, disgraced, deprived of his military retirement savings, and divorced by his wife. This officer is now a nearly broken man. It may seem inconceivable that any rational person would ever engage in such abusive behaviors, but it is important for us to recognize the power that situational and systemic forces have on our behaviors and choices.

WHEN ORDINARY PEOPLE DO EXTRAORDINARY THINGS

Zimbardo believes that the antidote to evil is heroism, and he has spearheaded the nonprofit Heroic Imagination Project, focusing his energy on understanding the nature of heroism. The Heroic Imagination Project "teaches people how to overcome the natural human tendency to watch and wait in moments of crisis" ("About HIP," 2011). Zimbardo and his colleagues suggest that in order to be considered heroic, an act must meet four criteria:

▸ It is engaged in voluntarily.

▸ It provides a service to one or more people in need, or the community as a whole.

▸ It involves potential risk/cost to physical comfort, social stature, or quality of life.

▸ It is initiated without the expectation of material gain. ("Defining Heroism," 2011)

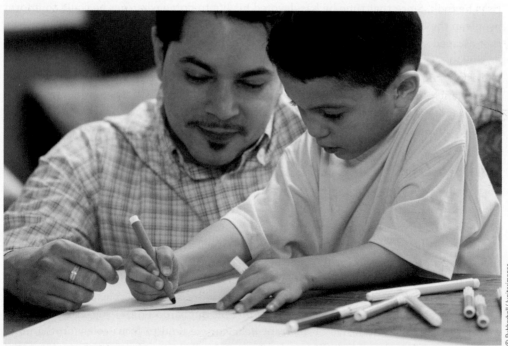

© Rubberball/Jupiterimages

≫ Meaning in life is found in relationships with others.

Although children tend to believe that one must have supernatural powers to be a hero, we see evidence all around us that ordinary people are capable of heroic deeds. Although you may not view yourself as an extraordinary person, it is likely that at some point in your life you will have the opportunity to be someone's hero.

OUR SEARCH FOR MEANING AND PURPOSE

Meaning in life is found through intense relationships with others rather than through an exclusive and narrow pursuit of self-realization (Bellah, Madsen, Sullivan, Swidler, & Tipton, 1985). Healthy relationships are two-sided transactions characterized by reciprocal giving and taking, and many people Bellah and his colleagues interviewed expressed a desire to move beyond the isolated self. Sacrificing yourself, without getting anything in return, is not the way to achieve a meaningful life. We must find a balance between our concern for ourselves and our desire to further the interests of the community. Ideally, by using our gifts in the service of others, we also are giving to ourselves.

Although the world itself may appear meaningless, our challenge as human beings is to create meaning. To live without meaning and values provokes considerable distress, and in its most severe form may lead to suicide. We need clear ideals to which we can aspire and guidelines by which we can direct our actions.

What Is the Meaning of Life?

In 1988 the editors of *Life* magazine asked a wide spectrum of people from all walks of life the question "What is the meaning of life?" David Friend's (1991) *The Meaning of Life* is the product of 300 thoughtful people. This mosaic of responses offers a variety of approaches to understanding life. As you read, think about the responses that resonate most closely with your own values.

▸ "The meaning of life is to live in balance and harmony with every other living thing in creation. We must all strive to understand the interconnectedness of all living things and accept our individual role in the protection and support of other life forms on earth. We must also understand our own insignificance in the totality of things" (Wilma Mankiller, Chief of the Cherokee Nation, p. 13).

▸ "It's my belief that the meaning of life changes from day to day, second to second. We're here to learn that we can create a world and that we have a choice in what we create, and that our world, if we choose, can be a heaven or hell" (Thomas E. O'Connor, AIDS activist and lecturer, p. 20).

▸ "Since age two I've been waltzing up and down with the question of life's meaning. And I am obliged to report that the answer changes from week to week. When I know the answer, I know it absolutely; as soon as I know that I know it, I know that I know nothing. About seventy percent of the time my conclusion is that there is a grand design" (Maya Angelou, writer and actress, p. 20).

▸ "I believe we as humans have the great challenge of living in harmony with the planet and all its parts. If we achieve that harmony we will have lived up to our fullest potential" (Molly Yard, feminist activist, p. 27).

▸ "I believe we are here to do good. It is the responsibility of every human being to aspire to do something worthwhile, to make this world a better place than the one he found. Life is a gift, and if we accept it, we must contribute in return. When we fail to contribute, we fail to adequately answer why we are here" (Armand Hammer, industrialist, physician, and self-made diplomat, p. 29).

▶ "While we exist as human beings, we are like tourists on holiday. If we play havoc and cause disturbance, our visit is meaningless. If during our short stay—100 years at most—we live peacefully, help others and, at the very least, refrain from harming or upsetting them, our visit is worthwhile" (Dalai Lama, spiritual leader of Tibetan Buddhism, p. 49).

▶ "We believe that we are in fact the image of our Creator. Our response must be to live up to that amazing potential—to give God glory by reflecting His beauty and His love. That is why we are here and that is the purpose of our lives" (South African civil rights leader, Archbishop Desmond Tutu, p. 13).

▶ "The purpose of human life is to achieve our own spiritual evolution, to get rid of negativity, to establish harmony among our physical, emotional, intellectual and spiritual quadrants, to learn to live in harmony within the family, community, nation, the whole world and all living things, treating all of mankind as brothers and sisters—thus making it finally possible to have peace on earth" (Elisabeth Kübler-Ross, psychiatrist and author, p. 65).

What is the meaning of your life? How would you answer this complex question in a few brief sentences? To help you refine your answer, let's look at some of the dimensions of a philosophy of life.

Developing a Philosophy of Life

A **philosophy of life** is made up of the fundamental beliefs, attitudes, and values that govern a person's behavior. You may not have thought much about your philosophy of life, but the fact that you have never explicitly defined the components of your philosophy does not mean you are completely without one. All of us operate on the basis of general assumptions about ourselves, others, and the world. The first step in actively developing your philosophy of life is to formulate a clear picture of your present attitudes, assumptions, and beliefs.

We have all been developing an implicit philosophy of life since we first began to wonder about life and death, love and hate, joy and fear, and the nature of the universe. If we were fortunate, adults took time to engage in dialogue with us and fostered our innate curiosity, rather than discouraging us from asking questions.

During the adolescent years, the process of questioning usually assumes new dimensions. Adolescents who have been encouraged to question and to think for themselves as children begin to get involved in a more advanced set of issues. Many adolescents struggle with these questions:

▶ Are the values I've believed in all these years the values I want to continue to live by?

▶ Where did I get my values? Are they still valid for me? Are there additional sources from which I can derive new values?

▶ Is there a higher power? What is my perception of a higher power? What is the nature of the hereafter? What does religion (or spirituality) mean to me?

▶ What do I base my ethical and moral decisions on? Peer group standards? Parental standards? The normative values of my society? My culture? My religion? My spirituality?

▶ What explains the inhumanity I see in the world?

▶ What kind of future do I want? What can I do to help create this kind of future?

A philosophy of life is not something we arrive at once and for all during our adolescent years. Developing your own philosophy of life continues as long as you live. As long as you remain curious and open to new learning, you can revise and rebuild your conceptions of the world. Life may have a particular meaning for us during adolescence, a new meaning during early and middle adulthood, and still another meaning as we reach old age. Indeed, if we do not remain open to basic changes in our views of life, we may find it difficult to adjust to changed circumstances. Both Janelle and Henry demonstrate how their core values changed as their philosophy of life evolved.

JANELLE'S STORY

As a child and as a teenager, my thinking was black and white. I either won or I lost. When I was the runner-up in a regional spelling bee, I considered myself a loser. I once received a third place award in a state-level essay contest. Most people would be pretty satisfied with that. Not me. If I didn't win the top prize, I felt like I didn't accomplish anything. It didn't help that my older sister teased me mercilessly about my insecurities and self-doubt. I think her teasing contributed to my obsession with winning. As I grew older, I was uptight most of the time because I felt there was no margin for error. Being the best was the only option. That's a hard way to live.

Because I was so compulsive about winning throughout high school, I derived little pleasure from academics or extracurricular activities. When I entered college, I made a conscious effort to change my unhealthy mind-set. Being preoccupied with perfection was robbing me of a satisfying life. I began to seriously question my values and the importance I placed on achievement. What good was attaining a goal if the joy of winning was quickly replaced by a fear of failing at the next goal? I did a 180° and went through a phase in which I didn't care about outcomes at all. I abruptly shifted my focus to the process of learning and de-emphasized grades. This phase lasted quite a while, and although my GPA suffered a bit, I felt much happier. I felt more connected to what I was doing because I actually felt engaged in the process.

Years have passed and now I have a much more balanced perspective. I have become a firm believer in embracing the process while not losing sight of the goal or outcome. Winning for the sake of winning is no longer my goal. Engaging in meaningful activities and learning from experience matter most to me. This has become an integral part of my philosophy of life.

HENRY'S STORY

I always put off things that I wanted to do. I lived a relatively unexciting life that involved getting up in the morning and going to a job that was pretty mundane but paid the bills. Then I was in a boating accident and nearly died. My near-death experience reinforced the point that we don't have unlimited time to accomplish our goals and pursue our dreams. It made me reevaluate the way I was spending my time. I now live my life fully aware that I may not live to see tomorrow. Because of this change in my attitude, I decided to look for a job that was more fulfilling and that allowed me to use my talents. I took a slight cut in pay, but I love what I do and have more energy too. I don't waste much time anymore doing things that have little value to me. The accident nearly killed me, but it also woke me up. The saying "live life to the fullest" seems so cliché, but it is the philosophy by which I live today.

Now may a good time to consider what changes you would like to make in your philosophy of life. Consider what would be helpful for you in evaluating your core values and in motivating you to begin by making even small shifts in the way you approach the tasks of daily living. You may find the following suggestions helpful as you go about formulating and reforming your own philosophy:

▶ Create time to be alone in reflective thought.

▶ Reflect on the basic assumptions you have made about life that influence what you do. Are your assumptions and beliefs leading you to self-criticism or to self-acceptance?

▶ Consider what meaning the fact of your eventual death has for the way you are presently living.

▶ Listen to others who are willing to challenge your beliefs and the degree to which you live by them.

▶ Adopt an accepting attitude toward those whose belief systems differ from yours and develop a willingness to critically evaluate your own beliefs.

All of these suggestions require that you be willing to challenge yourself and the beliefs you hold. Keeping track of yourself can provide unexpected rewards.

TAKE TIME TO REFLECT

Complete the following sentences by writing down the first responses that come to mind:

1. My parents have influenced my values by _____

2. Life is worth living because of _____

3. One thing that I most want to say about my life at this point is _____

4. If I could change one thing about my life at this point, it would be _____

5. If I had to answer the question "Who am I?" in a sentence, I'd say _____

6. What I like best about me is _____

7. I keep myself vital by _____

8. I am unique in that _____

9. When I think of my future, I _____

10. I feel discouraged about life when _____

11. My beliefs and values have been influenced by _____

12. I feel most powerful when _____

13. If I don't change, _____

14. I feel good about myself when _____

15. To me, the essence of a meaningful life is _____

16. I suffer from a sense of meaninglessness when _____

Feel free to expand your responses on a separate piece of paper or in the journal pages at the end of this chapter.

RELIGION/SPIRITUALITY AND MEANING

Religious faith, or some form of personal spirituality, can be a powerful source of meaning and purpose. For some, religion does not occupy a key place, yet personal spirituality may be a central force. Spiritual values help many people make sense out of the universe and the purpose of their life on this earth. Like any other potential source of meaning, religious faith or spirituality seems most authentic and valuable when it enables us to become as fully human as possible. It can help us get in touch with our own powers of thinking, feeling, deciding, willing, and acting.

There are many ways to define spirituality; Kottler and Carlson (2007) provide this thoughtful description: **Spirituality** is "a set of beliefs and practices that can result in a life-changing path that gives greater meaning, purpose, and fulfillment to a person's life" (p. 3). They expand on this theme in this way:

> Spirituality is often viewed as a journey, an odyssey, quest, pilgrimage, process, a wandering or movement, an expedition into the meaning of life. It is a way of experiencing life, one that is intended to increase awareness and help you to become more fully alive, as well as to appreciate better the heaven that exists on this earth. (p. 3)

Spirituality is at the foundation of healing in Twelve Step programs for people struggling with addictions to alcohol and mood-altering substances. Alcoholics Anonymous (AA) teaches individuals struggling with addictions that they must accept the reality that their lives have become unmanageable and that they need to rely on a higher power to find a path to healing. Although AA does not endorse a particular religion or form of spirituality, spiritual values are fundamental to the philosophy of the program.

In *The Art of Happiness: A Handbook for Living,* the Dalai Lama and Howard Cutler (1998) offer some thought-provoking ideas about basic spiritual values and the subject of religion:

▶ Spiritual pursuits and religions are aimed at nourishing the human spirit.

▶ Diversity in religions can be celebrated, and it is important to respect and appreciate the value of the different major world religions.

▶ Religion can be used to help reduce conflict and suffering in the world, not as a source to divide people.

▶ Involvement in any form of spirituality or religion can create a feeling of belonging and a caring connection with others.

▶ Spiritual/religious beliefs can provide a deep sense of purpose and meaning in life. These beliefs can offer hope in the face of adversity and suffering and can offer a perspective when we are overwhelmed by life's problems.

The Dalai Lama believes that the ultimate goal of all religions is to produce better human beings who will demonstrate caring and acceptance of others. We agree with the Dalai Lama's position and are convinced that religious teachings should be evaluated by the degree to which the faithful act more loving toward others. Religions have sometimes been a force for dividing people into antagonistic camps and have resulted in great harm. We are bombarded daily with examples of religious fanaticism aimed at overpowering, dominating, and eliminating entire groups of people. History is replete with religious wars, and it seems that the lessons from the past have not been learned. Instead of being a divisive force, there can be unity in diversity. Despite our differences, we can be unified in striving to make this world a better place by treating one another with compassion and kindness.

The Dalai Lama (2001) teaches that religious beliefs are but one level of spirituality, and he talks about **basic spiritual values,** which include qualities of goodness, kindness, love, compassion, tolerance, forgiveness, human warmth, and caring. All religions have the same basic message in that they all advocate these basic human values. Love, compassion, and forgiveness are not luxuries; rather, they are essential values for our survival. **Compassion,** an essential part of one's spiritual development, involves caring about another's suffering and doing something about it. Whether we are believers or nonbelievers, this kind of spirituality is essential. True spirituality results in making people calmer, happier, and more peaceful, and it is a mental attitude that can be practiced at any time. The Dalai Lama has consistently emphasized that inner discipline offers the foundation of a spiritual life, which is also the fundamental pathway to achieving happiness.

Mother Teresa, who became known to the world for her selfless work with the poor people in Calcutta, India, talks about compassion in action. She believes that God and compassion are one and the same. Much like the Dalai Lama, Mother Teresa views compassion as attempting to share and understand the suffering of people. Mother Teresa states: "Religion has nothing to do with compassion; it is our love for God that is the main thing because we have all been created for the sole purpose to love and be loved" (cited in Shield & Carlson, 1999, p. 181).

Rabbi Harold Kushner believes that encountering God consists in doing the right thing (cited in Shield & Carlson, 1999). For Rabbi Kushner, we make room in our lives for God when we do things that make us truly human, such as helping the poor, working for social justice, and keeping in check our exaggerated sense of self-importance. The Dalai Lama, Mother Teresa, and Rabbi Kushner seem to agree that leading a religious life is characterized by action that leads to bettering ourselves and treating others with kindness and dignity. Acting on our beliefs is what matters.

Andrew Harvey writes that there are three ways in which we can have a relationship with the divine: through prayer, meditation, and service (cited in Shield & Carlson, 1999). It is essential to combine prayer (talking to God) with a simple daily practice of meditation (listening to God). But Harvey says that prayer and meditation are not enough. We need to put what we learn about divine love into practice through service to others. Harvey points to a common

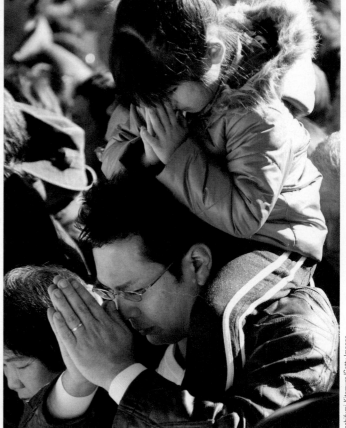

Toshifumi Kitamura/Getty Images

» Religious or spiritual beliefs can provide a deep sense of purpose and meaning in life.

message from all the great figures—from Lao Tzu to Buddha to Confucius to Jesus—we must give our love to those around us. Harvey writes: "Prayer, meditation, and service, lived together, can engender the divine life if they are pursued with humility, reverence, and simplicity of heart" (p. 76).

People of diverse religious faiths are able to establish a connection with a personal God by reading and reflecting on sacred texts. Some of these texts include *The Torah* (Judaism), *The Bible* (Christianity), *Dharma* (Buddhism), *Tao Te Ching* (Taoism), *Qur'an* (Islam), and *The Vedas* (Hinduism). Boenisch and Haney (2004) claim that the wisdom in the various sacred texts shared by diverse groups of people has a common theme, which is a message of hope.

At this point, what do you think is the heart of your spirituality or religion? Reflect on the following questions about your religion or your spirituality to determine the degree to which it is a constructive force in your life:

▶ Is the way that I live my life congruent with the religion or spirituality that I profess?

▶ Does my religion or spirituality assist me in better understanding the meaning of life and death?

▶ Does my religion or spirituality allow acceptance for others who see the world differently from me?

▶ Does my religion or spirituality encourage me to put my beliefs into action?

▶ Does my religion or spirituality provide me with a sense of peace and serenity?

▶ Is my religious faith or my spiritual path something I actively chose or uncritically accepted?

▶ Do my core religious and spiritual values help me live life fully and treat others with respect and concern?

▶ Does my religion or spirituality help me integrate my experiences and make sense of the world?

▶ Does my religion or spirituality encourage me to exercise my freedom and to assume responsibility for the direction of my own life?

▶ Are my religious or spiritual beliefs and practices helping me to become more the person I would like to be?

▶ Does my religion or spirituality encourage me to question life and keep myself open to new learning?

As you take time for self-examination, how able are you to answer these questions in a way that is meaningful and satisfying to you? If you are honest with yourself, perhaps you will find that you have not critically evaluated the sources of your spiritual and religious beliefs. Although you may hesitate to question your belief system out of a fear of weakening or undermining your faith, the opposite might well be true; demonstrating the courage to question your beliefs and values might strengthen them.

Religious faith or personal spirituality can help you define meaning in your life, but many people do not have a religious or spiritual orientation. For them, meaning is found in other endeavors. Irvin Yalom writes about his absence of belief in a hereafter and claims to be an atheist. When people ask how he is able to find meaning in life without a belief in God, he replies that for him doing good therapy and writing books are sources of meaning in his life. Indeed, there are many routes to a meaningful life.

OUR VALUES IN ACTION

Values for Our Daughters

When our daughters Heidi and Cindy were growing up, we hoped they would come to share these important values with us:

▶ Have a positive and significant impact on the people in their lives

▶ Be willing to take risks and make mistakes

▶ Form their own values rather than unquestioningly adopting ours

▶ Like and respect themselves and feel good about their abilities and talents

▶ Be open and trusting rather than fearful or suspicious

▶ Respect and care for others

▶ Continue to have fun as they grew older

▶ Be able to express their feelings and always feel free to come to us and share meaningful aspects of their lives

▶ Remain in touch with their power and refuse to surrender it

▶ Be independent and have the courage to be different from others if they want to be

▶ Have a belief in spirituality that guides their actions

▶ Be proud of themselves, yet humble

▶ Respect the differences in others

▶ Strive to live in accordance with their values and principles

▶ Develop a flexible view of the world and be willing to modify their perspective based on new experiences

▶ Give back to the world by contributing to make it a better place to live in

Our daughters are now independent adults, yet they continue to value time with us and to invite us to be involved in their lives. Although their lives are not problem-free, they typically show a willingness to face and deal with their struggles and are succeeding in making significant choices for themselves. If you have children or expect to have children someday, think about the values you would like them to develop, as well as the part you will need to play in offering them guidance.

Becoming Aware of How Your Values Operate

Your values influence what you do; your daily behavior is an expression of your basic values. We ask you to take time to examine the source of your values to determine if they are appropriate for you at this time in your life. Furthermore, it is essential that you be aware of the significant impact your value system has on your relationships with others. In our view, it is not appropriate for you to push your values on others, to assume a judgmental stance toward those who have a different view, or to strive to convert others to adopt your perspective on life. Indeed, if you are secure in your values and basic beliefs, you will not be threatened by those who have a different set of beliefs and values.

In *God's Love Song*, Maier (1991) wonders how anyone can claim to have found the only way, not only for him- or herself, but also for everyone else. As a minister, Sam Maier teaches that diversity shared is not only beautiful but also fosters understanding,

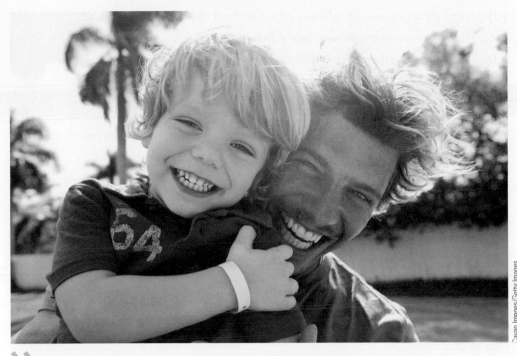

Cavan Images/Getty Images

>> We want to know that we have touched the lives of others and that somehow we have contributed to helping others live more fully.

caring, and the creation of community. He puts this message in a powerful and poetic way:

▶ It is heartening to find communities where the emphasis is placed upon each person having the opportunity to:

▶ share what is vital and meaningful out of one's own experience;

▶ listen to what is vital and meaningful to others;

▶ not expect or demand that anyone else do it exactly the same way as oneself. (p. 3)

Reverend Maier's message is well worth contemplating. Although you might clarify a set of values that seem to work for you, we hope you will respect the values of others that may be quite different from yours. One set of values is not right and the other wrong. The diversity of cultures, religions, and worldviews provides a tapestry of life that allows us the opportunity to embrace many paths toward meaning in life. Whatever your own values are, they can be further clarified and strengthened if you entertain open discussion of various viewpoints and cultivate a nonjudgmental attitude toward diversity. Ask yourself these questions:

▶ Where did I develop my values?

▶ Have I questioned my values?

▶ Do I have a need for everything to remain the same without changes?

▶ Are my values and practices open to modification?

▶ Do I find a consistency between what I say I believe in and what I do?

▶ Do I feel so deeply committed to any of my values that I am likely to push my friends and family members to accept them?

▸ How can I communicate my values to others without imposing those values?

▸ Am I willing to accept people who hold different values?

▸ Do I avoid judging others even if they think, feel, or act in different ways from me?

TAKE TIME TO REFLECT

1. At this time, what are some of the principal sources of meaning and purpose in your life?

_____

_____

2. Have there been occasions in your life when you have allowed other people or institutions to make key choices for you? If so, give a couple of examples.

_____

_____

3. What role, if any, does religion or spirituality play in your life?_____

_____

_____

4. If you were to create a new religion or a spiritual path, what virtues and values would you include? What would be the vices?

_____

_____

5. What are some of the values you would most like to see your children adopt?

_____

_____

EMBRACING DIVERSITY

We are a people of many diverse backgrounds. One barrier to forming meaningful connections with others is the tendency to hold negative attitudes toward those who are different from us. It is not an easy task to learn to embrace and appreciate diversity rather than be threatened by it. If we are unwilling or unable to accept this challenge, we remain isolated and separate from one another.

Many people incorrectly assume that cultural diversity relates only to one's race or ethnicity. Broadly conceived, **culture** pertains to the knowledge, language, values, and customs that are passed from person to person and from one generation to the next generation. We possess both an individual cultural identity and a group identity with a variety of cultures. Culture is one aspect of our experience that makes us similar to some people and different from others. It is clear that in the United States we are affected by the ever-changing and increasing diversity of our culture. The global community will continue to become more interdependent, creating a need to understand and build connections with diverse cultures. It is relatively easy to get caught in the trap of an **ethnocentric bias,** using our own culture or country as a standard of what is right and good and judging other cultures or countries by our own frame of reference. Our central challenge is to welcome and embrace diversity.

We sometimes choose to live in an **encapsulated world,** ignoring consideration of the diversity of worldviews and seeking support from those who think and value as we do. This disinterest prevents us from learning from those who may have a different worldview and allows us to remain unchallenged in our own views. Many times our attitudes come not from personal experience of others but from stereotypes of others. When we make no attempt to get to know people different from ourselves, we are likely to retain our prejudicial attitudes.

I (Marianne) frequently travel between the United States and Germany, and to other countries as well. I view myself as an ambassador in many respects. When I am in the United States, I share my thoughts, perceptions, and experiences with people from other countries. When I am away from the United States, I talk about life in this country. Over the years I have encouraged many people to take another look at misconceptions or negative attitudes they hold about people who are different from themselves or who live in a different region of the world.

Meaning in life can be found by paying attention to the common ground we all share and by becoming aware of universal themes that unite us in spite of our differences. In the early chapters of this book, we emphasized that a meaningful life is not lived alone but is the result of connectedness to others in love, work, and community. In accepting and understanding others, we discover deeper meanings in life. If we live in isolation, we are placing a barrier between ourselves and those who are different from us.

We invite you to reflect on a philosophy of life that embraces understanding and acceptance of diverse worldviews. Consider those attitudes and behaviors you are willing to change that will allow you to increasingly accept and respect others, whether they are like or different from you.

Embracing Versus Denying Our Cultural Heritage

If you have a sense of your own cultural background and values, and of how your culture has evolved, you have a framework for appreciating the values of people in another culture. The more you know about people from diverse cultures, the more able you will be to connect with them in a positive way.

I (Jerry) am a first-generation Italian American. Both of my parents were from Italy, yet neither of them seemed to think it important that I learned to speak Italian, nor did they teach me much about my cultural heritage. When I was a child, we spent almost every Sunday at a family gathering at my maternal grandparents' house. Most of the conversation was in Italian, and I felt lost and separate from my extended family because I could not understand what was being said. Not passing on family history or Italian customs was a common practice among recent immigrants at that time. They believed it was best for their offspring to blend into the dominant society and not stand out by being different. This was also encouraged by the dominant culture.

My father, Guiseppi Cordileone, came to the United States from Italy when he was 7 years old, not knowing a word of English. He had an extremely hard life and grew up in an orphanage. He did not have any contact with his father, and his mother had died in Italy when he was young. In spite of many odds against him, he eventually managed to become a dentist. Once he began his dental practice, he was concerned that people might not want to come to an Italian dentist, so he changed his name from *Cordileone* (meaning "heart of the lion") to *Corey*. It was likely that my father had some shame about his roots, and he also wanted to prevent his children from experiencing the prejudice and discrimination that he had experienced.

Being around a nuclear and extended immigrant Italian family, I learned at an early age that people see the world through different eyes and express themselves in different ways. I came to appreciate differences rather than judge them. Because of my father's experiences,

I became aware that people were discriminated against because of their ethnicity. Today, immigrants might still be encouraged to blend into the mainstream, but I hope not to the degree I experienced as a child.

Not all immigrants actively deny their cultural roots. Many take pride in passing on their language, customs, and values to their children. I (Marianne) earlier mentioned that I emigrated from Germany to the United States as a young adult. I was surprised that many first-generation offspring did not speak their parents' language and knew very little about their ancestors. I made a decision that I wanted our daughters to learn as much as possible about their German heritage and language. So that Heidi and Cindy would not be teased by their friends for speaking German, I taught some of the neighborhood children German lessons. This proved to be a fun experience and was positive for all concerned. Living in a typical middle-class neighborhood, I had observed that people oftentimes did not know how to react when they were in the presence of others who spoke a foreign language.

Most Americans speak English only, and people speaking another language are sometimes viewed as being secretive, impolite, exclusionary, and cliquish—even when English speakers are not part of the interaction. I (Marianne) will sometimes speak to fellow Germans in my own language, even among Germans who also understand English. Doing so is not aimed at excluding others who do not understand German; rather, it is a way of being more intimate and forming a more meaningful connection. During such encounters, speaking English may lose the meaning and feeling of what I want to convey.

When I (Marianne) am working with a client in a group counseling situation, I may ask the person to role-play with a significant person in her life. If English is her second language, I often invite her to speak in her primary language. Doing so is typically very powerful for the group member, and it assists her in becoming emotionally connected with her therapeutic work. This is well described in the book (not the movie) *Lost in Translation* (Hoffman, 1990). The emotional quality and connection can easily be lost when translating from one's primary language. In our DVD *Groups in Action: Evolution and Challenges* (Corey, Corey, & Haynes, 2014), I demonstrate how I work with Casey by encouraging her to talk in a symbolic way to her mother in Vietnamese in a role-playing scenario in a group. This was powerful not only for Casey but for everyone in the group. In another *Groups in Action* video, I facilitate working with Maria by speaking in Spanish when she informs the group that it is difficult for her to think and speak in English when she is struggling with a personal concern. These women are not unique in finding it a freeing experience to do therapeutic work by speaking in their primary language. It was not essential that others understood the content of what was said. It was more important that each woman, by speaking in her primarily language, derived meaning and experienced healing from this therapeutic work.

Stereotypes as Barriers to Understanding Others

A **stereotype** is a judgmental generalization applied to an individual without regard to his or her own uniqueness; it is also a set of beliefs about characteristics of members of a social group (Miller & Garran, 2008). Gender-role stereotypes can result in isolating an individual, and they often put a distance between women and men (see Chapter 8). Stereotypes also create boundaries that prevent us from seeing our interconnectedness as members of the human race. This social isolation limits our capacity to experience the richness that can be part of diverse human relationships. Stereotypes can be either positive or negative. Here are a few examples of stereotypes: "Men are unemotional and uncaring." "Lesbians hate men." "Asians are talented in mathematics and are aggressive drivers." "Italians are emotional." "Most Irish are alcoholics." "Most old people are sad and lonely." "Women are emotional."

Stereotypes stem from the need to generalize and put social groups in categories as we navigate the world (Miller & Garran, 2008). Stereotypes have been used to discredit victims of racism, to justify mistreatment of groups, and to mask privilege. If we view ourselves as being fair, open-minded, enlightened, and without prejudices, a recurring negative stereotype about people can be disturbing and we may reject it because it does not fit our self-perception. Stereotypes are very common in our society, partly because they make complex problems seem simple. But putting people in boxes is hardly treating them as individuals, and most of us would resist being categorized this way.

Prevailing assumptions are generally held onto tenaciously. Once people have made an assumption, they are often interested in whatever proves it. People are likely to call someone an "exception" rather than change a stereotype. For example, if you believe all men are "macho," you are likely to look for and find macho men. However, if you take on the challenge of examining this generalization, you will likely find many exceptions to a generalized view. If you become aware of making any unexamined assumptions or generalizations, look for evidence that will disconfirm the expectations you have about a particular group of people. It takes a concerted effort to move beyond the stereotypes and prejudices that set people apart and strive to understand each individual in his or her subjective world. Unless they are critically examined, stereotypes can keep you separate and prevent you from getting to know people who could enhance your life.

Many of the people in our lives have diverse cultural backgrounds, belief systems, life experiences, and ethnicities. We find that diversity has enhanced our lives and that we can greatly benefit from interacting with a wide range of people different from ourselves. Furthermore, our daughters share this value and have learned that they are enriched by interacting and communicating with people who are very different from themselves. The United States is unique in its embrace of diverse cultural groups, which means you can reach out to diverse groups of individuals and enrich your own cultural experience without ever leaving home.

Think about stereotypes you may hold and reflect on ways that they serve as barriers in getting to know another person. Ask yourself how stereotypes get in your way of understanding people on an individual basis. How are you affected by having certain characteristics assigned to you, based on your gender, sexual orientation, ethnicity, culture, religion, age, or ability? How does the act of placing a label on you or on others affect your relationships?

Once you become aware of stereotypes, explore where you acquired those beliefs. Did you get messages from your parents? From people in your community? From your friends? From your teachers? From your religious background? The chances are that you have acquired stereotypes on a less than conscious level. Once you become aware of their existence, you can modify them and begin to act differently based on your new awareness and your revised perceptions.

Becoming Aware of Our Prejudices and Responding to Racism

Prejudice, discrimination, hatred, and intolerance, especially toward those who are different from us, are all paths toward an ever-narrowing existence. **Prejudice,** a preconceived notion or opinion about someone, can be overt or covert. Prejudice refers to negative attitudes; **discrimination** refers to biased behavior (Matlin, 2012). People can be obvious and blatant about their particular prejudices, or they can hide them. Prejudice can be a very subtle thing, and it may occur outside of conscious awareness. Ridley (2005) contends that **unintentional racism,** such as being convinced that we are free of any traces of prejudice, can be as harmful as intentional racism.

Becoming aware of our own subtle prejudice and unintentional racism is the first step toward change. Laughing at or being impatient with someone who has an accent, telling or laughing at racial jokes, speaking in generalities about a whole group of people as though they are all the same, and assuming that our culture is superior to any other are all signs of prejudice founded on racist attitudes. If you want to become more accepting of others, reflect on some of the ways you have acquired your beliefs about particular groups of people and begin to question the source of those beliefs. Although we may not be responsible for systemic racism, we are responsible for how we respond to racism in our own lives. Miller and Garran (2008) suggest striking a balance between pushing ourselves to do more and being gentle with ourselves and others. Self-awareness and self-monitoring are important, but excessive self-criticism can be detrimental. It is important to "press ourselves past our comfort zone to our learning edge and be open to absorbing new content, skills, and insights about ourselves and society" (p. 3). Being interested in other cultures opens up the world to us and makes us that much more interesting.

For the victims, prejudice often results in acts of discrimination and oppression that keep them from participating fully in the mainstream of society. People often feel intimidated by differences, rather than being drawn to the positive aspects of understanding those who are different. At the root of prejudice is fear of those who are different, low self-esteem, ignorance, and feelings of inferiority. Prejudice is a defense mechanism that protects individuals from facing undesirable aspects of themselves by projecting them onto others. Treating others in a demeaning way may give these people an illusion of superiority.

Each of us can take steps to address racism and overcome its insidious effects. Miller and Garran (2008) state the benefits of doing so: "Ultimately, dismantling racism will benefit us all individually and will support a better society and nation collectively" (p. 2). With honest self-examination, we can increase our awareness of the problems that prejudice, racism, and discrimination are causing to individuals and to society at large. The more we increase our awareness of these conditions, the more options we have for taking action. By changing your own attitudes, you can make a positive difference, and societal change can begin with you.

White Privilege

Racism in our society puts people of color at a disadvantage, but it is essential to recognize that **white privilege** puts Whites at an advantage. Although not all white people consciously discriminate against people of color, it is clear that Whites in general, especially white males, enjoy certain privileges. Those who are privileged tend to have a difficult time recognizing their privileged status, and this status may be in direct conflict with a person's belief that he or she is a good person who does not condone racism (Miller & Garran, 2008). White people may feel guilty or react with defensiveness when their unearned privileges are pointed out. If they feel blamed, they are not likely to reflect on the advantages of their privileged status. If you are White, we hope you will not quickly close your mind to what is implied by white privilege, but consider carefully the degree of truth in this concept.

According to Peggy McIntosh (1998), a professor at Wellesley College, North American culture is based on the hidden assumption that being White is normative. This white-as-normative concept implies that White people have certain privileges that they generally take for granted, and often are not aware of their privileged status. McIntosh describes white privilege as an "invisible knapsack" of unearned assets that White people enjoy that are not extended to people of color. White privilege is a phenomenon that is both denied and protected. Although she was taught about racism as something that puts others at a disadvantage, she was not taught the corollary: that white privilege gives White people distinct advantages. She lists 46 conditions in which being White is an unearned advantage, and McIntosh has experienced some of the following examples of unearned privileges that are not extended to people of color:

1. I can be in the company of people of my race most of the time.

2. I can go shopping alone and be assured that I will not be followed or harassed by store detectives.

3. If a traffic cop pulls me over or if the IRS audits my tax return, I can be sure I haven't been singled out because of my race.

4. I can criticize our government and talk about how much I fear its policies without being viewed as a cultural outsider.

5. I can do well in a challenging situation without being called a credit to my race.

6. I can be sure that my children will be given curricular materials that testify to the existence of their race.

7. I can be late to a meeting without having the lateness reflect on my race.

8. I can easily find academic courses and institutions that give attention only to people of my race.

9. I can be sure that if I need legal or medical help, my race will not work against me.

10. I can be concerned about racism without being seen as self-interested or self-seeking.

In unpacking the invisible knapsack of white privilege, McIntosh (1988, 1998) lists conditions of daily experience that she had once taken for granted as neutral, normal, and universally applicable to everybody. Once we realize that we benefit from this privileged and unearned race advantage, what might we be willing to do to lessen its effects? McIntosh indicates that one of our choices is to use our unearned advantage to reduce these invisible privilege systems and to use our conferred power to try to reconstruct power systems on a broader base. Do not judge or harshly criticize yourself if you realize that you do indeed have certain privileges based on skin color or gender. Give yourself credit for being open enough to recognize the position your socialization has created in your case, for this is the beginning of the change process.

In our educational DVD *Groups in Action: Evolution and Challenges* (Corey, Corey, & Haynes, 2014), one part of the program focuses on the challenges group counselors face in addressing diversity issues. Several of the members of color talk about negative experiences they have had with discrimination. They mention that when they were children in a store with a parent, they would be closely watched because of suspicion that they might steal goods. Eventually, another group member, George, says that he resents being stereotyped and put into a box because he is White. George talks about similar struggles he has had and becomes somewhat defensive, arguing against the notion that he has a privileged status in this society because he is a White male. He claims that nothing was given to him, that he has had many experiences living in several different countries, and that he has had plenty of struggles in growing up. In some ways, George was feeling accused and blamed, which made it difficult for him to reflect on and understand the experiences of some of the other members of this group. When he finally realized that he could walk into a store and not be a suspect because he was White or be mistaken for a bus boy because of his race, he began to recognize what other members were trying to communicate about white privilege. Through the process of exploring a range of feelings and attitudes being expressed by many of the group members, the group facilitators were able to intervene in a way that allowed George to lower his defenses and listen to the possibility that he did enjoy certain privileges that others do not always have. Many of these group members had diverse experiences and problems in society as a result of their cultural background, and they helped George recognize that privilege does exist and that discrimination is a reality.

In *Explorations in Diversity: Examining Privilege and Oppression in a Multicultural Society*, Sharon Anderson and Valerie Middleton (2011) challenge readers to dismantle privilege by acknowledging that it does exist, that oppression is a result of privilege, and that privilege is reinforced at institutional and societal levels. These authors contend that knowledge alone will not lead to change; rather, people need to act on what they know.

Breaking Down the Barriers That Separate Us

There are always barriers to understanding, regardless of how similar or different we are. Language difficulties and value differences can make intercultural communication challenging. Awareness of these obstacles is the first step toward increasing communication and breaking down the walls that separate people. Here are some ideas about how you can break down the barriers that keep you separate from other people:

▶ Acknowledge and understand your own biases and prejudices, no matter your race or culture.

▶ Critically examine your prejudices by looking for data that do not support your preconceived biases.

▶ Challenge your fears and anxieties about talking about racial or cultural differences.

▶ Participate in volunteer work in an agency that provides services to people who are culturally different from you.

▶ Be open to making friends with people who are culturally different from you.

▶ Look for similarities and universal themes that unite you with others who differ from you in certain ways.

▶ Avoid judging differences; view diversity as a strength.

▶ Be respectful of those who differ from you.

▶ Attempt to learn about cultures that differ from your own.

▶ Talk about yourself and your experience with people who differ from you. Try to keep it personal and not global.

▶ Be willing to test, adapt, and change your perceptions.

In relating to people who differ from us culturally, we will undoubtedly make mistakes. We can learn from our cultural blunders if we recognize them and admit them. In the process of working through a problem, we can recover from such blunders. It is crucial that we avoid becoming defensive, remain open and flexible, and focus on ways to resolve a conflict or a misunderstanding.

Unity in Diversity

Unity and diversity are related concepts, not polar opposites. It is not that diversity is good and right and homogeneity is bad and wrong. Both sameness and difference contribute to our connection to the common human experience. We share some common ground that enables us to understand one another despite our differences. Concerns about love, relationships, death and loss, and meaning in life are universal human themes that transcend culture.

Our experience of lecturing and conducting workshops in Korea revealed to us that regardless of our differences, we do share common ground that makes it possible to understand people from diverse cultures. We gave lectures on group counseling to graduate students in counseling, mental health practitioners, and university professors who taught counseling and social work; we also conducted workshops in group counseling and had many opportunities to interact with the participants and exchange ideas. Although our ideas and approach to group counseling were developed in the United States, this basic philosophy was well received by the students and professionals who made up the audience.

We felt that it was an honor and a privilege to be able to teach about group counseling in Korea. Rather than simply convey factual material, our main hope was to share an attitude toward counseling that might be useful to both students and professionals alike. During our interactions with people, it became apparent that there are many common life themes we share, even though we have our differences. This trip confirmed our belief that although it is essential to be aware of and respect cultural differences, it can be a mistake to make assumptions about any particular cultural group without making room for individual variances.

MAKING A DIFFERENCE

Each one of us can reach out to others and make a significant difference by our actions. Through our attitudes, choices, and actions, all of us have the capacity in our own way to make a difference in the world. Most of us want to know that we have influenced the lives of others and that somehow we have contributed to helping others live more fully. Although self-acceptance is a prerequisite for meaningful interpersonal relationships, there is a quest to go beyond self-centered interests. Ultimately, we want to establish connections with others in society, and we want to make a contribution. This is a pathway to finding meaning and purpose in life. This notion is captured by Alfred Adler's concept of social interest (see Chapter 1).

In the remainder of this chapter, we explore ways to make a difference. We can accomplish this by helping out a family member, friend, or neighbor in need just as we can make a difference by getting involved in human rights organizations; supporting social justice at the local, state, or national level; or taking steps to protect our planet. There are truly limitless possibilities about how we can make a positive difference in this world!

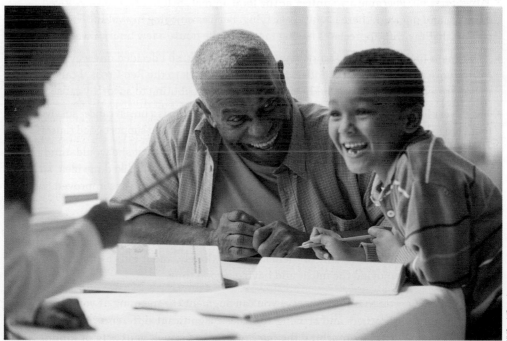

KidStock/Getty Images

≫ Each one of us can reach out to others and make a significant difference by our actions.

Making the World a Better Place

Bettering humanity may seem like an overwhelming task, but it is less staggering if we start with ourselves. It is easier to blame others for the ills of the world than to accept that we might be contributing to this malady. We might ask ourselves, "What am I doing, even in the smallest way, that contributes to the problems in our society? And what can I do to become part of the solution to these problems?"

One living example of the power to bring about change and make the world a better place can be found in Glide Memorial Church in San Francisco. The pastor of this church, the Reverend Cecil Williams, along with the executive director of the church, Janet Mirikitani, are committed to welcoming diverse people into their spiritual community, a community that truly embraces love and acceptance. Reverend Williams (1992) works to empower individuals who are recovering and provides assistance to troubled communities. The pastor does not see his congregation as a melting pot where all people are blended together. Instead, Glide Memorial Church is more akin to a salad bowl filled with different leaves. Reverend Williams does far more than preach about love to a packed congregation on Sunday; he is actively engaged in spreading the meaning of love. He demonstrates ways to find meaning and purpose in life through acts of love. Through the efforts of Glide, hundreds of homeless are fed each day, substance abusers are given hope of a new kind of life, and society's outcasts are welcomed into a loving community. By giving people unconditional love and acceptance, Reverend Williams and his people bring out the best in those they encounter.

People are making a difference in many ways through their choices and by reaching out to others. Here are a few examples of people who are making a difference:

▶ "My neighbor's wife passed away a year ago. I now make it a point to invite my neighbor over for dinner on Sundays. He didn't accept my invitation at first, but now he comes over regularly. It makes me feel good to know that he is not all alone."

▶ "After I retired, I became a volunteer at the local animal shelter. I have always loved animals, and my work there is quite satisfying. Besides enjoying my volunteer work, I am certain that my wife appreciates having me out of the house a few hours a week!"

▶ "My time is limited because I work many hours per week, so I decided one way I can make a difference is to donate a few dollars from each paycheck to the Red Cross. I can't afford to donate a lot, but I feel better knowing that I am contributing to a worthy cause."

▶ "Every year I participate in a fundraiser to support a friend who is a breast cancer survivor. Now that I am in better shape I plan to participate in other marathons to support good causes."

▶ "I am pretty outgoing and like to plan events, so I asked my boss if she would mind if we started doing something festive to celebrate special occasions. She liked my idea, so I am now in charge of planning our office parties. I think the morale has improved, which makes me feel like I've done a good deed."

▶ "I grew up in a musical family and cherished the time we spent together playing the guitar and singing songs. Now that I am grown, I go to nursing homes and play music for the older adults on weekends. Many of them seem very lonely, and it puts a smile on my face when I see them enjoying the music and having a good time."

We encourage you to reflect on ways you can augment the meaning of your life by making connections with others and striving to make a significant difference. You can change the world in small ways by touching the lives of others through your acts of kindness and generosity. The purpose of your life can take on expanded dimensions if you are interested in making the world a better place for all of us.

Protecting Our Planet

For most of this book we have encouraged you to make personal choices regarding the quality of your life and your interpersonal relationships. In this section we challenge you to extend your outlook to protecting and preserving your environment as well. The first step is for us to recognize that we are indeed in the midst of a growing global crisis, and the next step is to recognize that each of us can and must assume personal responsibility to bring about changes. It is easy to think that we are helpless in the face of a monumental crisis such as global warming, but this is a myth that only contributes to the inevitable destruction of our planet. Both collectively and as individuals, we can make a difference.

In his book *An Inconvenient Truth*, Al Gore (2006) forcefully makes the point that the world is witnessing undeniable evidence that nature's cycles are profoundly changing. Gore emphasizes that our climate crisis is extremely dangerous and that we are facing a true planetary emergency: "The voluminous evidence now strongly suggests that unless we act boldly and quickly to deal with the underlying causes of global warming, our world will undergo a string of terrible catastrophes, including more and stronger storms like Hurricane Katrina, in both the Atlantic and the Pacific" (p. 10). Gore believes that the climate crisis provides us with a generational mission, a moral purpose, and a shared and unifying cause. We are facing a moral, ethical, and spiritual crisis. We have the opportunity to find new hope and rise to the challenge.

Reflect on the kind of world you want your children, grandchildren, and great-grandchildren to inherit. Are you willing to make a few changes in your personal life at little cost to your lifestyle to secure the future of generations to come? Tim Flannery (2005), author of *The Weather Makers: How Man Is Changing the Climate and What It Means for Life on Earth,* provides many practical suggestions that you can incorporate in your daily life that will

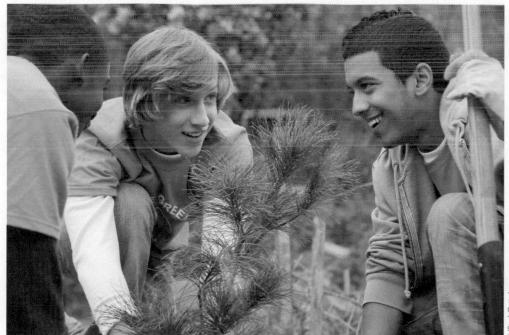

KidStock/Getty Images

》 Just one tree can absorb one ton of carbon dioxide over its lifetime.

make a difference in protecting the planet. Taking some simple steps can make a significant difference in the overall effort. Replacing the filters on your furnace and air conditioning units, turning off the television and lights when they are not in use, and washing dishes or clothes only when the machine is full, are but a few suggestions. No drastic lifestyle changes are necessary to make a collective difference in conserving our resources. Sometimes even the smallest changes have a surprisingly consequential effect on saving the planet. Each one of us can make choices to adopt a more Earth-friendly lifestyle. Reflect on some of the things you are already doing toward this goal.

TAKE TIME TO REFLECT

1. What value do you place on diversity as part of your philosophy of life?

_____

_____

2. How many, if any, of the important people in your life are culturally different from you?_____

_____

_____

3. What steps are you willing to take to move in the direction of challenging your prejudices or restricted ways of thinking?_____

_____

_____

4. What one action can you take to make a significant, even though small, difference in society? To what extent do you believe you are able to influence others?

_____

_____

5. What are your values concerning protecting and preserving the planet?

_____

_____

6. How committed are you to taking even small steps toward protecting the planet? What is one thing you are willing to do differently?_____

_____

_____

SUMMARY

Seeking meaning and purpose in life is an important part of being human. Meaning is not automatically bestowed on us; it is the result of active thinking and choosing. We have encouraged you to recognize your own values and to ask both how you acquired them and whether you can affirm them for yourself out of your own experience and reflection. This task of examining your values and purposes continues throughout your lifetime.

If you are secure about your value system, you will also be flexible and open to new life experiences. At various times in your life you may look at the world somewhat differently, which may lead you to modify some of your values after giving the matter considerable thought. Being secure about your values also implies that you do not need to impose them on other people. We hope you will be able to respect the values of others that may differ from your own. If you are clear about the meaning in your own life, and if you have developed a philosophy of life that provides you with purpose and direction, you will be more able to interact with others who might embrace different value systems.

In this chapter we have focused on the central role of values as a basis for meaning in life. In addition to finding meaning through projects that afford opportunities for personal growth, we have seen that meaning and purpose extend to the broader framework of forming linkages with others in the human community. Accepting others by respecting their right to hold values that may differ from yours is a fundamental dimension of a philosophy of life that embraces diversity. Prejudice, based on fear and ignorance, is often a barrier that separates us from others instead of uniting us. We hope you will welcome diversity as a bridge to link yourself with others who differ from you. It may be overwhelming to think of solving societal problems of prejudice and discrimination, but you can begin in smaller but still significant ways by changing yourself. Once you recognize the barriers within yourself that prevent you from understanding and accepting others, you can take steps to challenge these barriers.

Environmental problems such as global warming seem overwhelming, and you can easily conclude there is almost nothing you can do to make a difference. But your values and the choices you make can reduce the destructive forces that are endangering the planet; you can be instrumental in contributing to a better future for all.

Where Can I Go From Here?

1. Ask a few close friends what gives their lives meaning. How do they think their lives would be different without this source of meaning?

2. Make a list of what you consider to be the major accomplishments in your life. What did you actually do to bring about these accomplishments? What kinds of future accomplishments would enhance the meaning of your life?

3. What do you think makes good people engage in evil acts? Are people born predisposed to committing evil actions, or do they choose to do so? Now think about what makes ordinary people do extraordinary deeds. In your opinion, what makes a person a hero? Do you believe some people are inherently predisposed to behave heroically and that others are not? Are your ideas about why people are evil or good congruent?

4. Review the section on actions you can take to protect the environment and circle some of the suggestions you are willing to implement in your daily life. Consider talking to a close friend or family member about your concerns about the environment and how you can make a difference in protecting it.

5. Create a "bucket list" of all the things that you would like to accomplish before you die. What would be first on your list? What things can you start working on right now? What things would bring meaning to your life that you haven't made the time to do? Create a timeline for accomplishing these tasks.

6. Suggested Readings. The full bibliographic entry for each of these sources can be found in the References and Suggested Readings at the back of the book. For a compelling account of finding meaning even in the most dire of circumstances, see Frankl (1963). For accounts of the spiritual journeys of healers, see Kottler and Carlson (2007). For a collection of inspiring essays by various spiritual writers, see Carlson and Shield (1995, 1996). For a useful book on racism, see Miller and Garran (2008). For a comprehensive discussion of global warming and actions we can take to protect the planet, see Flannery (2005).

WEBSITE RESOURCES

Included here are some valuable websites. For access to these websites, video activities, and other supporting materials, visit Cengage Learning's Counseling CourseMate website for *I Never Knew I Had a Choice,* 10th Edition, at www.cengagebrain.com.

SPRITUALITY AND PRACTICE

www.sprituralityandpractice.com

Recommended Search Words: "spirituality and practice"

This site provides resources for spiritual journeys. The site's founders state: "The site's name reflects a basic understanding: *spirituality* and *practice* are the two places where all the world's religions and spiritual paths come together. With respect for the differences among them, we celebrate what they have in common."

GLOBAL CLIMATE-CHANGE RESOURCES

www.aaas.org/news/press_room/climate_ change

Recommended Search Words: "AAAS climate"

The American Association for the Advancement of Science is an excellent resource to consult for information about global climate change. This site offers leads on what you can do to stop global warming; it has reports on the impact of global climate change, publications, and trends.

STOP GLOBAL WARMING VIRTUAL MARCH

www. stopglobalwarming.org

Recommended Search Words: "stop global warming"

This is a nonpartisan effort to unite people who are concerned about global warming. You can add your voice to the hundreds of thousands of other people who are calling for action on this issue.

MARTIN LUTHER KING JR. CENTER FOR NONVIOLENT SOCIAL CHANGE

www.thekingcenter.org/

Recommended Search Words: "center for nonviolent social change"

This website offers information about the lives of Martin Luther King Jr. and Coretta Scott King. It includes a digital archive that you can browse. You can also learn about nonviolence education and training on this site. It offers a bibliography, news, and a blog.

LUCIFER EFFECT

http://lucifereffect.com/

Recommended Search Words: "Lucifer effect"

This is the official site of Philip Zimbardo's book *The Lucifer Effect: Understanding How Good People Turn Evil* (2007). It contains information about the infamous Stanford Prison Experiment, heroism, resisting influence, dehumanization, and more.

HEROIC IMAGINATION PROJECT

http://heroicimagination.org

Recommended Search Words: "heroic imagination project"

Based on Philip Zimbardo's work, this nonprofit organization "teaches people how to overcome the natural human tendency to watch and wait in moments of crisis and to create meaningful and lasting change in their lives." It offers news and information about events as well as links to resources and research.

THE INTERNATIONAL MOVEMENT AGAINST ALL FORMS OF DISCRIMINATION AND RACISM

http://www.imadr.org

Recommended Search Words: "international movement against discrimination"

This international nonprofit, nongovernmental human rights organization is dedicated to empowerment, solidarity, and advocacy. This site provides many links to resources and organizations that are working to stop discrimination and racism all over the world.

NATIONAL ASSOCIATION FOR THE ADVANCEMENT OF COLORED PEOPLE

www.naacp.org

Recommended Search Words: "naacp"

"Founded in 1909, the NAACP is the nation's oldest and largest civil rights organization." The site provides access to information about advocacy, information about legal milestones, and much more.

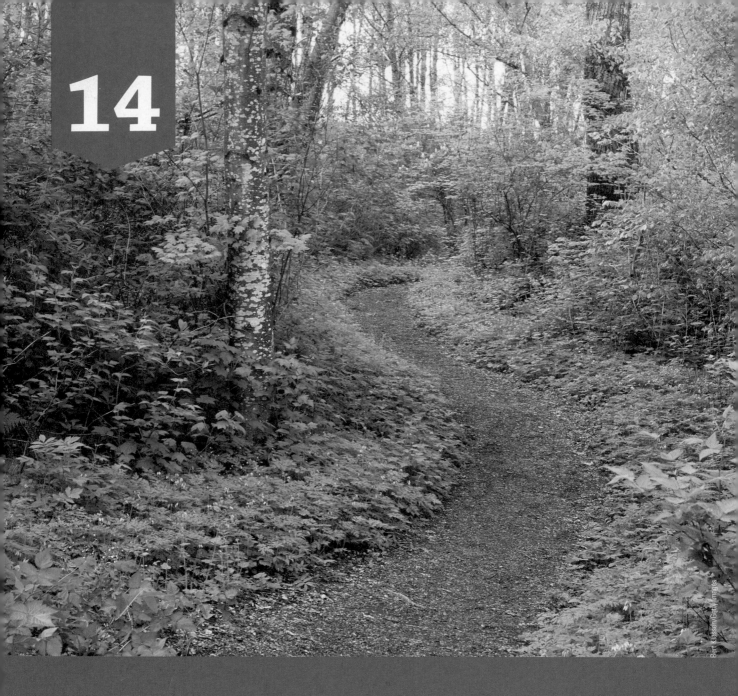

14

PATHWAYS TO PERSONAL GROWTH

› Where Am I Now?

› Self-Assessment as a Key to Personal Growth

› Overcoming Barriers, Opening Doors

› Pathways for Continued Self-Exploration

› Counseling as a Path to Self-Understanding

› Dreams as a Path to Self-Understanding

› Concluding Comments

› Where Can I Go From Here?

› Website Resources

Bert Klassen/Getty Images

WHERE AM I NOW?

Use this scale to respond to these statements:

4 = I *strongly agree* with this statement.
3 = I *agree* with this statement.
2 = I *disagree* with this statement.
1 = I *strongly disagree* with this statement.

1. I am motivated to keep up with regular journal writing.

2. I would like to begin meditation practices.

3. I intend to incorporate relaxation methods into my daily life.

4. At this point, I can see that I have more choices available to me than I realized.

5. Personal growth is a journey rather than a fixed destination.

6. I really intend to do what it takes to continue the self-exploration I have begun through this course and book.

7. If I had a personal problem I could not resolve by myself, I would seek professional counseling.

8. I dream a lot and am able to remember many of my dreams.

9. I see dreaming as a way to understand myself and to remain psychologically healthy.

10. I intend to develop an action plan to begin making the changes I most want for my life.

I n this relatively brief chapter, we invite you to review what you have learned and determine where you will go from here. If you have invested yourself in the process of reflecting on your life, now is a good time to make a commitment to yourself, and maybe to someone else, to actively implement your new learnings.

You can deliberately choose experiences that will help you become the person you want to be. As you consider what experiences for continued personal growth you are likely to choose at this time, be aware that as you change you may find that what brings meaning to your life will also change. Sometimes the projects you were deeply absorbed in at an earlier time in your life hold little meaning for you today. Where and how you discover meaning today may not be the pattern for some future period.

Often, we make resolutions about what we would like to be doing in our lives or about experiences we want to share with others, yet we fail to carry them out. Are there activities you value, yet rarely take the time to do? How would you like to be spending your time? What changes can you realistically see yourself making? What kind of plan can you devise that will enable you to make these changes? How will you deal with difficulties you may encounter in making the changes you desire? We encourage you to reflect on the previous chapters and identify some of the areas that stand out most for you.

SELF-ASSESSMENT AS A KEY TO PERSONAL GROWTH

Throughout this book you have been challenged to assess the ways you think, feel, and act on a variety of topics. Now is a good time to consolidate what you have learned and to review the decisions you have made about how you are living. Use your responses to the Where Am I Now? sections at the beginning of each chapter and your written responses to the Take Time to Reflect exercises to make a life assessment. Did you identify any persistent themes in your review of these exercises? In Chapter 1 you were introduced to choice theory, which emphasizes the role of self-assessment as a first step toward change. What are some areas of your life that are working well for you? Are there any aspects of your life that are not presently working for you? Did your review reveal any insights that may lead to changes in the future?

We are challenged to let go of old and familiar ways of being when we begin to live in new ways. For example, when you let go of the security of living with your parents in exchange for testing your independence you may have lost something that was valuable to you because it was incompatible with your further development and growth. You might stay in a relationship—even though you know it is unhealthy and maybe even harmful to you— because you are familiar with what you have and fear the unknown. Once you identify your strengths and resources and the specific aspects of your life you want to change, you will be better prepared to continue making changes that lead to a more satisfying life. Think about where you are now as you contemplate the following questions.

Are Your Roles Enhancing Your Life?

All of us play many different roles in daily living, but these roles are subject to change, especially as we make new choices. These roles may be life-affirming or life-limiting. We may get lost in our roles and in the patterns of thought, feeling, and behavior that go with them. As a result, we may neglect important aspects of ourselves, limiting our options of feeling and experiencing. We may feel lost when we are unable to play a certain role, such as when we lose a job or retire from a meaningful career. Parents may find life difficult when their children have moved away from home.

Can you identify the routines and roles of your daily life? Is today a copy of yesterday? Do you depend on being able to fill certain roles to feel alive and valuable? How would it affect you if these roles were taken from you? When roles lose meaning for you, are you open to pursuing a different path?

Are You Alive to Your Senses and Your Body?

Your body speaks to your vitality and reveals your tiredness with life. To a significant degree, your body expresses how alive you feel. Ask yourself these questions: "Do I like how my body feels? Am I taking good care of myself physically? What am I expressing by my posture? What does my facial expression communicate? How does my body react to stress?"

Are you alive to your senses? Perhaps you rarely stop to notice the details of your surroundings. If you take time to absorb the world through your senses, you may feel renewed and more interested in life. Ask yourself, "What sensations have I felt today? What have I experienced and observed? What sensory surprises have enlivened me? Am I willing to slow down and embrace life by being in tune with my senses?"

Can You Be Spontaneous and Playful?

Can you be playful, fun, curious, explorative, and spontaneous? Even as adults we can continue to be playful. Humor shakes us out of our patterned ways and promotes new perspectives. If you are typically realistic and objective to the point that it is difficult for you to be playful or light, examine the inner messages that are blocking your ability to let go. Are you inhibited by a fear of being silly or wrong? If you want to, you can begin to challenge the messages that say "Don't!" "You should!" "You shouldn't!" Experiment with new behaviors that increase your ability to be more spontaneous.

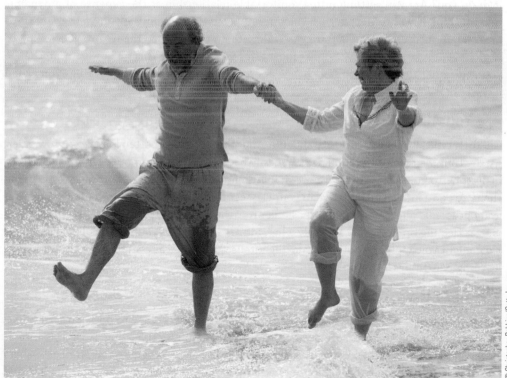

Are you alive to your senses and your body?

Do You Listen to Your Feelings?

We can numb ourselves to our feelings, both joyful and painful. We can decide that feeling involves too much risk of pain. In choosing to cut off one feeling, we may cut off other more pleasurable feelings. Closing ourselves to our sadness usually means closing ourselves to our joys as well. Sometimes we insulate ourselves emotionally and find it difficult to recognize our flat emotional state. To begin assessing how alive you are emotionally, ask yourself these questions:

▸ Do I let myself feel my sadness and grief over a loss?

▸ Do I try hard to cheer people up when they are sad instead of allowing them to experience their feelings?

▸ Do I let myself cry if I feel like crying?

▸ Am I ever really joyous?

▸ How many people have I let myself get close to in my life?

▸ Do I suppress certain emotions such as insecurity, fear, tenderness, or anger?

Are Your Relationships Alive?

Our relationships with the significant people in our lives can lose a sense of vitality. It is easy to become set in routine ways of being with another person and to lose any sense of surprise and spontaneity. Long-term relationships are vulnerable to this kind of predictability. Breaking out of routine patterns in relationships takes conscious effort and can be anxiety provoking. Look at the significant relationships in your life and think about how alive both you and the other person are in the relationship. Does the relationship energize you, or does it drain? Are you settling into a comfortable relationship at the expense of a dynamic relationship? If you recognize that you are not getting what you want in your friendships or intimate relationships, what are you willing to do to revitalize them? Are you willing to explore your relationships with those most affected by them? Focus on how you can change yourself rather than how you can change another. Consider what specific things you would like to ask from the other person.

Are You Alive Intellectually?

Children typically display curiosity about life, but this curiosity is often lost as we grow older. By the time we reach adulthood, we can easily become caught up in our activities, devoting little time to considering why we are doing them and whether we even want to be doing them. Are you intellectually active in your classes? In Chapter 1 we focused on ways to integrate academic and emotional dimensions of learning. One way of keeping mentally alert is by reflecting on how you can apply what you are learning to your personal development. How might you apply the notion of staying intellectually alive as a student? Are you open to learning new things? Are you changing as a learner?

Are You Alive Spiritually?

There is growing attention in the field of counseling and psychology to how spiritual values can enhance living and promote both psychological and physical healing. An abundance of books have been written on spirituality and our well-being. Religious and spiritual beliefs and practices affect many dimensions of human experience. To what degree do your spiritual beliefs enhance your life? How do you define spirituality for yourself? What moral, ethical, or spiritual values guide your life? Take time to reflect on this aspect of your life.

Are You Satisfied With the Way You Handle Life's Challenges?

We are constantly faced with stressors in today's world. Some may be minor irritations, whereas others may seem insurmountable. Part of becoming an autonomous person involves developing effective ways of coping with life's challenges that may arise at school, in the workplace, at home, or in your social life. They may be chronic or situational. How well do you deal with the tasks you encounter in the various domains of your life? How does your style of coping influence the way you interact with others? Does your style of coping typically affect the outcome of stressful situations? An important part of personal growth is examining how you sometimes get in your own way. Are you inclined to become defensive under particular circumstances? Can you develop more constructive ways of handling difficult situations?

Do You Like the Person You Are Today?

The existential view is that ultimately you are alone in this world. Only you are with yourself 24 hours a day, 7 days a week. Each of us is a work in progress. After reflecting on the ideas presented in this book and applying them to your own life, you should have greater clarity about who you are and areas in which you can improve. Do you enjoy the companionship of others and have an active social life? Are you happy with the person you have become? Have you identified issues you need or want to address in greater depth? Ask yourself, "Am I worthy of my own company?" The way you respond may indicate aspects of yourself that can be further developed.

Take a moment right now to give yourself credit for the work you have already done. Walking your own path takes courage and determination. Reward your successes as you begin to think about future changes. Remember, personal growth is a process, not a destination.

OVERCOMING BARRIERS, OPENING DOORS

Sometimes we limit our potential for personal growth by letting obstacles stop us from realizing our dreams and pursuing our goals. External and internal barriers do not have to block choices that can lead to success. Joseph's story illustrates how our beliefs can guide us to the open doors rather than to barriers to life's richest rewards.

JOSEPH'S STORY

I have always been fond of the phrase "the sky is the limit" because life provides people with different opportunities for self-improvement. It is my belief that each individual has a purpose and a function to leave this world in a somewhat better state than he or she found it, even if that means making a difference in the life of only one person.

Eleven years ago, I lost my sight. Needless to say, this event radically changed my life and inevitably changed my future and my plans. However, after much reflection and personal suffering, I came to the realization that I had to continue living. Although fulfilling my dreams would certainly be difficult, I assured myself that it would not be impossible. Now more than ever I believe I am capable of achieving anything I put my mind to. I am confident, constantly seeking ways to improve myself and my situation. I refuse to allow my blindness to excuse me from my responsibilities. I am convinced that a disability is not an exemption from a person's tasks in life. It is still my duty and my desire to leave this world having added something positive to it.

Two years ago I decided to travel to Europe, and as my best friend drove me to the airport he asked me, "Do you really want to spend money to travel? Although you are unable to see, you are interested in visiting Europe? You won't be able to appreciate the beautiful architecture or landscapes!" I answered immediately, "This is exciting for me; I see it as an adventure. I love trying new foods, touching new grounds, and using my other senses to experience something different. I want to learn about new places and engage in conversations with people. I believe I can do the same things a sighted person can do, just in different ways." Disabled or not, everyone is different and therefore unique. It depends on the lens through which you analyze your life.

I recognized that if I took appropriate steps in overcoming obstacles, the bumps on the road would eventually smooth out. I have chosen not to run in the opposite direction, but to move forward one step at a time and at a pace that I can handle. Being a person with a disability has helped me to become strong, to achieve my goals, and to be comfortable fitting into this world. I am confident that my life experiences will enabled me to do great things. I am committed to taking full advantage of the opportunities presented to me and to working as hard as I possibly can to succeed. If the sky is my limit, then I am more than ready to fly.

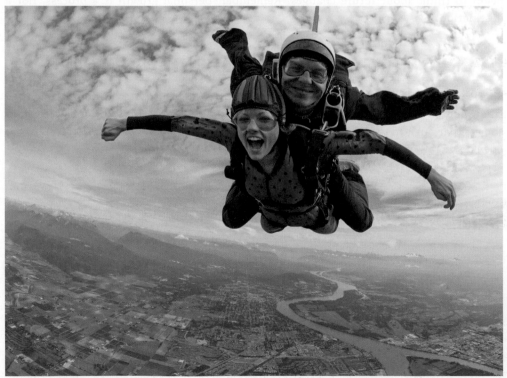

≫ You can choose experiences that will help you become the person you want to be.

PATHWAYS FOR CONTINUED SELF-EXPLORATION

Growth has no small steps. Every step is significant because it is a step in a new direction. You can choose to do many things on your own (or with friends or family) to continue your personal development. A few of the resources available to you for continued personal growth are outlined in the pages that follow. Different resources may fit your needs at different stages of your personal journey. We encourage you to investigate any avenues that you feel are appropriate for you at this time.

Develop a Reading Program

One excellent way to explore life is through reading, including selected self-help books. In each chapter we provided suggestions for further reading on many of the topics covered. In addition, the *References and Suggested Readings* section at the end of this book includes a variety of books that can give you a start on developing a personal reading program. Many students and clients tell us how meaningful selected books have been for them in putting into perspective some of the themes they have struggled with, and you may find this resource valuable. What books most interest you?

Continue Your Writing Program

Along with setting up a reading and reflection program for yourself, another way to build on the gains you have made up to this point is to continue the practice of journal writing. If you have begun a process of personal writing in this book or in a separate notebook, we hope you will continue this practice. Even devoting a short period a few times each week to reflecting on how your life is going and then recording some of your thoughts and feelings is useful in providing you with an awareness of patterns in your behavior. You can learn to observe what you are feeling, thinking, and doing; then you have a basis for determining the degree to which you are successfully changing old patterns that are not working for you. Have you gotten any insights as a result of journal writing?

Contemplate Self-Directed Behavior Change

Now that you have finished this book, you have probably identified a few specific areas where you could do further work. If you decide that you are frequently tense and that you do not generally react well to stress, for example, you might construct a self-change program that includes practicing relaxation methods and breathing exercises. Identify some target areas for personal change and set realistic goals. Then develop some specific techniques for carrying out your goals, and practice the behaviors that will help you make those changes. What changes do you most want to make? What might help you to begin and to maintain your program?

COUNSELING AS A PATH TO SELF-UNDERSTANDING

To wrestle with choices about life is human, and taking this course has probably shown you that you are not alone with your struggles. We hope you will remain open to the idea of seeking counseling for yourself at critical transition periods in your life or at times when you feel particularly challenged with life events or choices to be made. Even a few counseling sessions at the right time can assist you in clarifying your options and can provide you with the impetus to formulate action plans leading to change.

Counseling for Personal Enhancement

As you have seen, personal growth is a life-long process, and you have choices to make in many areas of your life. It is essential to attend to your physical, psychological, social, and spiritual well-being. When you find that you cannot give yourself the help you need or get needed assistance from your friends and family, you may want to seek out a professional counselor. When people are physically ill, they generally seek a physician's help. Yet when people are not psychologically well, they often hesitate to ask for assistance. Counseling does not necessarily involve a major revamping of your personality. Instead of getting a major overhaul, you might need only a minor tune-up! Many people refuse to take their car to a mechanic unless it breaks down because they do not want to take the time for preventive maintenance. Some will avoid a trip to the dentist until they are in excruciating pain with a toothache. Likewise, many people wait until they are unable to function at home, at work, or at school before they reach out for professional counseling. Your pathway to personal growth will be smoother if you opt for a few tune-ups along the way.

Many people are reluctant to seek counseling because they worry about the potential stigma of working with a counselor and being labeled psychologically unstable. For some people, their culture may not be supportive of counseling. If you are considering using counseling as a resource for personal growth, we hope you will not be stopped by the fear of what others might think if they found out that you were seeing a counselor. Perhaps even more important, do not allow fears of what you might think of yourself stop you from seeking counseling. Participating in counseling is a sign of strength; it takes courage to seek professional help in achieving your personal goals. You do not have to be in a crisis to benefit from either individual or group counseling. Counselors can work with people to develop a revised perspective on life when they feel stuck in some aspect of living. If you can identify with any of these statements, you might consider seeking counseling as a pathway for effective living:

▶ I feel my life is out of control sometimes.

▶ I am unhappy with where I am heading.

▶ I think that I make a lot of bad choices.

▶ I am the victim of a crime or a survivor of some form of abuse.

▶ I have no sense of what to do with my life.

▶ I am often depressed.

▶ I am in an unhappy relationship.

▶ I have several addictions.

▶ I don't like myself.

▶ I am experiencing a spiritual crisis.

▶ I am experiencing a significant loss.

▶ I am having problems related to work or school.

▶ I am under chronic stress and have stress-related ailments.

▶ I have been discriminated against and experienced oppression.

▶ I'm a recent immigrant and I often feel overwhelmed, lost, and unable to connect with others.

▶ I am ending a significant relationship.

▶ I am using only a fraction of my potential.

Counseling Resources on Your Campus

A good place to seek personal counseling at no fee is at the counseling center at your college or university. In a study of student problems in college counseling centers, Benton, Robertson, Tseng, Newton, and Benton (2003) found that many college students who seek counseling today have problems associated with normal developmental issues and relationship concerns. Others have more severe problems such as anxiety, depression, suicidal ideation, and personality disorders. College and university counseling centers typically offer group counseling as well as individual counseling, and both personal and academic counseling are resources that can benefit you. The wide variety of counseling groups and support groups for students will help you see that you are not alone in your struggles. Support groups may explore alternatives you had not considered, and group counseling can provide you with the tools for personal change.

Counselors are mentors who guide you in making use of your inner resources. Good counselors do not attempt to solve your problems for you. Instead, they teach you how to cope with your problems more effectively. In many respects counselors are psychological educators, teaching you how to get the most from living, how to create more joy in your life, and how to use your own strengths and resources.

A counselor's function is to teach you how to eventually become your own therapist. Counselors do not change your beliefs through brainwashing; rather, they assist you in examining how your thinking affects the way you feel and act. A counselor will help you identify specific beliefs that may be getting in the way of your living effectively. You will learn how to critically evaluate your values, beliefs, thoughts, and assumptions. Counseling can teach you how to substitute constructive thinking for self-destructive thinking. If you find it hard to identify and express feelings such as joy, anger, fear, or guilt, counseling can help you learn to do so. If your present behavior prevents you from getting where you want to go, counseling can assist you in exploring alternative ways of acting.

The Challenges of Seeking Counseling

Therapeutic work can be difficult for you *and* for the counselor. Being honest with yourself is not easy. Confronting and dealing with your problems takes courage. The Serenity Prayer (see Chapter 1) can be an appropriate foundation for some as a therapeutic practice: "God, grant me the serenity to accept the things I cannot change, courage to change the things I can, and wisdom to know the difference."

By seeking counseling, you have taken the first step in the healing process. Recognizing the need for help is itself significant in moving forward. Self-exploration requires discipline, patience, and persistence in working at those aspects of our life that we can change. There may be times when progress seems slow, for counseling does not work wonders. Indeed, at times you may feel worse before you get better because old wounds are brought to the surface and explored.

Selecting the counselor who is right for you is of the utmost importance. Just as it is important to go to a physician you trust, it is critical that you find a counselor whom you can trust. Ask questions about the counselor's training and background before you make a commitment to work with that person. In fact, ethical therapists feel a responsibility to inform their clients about the way counseling works. Another good way to find an effective therapist is to ask others who have been in counseling. A personal referral to a specific person can be useful. However you select a counselor, do some research and make an informed decision. Counseling is a highly personal matter, and you have a greater chance to benefit from this process if you trust your counselor.

Remember, counseling is a process of self-discovery aimed at empowerment. Counseling is not an end in itself, and effective counseling involves developing a collaborative partnership between yourself and your counselor. You will eventually stop seeing a counselor, but the process you have begun does not necessarily have to end. You can continue to apply in your daily life what you learned in your counseling experience. If your counseling is successful, you will learn far more than merely how to solve a specific problem. You will acquire skills of self-examination and assessment that you can use to confront new problems and challenges as they arise. Ultimately, you will be better equipped to make your own choices about how you want to live.

DREAMS AS A PATH TO SELF-UNDERSTANDING

Although all counselors do not work with their clients' dreams, exploring dreams is a vital part of the practice of some forms of counseling. Dreams can reveal significant clues to events that have meaning for us. If we train ourselves to recall our dreams—and this can indeed be learned—and discipline ourselves to explore their meanings, we can get a good sense of our struggles, wants, goals, purposes, conflicts, and interests. Dreams can shed a powerful light on our past, present, and future dynamics and on our attempt to construct meaning. Dreaming helps us deal with stress, work through loss and grief, resolve anger, and bring closure to painful life situations. Our dreams can provide us with a path toward greater understanding of ourselves and our relationships with others. If dreams are to be healing, it is essential that we learn to remember key aspects and patterns of our dreams. One of the best ways to keep track of your dreams is to record them in your journal. Sharing a dream with someone you trust can be self-revealing and helpful. If you journal around themes in your dreams, you may begin to see more parallels between your sleeping and waking life.

In the past, I (Jerry) rarely had dreams that I could remember. Some years ago I attended a conference that focused on exploring dreams. I began to record whatever fragments of dreams I could recall, and, interestingly, during this conference I started to recall some vivid and rich dreams. I have made it a practice to record in my journal any dreams upon awakening, along with my impressions and reactions to the dreams. It helps me to share my dreams with Marianne or other friends; especially useful is comparing impressions others have of my dreams.

All the images in my dreams are manifestations of some dimension within me. In Gestalt fashion, I typically allow myself to reflect on the ways the people in my dreams represent parts of me. "Becoming the various images" in the dream is one way for me to bring unconscious themes forward. I am finding that my dreams have a pattern and that they are shorthand ways of understanding conflicts in my life, decisions to be made at crossroads, and themes that recur from time to time. Even a short segment of a dream often contains layers of messages that make sense when I look at what is going on in my waking state.

Exploring the Meaning of Dreams

Dreams are not mysterious; they are avenues to self-understanding. People have been fascinated with dreams and have regarded them as significant since ancient times, but dreams have been the subject of scientific investigation only since the mid-19th century. When we give lectures on counseling, students are typically interested in learning about the purpose of dreams and pose many questions to us.

Recently we had a conversation with Elida, who was concerned about her dreams involving an uncle who had died a few years ago. Elida had not been able to work through the grief of missing her uncle, and she felt guilty because she had not talked with him more when he was alive. In a dream her uncle appeared to her and told her that he was alright and that she should not worry about him. After this dream Elida felt free and light, as though a burden had been lifted from her. When she shared this dream with her family, they reacted by saying she was "weird." We reassured Elida that her dreams were normal and healthy and that this dream was a healing experience. Elida was glad to hear that she was not weird after all, and she treasured this dream encounter with her uncle.

We believe in the healing capacity of dreams but recognize that a little knowledge can be a dangerous thing. A full understanding of the complexity of dream interpretation is necessary when analyzing dreams. Trying to analyze your own or friends' or family members' dreams without a foundation in dream analysis could have far more negative than positive outcomes.

Fritz Perls, a founder of Gestalt therapy, discovered some useful methods to assist people in better understanding themselves. He suggested that we become friends with our dreams. According to Perls (1969, 1970), the dream is the most spontaneous expression of the existence of the human being; it is a piece of art that individuals chisel out of their lives. It represents an unfinished situation, but it is more than an incomplete situation, an unfulfilled wish, or a prophecy. Every dream contains an existential message about oneself and one's current struggle. Gestalt therapy aims at bringing a dream to life by having the dreamer relive it as though it were happening now. This includes making a list of all the details of the dream, remembering each person, event, and mood in it, and then becoming each of these parts by acting and inventing dialogue. Perls saw dreams as "the royal road to integration." By avoiding analysis and interpretation and focusing instead on becoming and experiencing the dream in all its aspects, the dreamer gets closer to the existential message of the dream.

Rainwater (1979) offers some useful guidelines for dreamers to follow in exploring their dreams:

▶ Be the landscape or the environment.

▶ Become all the people in the dream. Are any of them significant people?

▶ Be any object that links and joins, such as telephone lines and highways.

▶ Identify with any mysterious objects, such as an unopened letter or an unread book.

▶ Assume the identity of any powerful force, such as a tidal wave.

▶ Become any two contrasting objects, such as a younger person and an older person.

▶ Be anything that is missing in the dream. If you do not remember your dreams, then speak to your missing dreams.

When you wake from a dream, is your feeling state one of fear, joy, sadness, frustration, surprise, or anger? Identifying the feeling tone may be the key to finding the meaning of the dream (Rainwater, 1979). As you play out the various parts of your dream, pay attention to what you say and look for patterns. By identifying your feeling tone and the themes that emerge, you will get a clearer sense of what your dreams are telling you.

Dreams are full of symbols. Gestalt therapists contribute to dream work by emphasizing the individual meaning of symbols. The person assigns meaning to his or her own dream. For example, an unopened letter could represent a person who is clinging to secrets. An unread book might symbolize an individual's fear of not being noticed or of being insignificant. A Gestalt therapist might ask the person, "What is the first thing that comes to you when you think about an unopened letter?" One person replies, "I want to hide. I don't want anyone to know me." Another individual says, "I wish somebody would open me up." To understand the personal meaning of a dream, a therapist often asks, "What might be going on in your life now where what you just said would make sense?" In Gestalt therapy no established meaning fits everyone; rather, meaning is deciphered by each individual.

Dreams are a rich source of meaning. Dreams are the link between our inner and outer lives, and they give us a unique opportunity to listen to and learn from our inner wisdom. Your dreams can provide you with a direction in making better choices and living more fully.

Dare to Dream

Dreams can reveal significant aspects of our past and present struggles. As a gateway to the unconscious, dreaming can also inform us of our future strivings. To better design a personal vision for your future, we encourage you to dream when you are awake as well as when you are asleep. Don Quixote dared "to dream the impossible dream." We encourage you to follow a similar path.

The greatest hindrance to your growth may be allowing your fear of failing to stop you from doing what you most want to do. My (Jerry) fear of failing and feelings of inadequacy have been my best teachers. I have learned that failure isn't fatal, that much can be gained from reflecting on mistakes, and how essential it is to have a personal vision. You may have restricted your vision of what you might become by not allowing yourself to formulate a vision or pursue your dreams. At age 8 when I (Marianne) decided to come to America, I did not fully realize what an unrealistic dream this was. I was challenged many times to give up my dream, yet I did not let obstacles stop me. The choice I made when I was 8 greatly influenced my life and the lives of many others as well.

If you reflect thoughtfully on the messages in your dreams, a range of choices will unfold for you. We have met many people who continue to surprise themselves with what they have in their lives. At one time they would not have imagined such possibilities—even in their wildest dreams—but their dreams became reality for them. We encourage you to dare to dream what may seem like impossible dreams, to believe in yourself in spite of your self-doubts, and then to work hard to make your dreams become a reality. Dare to dream, and then have the courage to follow your passions.

CONCLUDING COMMENTS

If you have become more aware of personal aspects of your life than you were when you began the course, and if you decide that you want to continue on the path of self-reflection, you have already taken the first steps toward making changes in your life. Sometimes people expect dramatic transformations and feel disappointed if they do not make major changes in their lives. Remember that it is not the big changes that are necessarily significant; rather, it is your willingness to take small steps that will lead to continued growth. Only you can change your own ways of thinking, feeling, and doing. Look for subtle ways you are changing.

The knowledge and skills that you have gained from both the course and the book can be applied to virtually all of your future experiences. Recognize that there is no one path for you to follow. You will encounter many paths and make critical decisions at various transition points in your life. Remain open to considering new paths.

At this point you may have a clearer vision of the personal goals that you want to pursue. Although we encourage you to make plans that will help you achieve your new goals, avoid overwhelming yourself and do not expect change to happen easily and quickly. Personal change is an ongoing process that really does not come to an end until you do. We sincerely

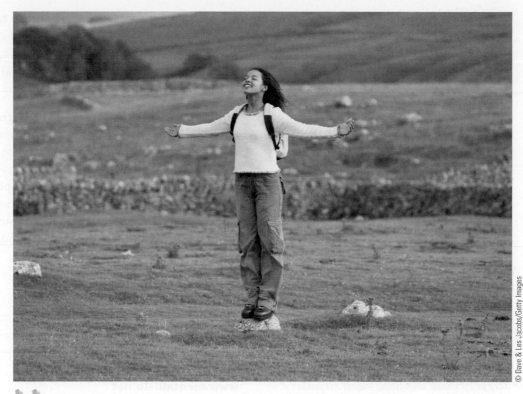

There is no one path for you to follow in increasing your personal freedom.

© Dave & Les Jacobs/Getty Images

wish you well in your commitment to take the steps necessary, no matter how small, in your journey to becoming the person you want to be. Remember that even a journey of a thousand miles begins with the first step—so start walking!

Where Can I Go From Here?

1. If you have trouble remembering your dreams, before you go to sleep (for about a month) repeat this statement: "I will have a dream tonight, and I will remember it." Keep a paper and a pen near your bed, and jot down even brief dream fragments you may recall when you wake up. If you do not recall dreaming, at least write that down. This practice may increase your ability to remember your dreams.

2. If you are aware of dreaming fairly regularly, develop the practice of writing your dreams in your journal as soon as possible upon awakening. Look at the pattern of your dreams; become aware of the kinds of dreams you are having and what they might mean to you. Simply reading your descriptions of your dreams can be of value to you.

3. Make a list of all the reasons you would not want to seek out a counselor when you are in

psychological pain or coping with a problem that hampers your personal effectiveness. Apply this same list to whether you would seek out a physician when you are in physical pain. Compare your answers to determine your attitudes regarding psychological health and physical health.

4. If you have invested yourself in this book and in this course, you have acquired a set of skills that you can continue to use, one being the art of self-assessment. Respond to each of the following questions in your journal. Do not check off the question until you feel you have responded as fully as you can.

   a. Have you felt good about the kind of student you have been this term? If the rest of your college career will be much like this term, what will that be like for you?

b. Go back to the discussion of becoming an active learner in Chapter 1. To what degree have you become more involved and active as a student and as a learner?

c. You were invited to become a coauthor of this book by writing in it and personalizing the material. Take time to reread some of what you wrote in the Take Time to Reflect sections and in the journal pages at the end of each chapter. What patterns do you see in your thoughts?

d. Describe the student and person you would like to be one year from today. Consider these questions as you imagine pursuing different pathways:

▸ What might be getting in my way of being the kind of person and student I would like to be?

▸ What are a few specific actions I need to take if I want to accomplish new goals?

▸ What will help me to stick with a plan aimed at becoming more of the person and student I want to become?

5. Suggested Readings. The full bibliographic entry for each of these sources can be found in the References and Suggested Readings at the back of the book. For specific suggestions on how to design and implement an action plan aimed at making the changes you want, see Wubbolding (2000, 2011). For ideas on understanding the meaning of dreams, see Fontana (1997) and Perls (1969).

WEBSITE RESOURCES

Included here are some valuable websites. For access to these websites, video activities, and other supporting materials, visit Cengage Learning's Counseling CourseMate website for *I Never Knew I Had a Choice,* 10th Edition, at www.cengagebrain.com.

AMERICAN COLLEGE COUNSELING ASSOCIATION

http://collegecounseling.org/

Recommended Search Words: "American college counseling association"

ACCA, is a division of the American Counseling Association. Visit this site to access resources about career fields in college counseling as well as information that is relevant to the lives of college students.

AMERICAN ASSOCIATION OF MARRIAGE AND FAMILY THERAPY

www.aamft.org

Recommended Search Words: "AAMFT"

This site explains how professional therapy can help couples and families experiencing difficulty. The site also offers links to important family and marriage-related resources including their TherapistLocator.net service.

MENTAL HEALTH NET

www.mentalhelp.net

Recommended Search Words: "mental help net"

This is an excellent site that explores all aspects of mental health. Many psychological disorders and treatments are discussed along with professional issues. There are links to thousands of mental health resources.

APA BROCHURES

www.apa.org/pubs/info/brochures/index.aspx

Recommended Search Words: "APA brochures"

This portion of the site, designed by the American Psychological Association, offers brochures about a wide range of issues and problems.

INTERNATIONAL ASSOCIATION FOR THE STUDY OF DREAMS

http://asdreams.org/idxaboutus.htm

Recommended Search Words: "association for dreams"

This is a nonprofit, international, multidisciplinary organization devoted to the pure and applied investigation of dreams and dreaming. Visit it to learn about dreams and nightmares, the science of dreaming, films and dreams, and more.

REFERENCES AND
SUGGESTED READINGS

REFERENCES AND SUGGESTED READINGS

ABELES, N., VICTOR, T. L., & DELANO-WOOD, L. (2004). The impact of an older adult's death on the family. *Professional Psychology: Research and Practice, 35*(3), 234–239.

ABOUT DR. KING. (2012). Martin Luther King Jr. center for nonviolent social change. Retrieved from www.thekingcenter.org/about-dr-king

ABOUT HIP. (2011). Heroic imagination project. Retrieved from http://heroicimagination.org/welcome/about-us/

ADLER, A. (1958). *What life should mean to you.* New York: Capricorn.

ADLER, A. (1964). *Social interest: A challenge to mankind.* New York: Capricorn.

ADLER, A. (1969). *The practice and theory of individual psychology.* Paterson, NJ: Littlefield.

AINSWORTH, M. D. S., BLEHAR, M. C., WATERS, E., & WALL, S. (1978). *Patterns of attachment: A psychological study of the strange situation.* Hillsdale, NJ: Erlbaum.

ALBOM, M. (1997). *Tuesdays with Morrie.* New York: Doubleday.

ALCOHOLICS ANONYMOUS WORLD SERVICES. (2001). *Alcoholics anonymous.* New York: Author.

AMERICAN PSYCHIATRIC ASSOCIATION. (2000). *Diagnostic and statistical manual of mental disorders: Text revision* (4th ed.). Washington, DC: Author.

AMERICAN PSYCHOLOGICAL ASSOCIATION. (2004). Guidelines for psychological practice with older adults. *American Psychologist, 59*(4), 236–260.

ANDERSON, J. (2000). *A year by the sea: Thoughts of an unfinished woman.* New York: Broadway Books.

ANDERSON, J. (2004). *A walk on the beach.* New York: Broadway Books.

ANDERSON, M., KAUFMAN, J., SIMON, T. R., BARRIOS, L., PAULOZZI, L., RYAN, G., . . . POTTER, L. (2001). School-associated violent deaths in the United States, 1994–1999. *Journal of the American Medical Association, 286*(21), 2695–2703.

ANDERSON, S. K., & MIDDLETON, V. A. (2011). *Explorations in diversity: Examining privilege and oppression in a multicultural society* (2nd ed.). Belmont, CA: Brooks/Cole, Cengage Learning.

*ARMSTRONG, T. (1993). *7 kinds of smart: Identifying and developing your many intelligences.* New York: Plume.

ARMSTRONG, T. (1994). *Multiple intelligences in the classroom.* Alexandria, VA: Association for Supervision and Curriculum Development.

*ARMSTRONG, T. (2007). *The human odyssey: Navigating the twelve stages of life.* New York: Sterling

ARNETT, J. J. (2000). Emerging adulthood: A theory of development from the late teens through the twenties. *American Psychologist, 55*(5), 469–480.

ARNETT, J. J. (2011). Emerging adulthood(s): The cultural psychology of a new life stage. In L. A. Jensen (Ed.), *Bridging cultural and developmental approaches to psychology: New syntheses in theory, research, and policy* (pp. 255–275). New York: Oxford University Press.

ARONSON, E. (2000, May 28). *The social psychology of self-persuasion.* Keynote address at the Evolution of Psychotherapy Conference, Anaheim, CA.

BAKER, R. K., & WHITE, K. M. (2010). Predicting adolescents' use of social networking sites from an extended theory of planned behavior perspective. *Computers in Human Behavior, 26,* 1591–1597.

*BASOW, S. A. (1992). *Gender: Stereotypes and roles* (3rd ed.). Pacific Grove, CA: Brooks/Cole, Cengage Learning.

423

REFERENCES

An asterisk before an entry indicates a source that we highly recommend as supplementary reading.

BATESON, M. C. (1990). *Composing a life.* New York: Plume.

BAUMRIND, D. (1967). Child care practices anteceding three patterns of preschool behavior. *Genetic Psychology Monographs, 75,* 43–88.

BAUMRIND, D. (1971). Current patterns of parental authority. *Developmental Psychology Monographs, 4*(1, Part 2).

BAUMRIND, D. (1978). Parental disciplinary patterns and social competence in children. *Youth and Society, 9,* 239–276.

BAYES, A., & MADDEN, S. (2011). Early onset eating disorders in male adolescents: A series of 10 inpatients. *Australasian Psychiatry, 19*(6), 526–530.

*BECK, A. T., & WEISHAAR, M. E. (2011). Cognitive therapy. In R. J. Corsini & D. Wedding (Eds.), *Current psychotherapies* (9th ed., pp. 276–309). Belmont, CA: Brooks/Cole, Cengage Learning.

*BECK, J. S. (2008). *The complete Beck diet for life.* New York: Oxmoor House.

*BECK, J. S. (2011). *Cognitive behavior therapy: Basics and beyond* (2nd ed.). New York: Guilford Press.

BECK, R., TAYLOR, C., & ROBBINS, M. (2003). Missing home: Sociotropy and autonomy and their relationship to psychological distress and homesickness in college freshmen. *Anxiety, Stress, & Coping, 16*(2), 155–166.

BEISSER, A. R. (1970). The paradoxical theory of change. In J. Fagan & I. L. Shepherd (Eds.), *Gestalt therapy now* (pp. 77–80). New York: Harper & Row (Colophon).

BELLAH, R. N., MADSEN, R., SULLIVAN, W. M., SWIDLER, A., & TIPTON, S. M. (1985). *Habits of the heart: Individualism and commitment in American life.* New York: Harper & Row (Perennial).

BEN-SHAHAR, T. (2007). *Happier: Learn the secrets to daily joy and lasting fulfillment.* New York: McGraw-Hill.

BEN-SHAHAR, T. (2011). *Being happy: You don't have to be perfect to lead a richer, happier life.* New York: McGraw-Hill.

BENJAMIN, J. C. (2008, July/August). Tips on avoiding yoga injuries. *American Fitness,* 11.

*BENSON, H. (1976). *The relaxation response.* New York: Avon.

BENSON, H. (1984). *Beyond the relaxation response.* New York: Berkeley Books.

BENTON, S. A., ROBERTSON, J. M., TSENG, W., NEWTON, F. B., & BENTON, S. L. (2003). Changes in counseling center client problems across 13 years. *Professional Psychology: Research and Practice, 34*(1), 66–72.

BERMAN, J., & BERMAN, L. (2001). *For women only: A revolutionary guide to overcoming sexual dysfunction and reclaiming your sex life.* New York: Henry Holt.

BERNE, E. (1975). *What do you say after you say hello?* New York: Bantam.

*BLOOMFIELD, H. H. (with FELDER, L.). (1983). *Making peace with your parents.* New York: Ballantine.

*BLOOMFIELD, H. H. (with FELDER, L.). (1985). *Making peace with yourself: Transforming your weaknesses into strengths.* New York: Ballantine.

*BLY, R. (1990). *Iron John: A book about men.* New York: Random House (Vintage).

BOENISCH, E., & HANEY, M. (2004). *The stress owner's manual: Meaning, balance and health in your life* (2nd ed.). Atascadero, CA: Impact.

*BOK, F. (with TIVNAN, E.). (2003). *Escape from slavery.* New York: St. Martin's Press.

*BOLLES, R. N. (2012). *The 2012 what color is your parachute? A practical manual for job hunters and career-changers.* Berkeley, CA: Ten Speed Press.

BOWLBY, J. (1969). *Attachment and loss: Vol. 1. Attachment.* London: Hogarth Press.

BOWLBY, J. (1973). *Attachment and loss: Vol. 2. Separation.* New York: Basic Books.

BOWLBY, J. (1980). *Attachment and loss: Vol. 3. Loss, sadness, and depression.* New York: Basic Books.

BOWLBY, J. (1988). *A secure base.* New York: Basic Books.

BRANNON, L., & FEIST, J. (2004). *Health psychology: An introduction to behavior and health* (5th ed.). Belmont, CA: Wadsworth, Cengage Learning.

*BRENNER, P. (2002). *Buddha in the waiting room: Simple truths about health, illness, and healing.* Hillsboro, OR: Beyond Words.

BRODY, S. (2010). The relative health benefits of different sexual activities. *Journal of Sexual Medicine, 7*, 1336–1361.

BROOKS, K. P., ROBLES, T. F., & DUNKEL SCHETTER, C. (2011). Adult attachment and cortisol responses to discussions with a romantic partner. *Personal Relationships, 18*, 302–320.

BURDEN, R. (2008). Is dyslexia necessarily associated with negative feelings of self-worth? A review and implications for future research. *Dyslexia, 14(3)*, 188–196.

*BURNS, D. D. (1981). *Feeling good: The new mood therapy.* New York: New American Library (Signet).

BURNS, D. D. (1999). *The feeling good handbook* (Rev. ed.). New York: Penguin Putnam (Plume).

BURSTEIN, M., AMELI-GRILLON, L., & MERIKANGAS, K. R. (2011). Shyness versus social phobia in U.S. youth. *Pediatrics, 128*, 917–925.

*BUSCAGLIA, L. (1972). *Love.* Thorofare, NJ: Charles B. Slack.

BUSCAGLIA, L. (1992). *Born for love: Reflections on loving.* New York: Fawcett (Columbine).

BUSCAGLIA, L. (1996). Celebration of love. In R. Carlson & B. Shield (Eds.), *Handbook for the heart: Original writings on love* (pp. 133–139). Boston: Little, Brown.

*CACIOPPO, J. T., & PATRICK, W. (2008). *Loneliness: Human nature and the need for social connection.* New York: Norton.

CANFIELD, J. (1995). Rekindling the fires of your soul. In R. Carlson & B. Shield (Eds.), *Handbook for the soul* (pp. 87–94). Boston: Little, Brown.

CAPUZZI, D. (Ed.). (2004). *Suicide across the life span: Implications for counselors.* Alexandria, VA: American Counseling Association.

CARDUCCI, B. J. (1999). *The pocket guide to making successful small talk: How to talk to anyone anytime anywhere about anything.* New Albany, IN: Pocket Guide.

*CARDUCCI, B. J. (2000a). *Shyness: A bold new approach.* New York: Harper Perennial.

CARDUCCI, B. J. (2000b). What shy individuals do to cope with their shyness: A content analysis. In W. Ray Crozier (Ed.), *Shyness: Development, consolidation and change* (pp. 171–185). New York: Routledge.

CARDUCCI, B. J. (2005). *The shyness workbook: 30 days to dealing effectively with shyness.* Champaign, IL: Research Press.

CARDUCCI, B. J. (2008). Shyness. In W. A. Darity Jr. (Ed.), *International encyclopedia of the social sciences Vol. 4* (2nd ed., pp. 504–505). Detroit: Macmillan Reference.

CARDUCCI, B. J. (2009). What shy individuals do to cope with their shyness: A content analysis and evaluation of self-selected coping strategies. *Israel Journal of Psychiatry and Related Sciences, 46*, 45–52.

CARDUCCI, B. J., & Fields, T. H. (2007). *The shyness workbook for teens.* Champaign, IL: Research Press.

CARDUCCI, B. J., STUBBINS, Q. L., & BRYANT, M. L. (2008, August). *Still shy after all these (30) years: 1977 versus 2007.* Poster presentation at the meeting of the American Psychological Association, San Francisco.

CARDUCCI, B. J., & ZIMBARDO, P. G. (1995, November/December). Are you shy? *Psychology Today, 34*–41, 64, 66, 68, 70, 78, 82.

CARLSON, R. (1997). *Don't sweat the small stuff . . . and it's all small stuff.* New York: Hyperion.

*CARLSON, R., & SHIELD, B. (Eds.). (1989). *Healers on healing.* Los Angeles, CA: Jeremy P. Tarcher.

*CARLSON, R., & SHIELD, B. (Eds.). (1995). *Handbook for the soul.* Boston: Little, Brown.

*CARLSON, R., & SHIELD, B. (Eds.). (1996). *Handbook for the heart: Original writings on love.* Boston: Little, Brown.

CARNES, P. (2003). Understanding sexual addiction. *SIECUS Report, 31*(5), 5–7.

*CARROLL, J. L. (2013). *Sexuality now: Embracing diversity* (4th ed.). Belmont, CA: Wadsworth, Cengage Learning.

CASEY, L. (2011, October 13). *100-year-old man sets eight world track records in Toronto*. Retrieved from http://www.thestar.com/news/article/ 1069610--100-year-old-man-sets-eight-world-track-records-in-toronto

CHAMBERLAIN, L. J., & HODSON, R. (2010). Toxic work environments: What helps and what hurts. *Sociological Perspectives, 53*(4), 455–477.

CHAPMAN, A. B. (1993). Black men do feel about love. In M. Golden (Ed.), *Wild women don't wear no blues: Black women writers on love, men and sex*. New York: Doubleday.

CHAPMAN, G. (2010). *The 5 love languages: The secret to love that lasts*. Chicago, IL: Northfield.

COREY, G. (2012). *Theory and practice of group counseling* (8th ed.). Belmont, CA: Brooks/Cole, Cengage Learning.

COREY, G., COREY, C., & COREY, H. (1997). *Living and learning*. Belmont, CA: Wadsworth, Cengage Learning.

COREY, M. S., COREY, G., & COREY, C. (2014). *Groups: Process and practice* (9th ed.). Belmont, CA: Brooks/Cole, Cengage Learning.

COREY, G., COREY, M. S., & HAYNES, R. (2014). *Groups in action: Evolution and challenges, DVD and workbook*. Belmont, CA: Brooks/Cole, Cengage Learning.

CORNUM, R., MATTHEWS, M. D., & SELIGMAN, M. E. P. (2011). Comprehensive soldier fitness: Building resilience in a challenging institutional context. *American Psychologist, 66*(1), 4–9.

CORR, C. A. (1992). A task-based approach to coping with dying. *Omega, 24*, 81–94.

*CORR, C. A., & CORR, D. M. (2013). *Death and dying, life and living* (7th ed.). Belmont, CA: Wadsworth, Cengage Learning.

COURTNEY-CLARKE, M. (1999). *Maya Angelou: The poetry of living*. New York: Clarkson Potter.

*CROOKS, R., & BAUR, K. (2011). *Our sexuality* (11th ed.). Belmont, CA: Wadsworth, Cengage Learning.

CROSBY, A. E., HAN, B., ORTEGA, L. A. G., PARKS, S. E., & GFROERER, J. (2011). Suicidal thoughts and behaviors among adults aged ≥18 years— United States, 2008–2009. *MMWR Surveillance Summaries, 60*(13), 1–23.

CULVER, L. M., MCKINNEY, B. L., & PARADISE, L. V. (2011). Mental health professionals' experiences of vicarious traumatization in post-Hurricane Katrina New Orleans. *Journal of Loss & Trauma, 16*(1), 33–42.

*DALAI LAMA. (1999). *Ethics for the new millennium*. New York: Riverhead.

DALAI LAMA. (2001). *An open heart: Practicing compassion in everyday life*. Boston: Little Brown.

*DALAI LAMA, & CUTLER, H. C. (1998). *The art of happiness: A handbook for living*. New York: Riverhead.

DANHAUER, S. C., TOOZE, J. A., FARMER, D. F., CAMPBELL, C. R., MCQUELLON, R. P., BARRETT, R., & MILLER, B. E. (2008). Restorative yoga for women with ovarian or breast cancer: Findings from a pilot study. *Journal of the Society for Integrative Oncology, 6*(2), 47–58.

DARCY, A. M., DOYLE, A. C., LOCK, J., PEEBLES, R., DOYLE, P., & LE GRANGE, D. (2012). The eating disorders examination in adolescent males with anorexia nervosa: How does it compare to adolescent females? *International Journal of Eating Disorders, 45*(1), 110–114.

DEFINING HEROISM. (2011). The heroic imagination project. Retrieved from http://heroicimagination. org/welcome/psychology-and-heroism

*DELANY, S. L., & DELANY, A. E. (with HEARTH, A. H.). (1993). *Having our say: The Delany sisters' first 100 years*. New York: Dell (Delta).

DE PAUW, S. W., & MERVIELDE, I. (2010). Temperament, personality, and developmental psychopathology: A review based on the conceptual dimensions underlying childhood traits. *Child Psychiatry Human Development, 41*, 313–329.

DEUTSCH, B. (2010). The male privilege checklist. In M. S. Kimmel & M. A. Messner (Eds.), *Men's lives* (8th ed., pp. 14–16). Boston: Allyn & Bacon (Pearson).

DIBIASE, R., & GUNNOE, J. (2004). Gender and culture differences in touching behavior. *The Journal of Social Psychology, 144*(1), 49–62.

*DWECK, C. S. (2006). *Mindset: The new psychology of success: How we can learn to fulfill our potential.* New York: Ballantine Books.

*EASWARAN, E. (1991). *Meditation.* Tomales, CA: Nilgiri Press.

EDLIN, G., GOLANTY, E., & BROWN, K. (2000). *Essentials for health and wellness* (2nd ed.). Sudbury, MA: Jones & Bartlett.

EIDE, E. R., & SHOWALTER, M. H. (2012, February 9). *High school students test best with seven hours of rest* [Brigham Young University News Release]. Retrieved from http://news.byu.edu/archive12-feb-sleep.aspx

*ELLIS, A. (2001). *Overcoming destructive beliefs, feelings, and behaviors.* Amherst, NY: Prometheus Books.

* EPSTEIN, M. (1998). *Going to pieces without falling apart: A Buddhist perspective on wholeness.* New York: Broadway Books.

ERIKSON, E. (1963). *Childhood and society* (2nd ed.). New York: Norton.

ERIKSON, E. (1968). *Identity: Youth and crisis.* New York: Norton.

ERIKSON, E. (1982). *The life cycle completed.* New York: Norton.

EVERLY, G. S., & MITCHELL, J. T. (1997). *Critical Incident Stress Management (CISM): A new era and standard of care in crisis intervention.* Ellicott City, MD: Chevron.

EVERLY, G. S., & MITCHELL, J. T. (2008). *A primer on Critical Incident Stress Management (CISM).* Retrieved from http://www.icisf.org/inew_era.htm

FADIMAN, A. (1997). *The spirit catches you and you fall down.* New York: Farrar, Straus & Giroux.

FENTON, M. C., KEYES, K. M., MARTINS, S. S., & HASIN, D. S. (2010). The role of a prescription in anxiety medication use, abuse, and dependence. *The American Journal of Psychiatry, 167*(10), 1247–1253.

FEUERSTEIN, G., & BODIAN, S. (Eds.). (1993). *Living yoga: A comprehensive guide for daily life.* New York: Jeremy P. Tarcher (Putnam).

*FISHER, B. (2005). *Rebuilding: When your relationship ends* (3rd ed.). Atascadero, CA: Impact.

*FLANNERY, T. (2005). *Weather makers: How man is changing the climate and what it means for life on earth.* New York: Grove Press.

*FONTANA, D. (1997). *Teach yourself to dream: A practical guide.* San Francisco: Chronicle Books.

*FONTANA, D. (1999). *Learn to meditate: A practical guide to self-discovery and fulfillment.* San Francisco: Chronicle Books.

*FORREST, A. T. (2011). *Fierce medicine: Breakthrough practices to heal the body and ignite the spirit.* New York: HarperOne.

*FORWARD, S., & BUCK, C. S. (1988). *Betrayal of innocence: Incest and its devastation.* New York: Penguin.

FOWLER, J. (1981). *Stages of faith.* San Francisco, CA: Harper & Row.

*FRANKL, V. (1963). *Man's search for meaning.* New York: Washington Square Press.

FRANKL, V. (1965). *The doctor and the soul.* New York: Bantam.

FRANKL, V. (1969). *The will to meaning: Foundation and applications of logotherapy.* New York: New American Library.

*FRANKL, V. (1978). *The unheard cry for meaning.* New York: Bantam.

*FREEMAN, S. J. (2005). *Grief and loss: Understanding the journey.* Belmont, CA: Brooks/Cole, Cengage Learning.

FRIEND, D. (1991). *The meaning of life.* Boston: Little, Brown.

FRIEDMAN, M. J. (2006). Posttraumatic stress disorders among military returnees from Afghanistan and Iraq. *American Journal of Psychiatry, 163*, 586–593.

*FROMM, E. (1956). *The art of loving*. New York: Harper & Row (Colophon). (Paperback edition 1974)

FULLERTON, D. S. (2011). A collaborative approach to college and university student health and wellness. *New Directions for Higher Education, 153*, 61–69.

GANIBAN, J. M., ULBRICHT, J., SAUDINO, K. J., REISS, D., & NEIDERHISER, J. M. (2011). Understanding child-based effects on parenting: Temperament as a moderator of genetic and environmental contributions to parenting. *Developmental Psychology, 47*(3), 676–692.

GARDNER, H. (1983). *Frames of mind: The theory of multiple intelligences*. New York: Basic Books.

GARDNER, H. (1993). *Multiple intelligences: The theory in practice*. New York: Basic Books.

GARDNER, H. (2000). *Intelligence reframed: Multiple intelligences for the 21st century*. New York: Basic Books.

GENEVAY, B. (2000). There is life after work: Re-creating yourself in the later years. In N. Peterson & R. C. Gonzalez (Eds.), *Career counseling models for diverse populations* (pp. 258–269). Belmont, CA: Wadsworth, Cengage Learning.

*GEORGE, M. (1998). *Learn to relax: A practical guide to easing tension and conquering stress*. San Francisco: Chronicle Books.

GERMER, C. K., SIEGEL, R. D., & FULTON, P. R. (Eds.). (2005). *Mindfulness and psychotherapy*. New York: Guilford Press.

*GIBRAN, K. (1923). *The prophet*. New York: Knopf.

GILBERT, E. (2006). *Eat, pray, love*. New York: Penguin Books.

GILLHAM, J., ADAMS-DEUTSCH, Z., WERNER, J., REIVICH, K., COULTER-HEINDL, V., LINKINS, M., . . . SELIGMAN, M. E. P. (2011). Character strengths predict subjective well-being during adolescence. *Journal of Positive Psychology, 6*(1), 31–44.

GLASSER, W. (1998). *Choice theory: A new psychology of personal freedom*. New York: Harper & Row.

*GLASSER, W. (2000). *Counseling with choice theory: The new reality therapy*. New York: Harper & Row.

GLIONNA, J. M. (1992, January 12). Dance of life. *Los Angeles Times*.

GOLDBERG, A. E., & SMITH, J. Z. (2011). Stigma, social context, and mental health: Lesbian and gay couples across the transition to adoptive parenthood. Journal of Counseling Psychology, 58(1), 139–150.

GOLDBERG, H. (1983). *The new male–female relationship*. New York: New American Library.

*GOLDBERG, H. (1987). *The inner male: Overcoming roadblocks to intimacy*. New York: New American Library (Signet).

*GOLEMAN, D. (1995). *Emotional intelligence*. New York: Bantam.

*GOLEMAN, D. (2000). *Working with emotional intelligence*. New York: Bantam.

*GOLEMAN, D. (2006). *Emotional intelligence, 10th anniversary edition: Why it can matter more than IQ*. New York: Bantam.

*GOLEMAN, D. (2007). *Social intelligence*. New York: Bantam.

GOLEMAN, D. (2011). *The brain and emotional intelligence: New insights*. Northampton, MA: More Than Sound.

GOOD, M., & GOOD, P. (1979). *20 most asked questions about the Amish and Mennonites*. Lancaster, PA: Good Books.

GORE, A. (2006). *An inconvenient truth*. New York: Rodale.

GOTTMAN, J. M., LEVENSON, R. W., GROSS, J., FREDRICKSON, B., McCOY, K., ROSENTAHL, L., et al. (2004). Correlates of gay and lesbian couples' relationship satisfaction and relationship dissolution. *Journal of Homosexuality, 45*(1), 23–43.

*GOTTMAN, J. M., & SILVER, N. (1999). *The seven principles for making marriage work*. New York: Three Rivers Press.

GOULDING, M., & GOULDING, R. (1979). *Changing lives through redecision therapy*. New York: Brunner/Mazel.

GOULDING, R., & GOULDING, M. (1978). *The power is in the patient.* San Francisco: TA Press.

GROV, C., GILLESPIE, B. J., ROYCE, T., & LEVER, J. (2011). Perceived consequences of casual online sexual activities on heterosexual relationships. *Archives of Sexual Behavior, 40,* 429–439.

GUINDON, M. H. (2002). Toward accountability in the use of the self-esteem construct. *Journal of Counseling & Development, 80,* 204–214.

GUINDON, M. H. (2010). *Self-esteem across the lifespan: Issues and interventions.* New York: Taylor & Francis.

GUO, Y. J., WANG, S. C., JOHNSON, V., & DIAZ, M. (2011). College students' stress under current economic downturn. *College Student Journal, 45*(3), 536–543.

HALDEMAN, D. C. (2001). Psychotherapy with gay and bisexual men. In G. R. Brooks & G. E. Good (Eds.), *The new handbook of psychotherapy and counseling with men, Volume 2* (pp. 796–815). San Francisco: Jossey-Bass.

*HALES, D. (2012). *An invitation to health: Choosing to change* (Brief, 7th ed.). Belmont, CA: Wadsworth, Cengage Learning.

*HALES, D. (2013). *An invitation to health: Build your future* (15th ed.). Belmont, CA: Wadsworth, Cengage Learning.

HARLOW, H. F., & HARLOW, M. K. (1966). Learning to love. *American Scientist, 54,* 244–272.

HARRIS, A. S. (1996). *Living with paradox: An introduction to Jungian psychology.* Pacific Grove, CA: Brooks/Cole, Cengage Learning.

HARRIS, I. M. (1995). *Messages men hear: Constructing masculinities.* Bristol, PA: Taylor & Francis.

HARRIS, K. J., HARVEY, P., & BOOTH, S. L. (2010). Who abuses their coworkers? An examination of personality and situational variables. *Journal of Social Psychology, 150*(6), 608–627.

HAZAN, C., & SHAVER, P. R. (1987). Romantic love conceptualized as an attachment process. *Journal of Personality and Social Psychology, 52,* 511–524.

*HEDTKE, L., & WINSLADE, J. (2004). *Re-membering conversations: Conversations with the dying and bereaved.* Amityville, NY: Baywood.

HENDERSON, L. (2011). *Improving social confidence and reducing shyness: Using compassion focused therapy.* Oakland, CA: New Harbinger.

HINDUJA, S., & PATCHIN, J. W. (2010). Bullying, cyberbullying, and suicide. *Archives of Suicide Research, 14*(3), 206–221.

*HIRSHMANN, J. R., & MUNTER, C. H. (1995). *When women stop hating their bodies: Freeing yourself from food and weight obsession.* New York: Fawcett (Columbine).

HODGE, M. (1967). *Your fear of love.* Garden City, NY: Doubleday.

HOFFMAN, E. (1990). *Lost in translation: A life in a new language.* New York: Penguin Books.

HOLLAND, J. L. (1994). *Self-directed search (form R).* Odessa, FL: Psychological Assessment Resources, Inc.

HOLLAND, J. L. (1997). *Making vocational choices: A theory of vocational personalities and work environments* (3rd ed.). Odessa, FL: Psychological Assessment Resources, Inc.

HOLLON, S. D., & DiGIUSEPPE, R. (2011). Cognitive theories in psychotherapy. In J. C. Norcross, G. R. Vandenbos, & D. K. Freedheim (Eds.), *History of psychotherapy* (2nd ed., pp. 203–242). Washington, DC: American Psychological Association.

HOLMES, T. H., & RAHE, R. H. (1967). The social readjustment rating scale. *Journal of Psychosomatic Research, 11,* 213–218.

HORVATIN, T., & SCHREIBER, E. (2006). *The quintessential Zerka: Writings by Zerka Toeman Moreno on psychodrama, sociodrama and group psychotherapy.* New York: Routledge.

HOULIHAN, D., RIES, B. J., POLUSNY, M. A., & HANSON, C. N. (2008). Predictors of behavior and level of life satisfaction of children and adolescents after a major tornado. *Journal of Psychological Trauma, 7*(1), 21–36.

HOW DID WE GET HERE? (2012). Learn the facts. Retrieved from www.letsmove.gov

HUSSAIN, A., WEISAETH, L., & HEIR, T. (2011). Psychiatric disorders and functional impairment among disaster victims after exposure to a natural disaster: A population based study. *Journal of Affective Disorders, 128*(1–2), 135–141.

*HWANG, P. O. (2000). *Other-esteem: Meaningful life in a multicultural society.* Philadelphia, PA: Accelerated Development (Taylor & Francis).

*JACKSON, M. (2008a). *Distracted: The erosion of attention and the coming dark age.* Amherst, NY: Prometheus Books.

JACKSON, M. (2008b, Winter). Distracted: The new news world and the fate of attention. *Nieman Reports,* 26–27.

JAKUPCAK, M., & VARRA, E. M. (2011). Treating Iraq and Afghanistan war veterans with PTSD who are at high risk for suicide. *Cognitive and Behavioral Practice, 18*(1), 85–97.

*JAMPOLSKY, G. G. (1981). *Love is letting go of fear.* New York: Bantam.

*JAMPOLSKY, G. G. (1999). *Forgiveness: The greatest healer of all.* Hillsboro, OR: Beyond Words.

JANNINI, E. A., FISHER, W. A., BITZER, J., & MCMAHON, C. G. (2009). Is sex just fun? How sexual activity improves health. *Journal of Sexual Medicine, 6,* 2640–2648.

JOEL, S., MACDONALD, G., & SHIMOTOMAI, A. (2011). Conflicting pressures on romantic relationship commitment for anxiously attached individuals. *Journal of Personality, 79*(1), 51–74.

JOHNSON, E. M. (1992). *What you can do to avoid AIDS.* New York: Times Books.

JORDAN, J. V., KAPLAN, A. G., MILLER, J. B., STIVER, I. P., & SURREY, J. L. (1991). *Women's growth through connection: Writings from the Stone Center.* New York: Guilford.

JOURARD, S. (1971). *The transparent self: Self-disclosure and well-being* (Rev. ed.). New York: Van Nostrand Reinhold.

JUDY, R., & D'AMICO, C. (1997). *Workforce 2020: Work and workers in the 21st century.* Indianapolis, IN: Hudson Institute.

*JULIA, M. (2000). *Constructing gender: Multicultural perspectives in working with women.* Pacific Grove, CA: Brooks/Cole, Cengage Learning.

JUNG, C. G. (1961). *Memories, dreams, reflections.* New York: Vintage Books.

KABAT-ZINN, J. (1990). *Full catastrophe living.* New York: Delacorte.

*KABAT-ZINN, J. (1994). *Wherever you go, there you are: Mindfulness meditation in everyday life.* New York: Hyperion.

KABAT-ZINN, J. (1995). Soul work. In R. Carlson & B. Shield (Eds.), *Handbook for the soul* (pp. 108–115). Boston: Little, Brown.

KASLOW, F. W. (2004). Death of one's partner: The anticipation and the reality. *Professional Psychology: Research and Practice, 35*(3), 227–233.

KASLOW, N. J., & ARONSON, S. G. (2004). Recommendations for family interventions following suicide. *Professional Psychology: Research and Practice, 35*(3), 240–247.

KAWALA, Y. (2011). *Consoled by the light.* Idyllwild, CA: Author.

KAYE, W. H., WAGNER, A., FUDGE, J. L., & PAULUS, M. (2011). Neurocircuitry of eating disorders. *Behavioral Neurobiology of Eating Disorders, 6,* 37–57.

KEEN, S. (1991). *Fire in the belly: On being a man.* New York: Bantam.

KIAZAD, K., RESTUBOG, S. L. D., ZAGENCZYK, T. J., KIEWITZ, C., & TANG, R. L. (2010). In pursuit of power: The role of authoritarian leadership in the relationship between supervisors' Machiavellianism and subordinates' perceptions of abusive supervisory behavior. *Journal of Research in Personality, 44,* 512–519.

KIMMEL, M. (1996). *Manhood in America: A cultural history.* New York: Free Press.

KIMMEL, M. S. (2010). Guyland: Gendering the transition to adulthood. In M. S. Kimmel & M. A. Messner (Eds.), *Men's lives* (8th ed., pp. 119–133). Boston: Allyn & Bacon (Pearson).

*KIMMEL, M. S., & MESSNER, M. A. (Eds.). (2010). *Men's lives* (8th ed.). Boston: Allyn & Bacon (Pearson).

KINOSIAN, J. (2000, May–June). Right place, write time. *Modern Maturity.*

KLEESPIES, P. M. (2004). *Life and death decisions: Psychological and ethical consideration in end-of-life care.* Washington, DC: American Psychological Association.

KNIGHT, C. (2009). *Introduction to working with adult survivors of childhood trauma.* Belmont, CA: Brooks/Cole, Cengage Learning.

KOBASA, S. C. (1979a). Personality and resistance to illness. *American Journal of Community Psychology, 7,* 413–423.

KOBASA, S. C. (1979b). Stressful life events, personality and health: An inquiry into hardiness. *Journal of Personality and Social Psychology, 37,* 1–11.

KOBASA, S. C. (1984, September). How much stress can you survive? *American Health, 64 67.*

*KOTTLER, J., & CARLSON, J. (2007). *Moved by the spirit: Discovery and transformation in the lives of leaders.* Atascadero, CA: Impact.

*KÜBLER-ROSS, E. (1969). *On death and dying.* New York: Macmillan.

KÜBLER-ROSS, E. (1975). *Death: The final stage of growth.* Englewood Cliffs, NJ: Prentice-Hall (Spectrum).

KWOK, J. (2010). *Girl in translation.* New York: Riverhead Books.

LAWYER, S., RESNICK, H., BAKANIC, V., BURKETT, T., & KILPATRICK, D. (2010). Forcible, drug-facilitated, and incapacitated rape and sexual assault among undergraduate women. *Journal of American College Health, 58*(5), 453–460.

LeMOYNE, T., & BUCHANON, T. (2011). Does "hovering" matter? Helicopter parenting and its effect on well-being. *Sociological Spectrum, 31*(4), 399–418.

LENHART, A., PURCELL, K., SMITH, A., & ZICKUHR, K. (2010). *Social media and young adults.* Washington, DC: Pew Internet & American Life Project.

*LERNER, H. G. (1985). *The dance of anger: A woman's guide to changing the patterns of intimate relationships.* New York: Harper & Row (Perennial).

LERNER, H. G. (1989). *The dance of intimacy: A woman's guide to courageous acts of change in key relationships.* New York: Harper & Row (Perennial).

LEVANT, R. F. (1996). The new psychology of men. *Professional Psychology: Research and Practice, 27*(3), 259–265.

*LEVINSON, D. J. (1978). *The seasons of man's life.* New York: Knopf.

LEVINSON, D. J. (with LEVINSON, J. D.). (1996). *The seasons of woman's life.* New York: Ballantine.

LINCOLN, A. J., & SWEETEN, K. (2011). Considerations for the effects of military deployment on children and families. *Social Work in Health Care, 50,* 73–84.

*LINDBERGH, A. (1975). *Gift from the sea.* New York: Pantheon. (Original work published 1955)

*LOCK, R. D. (2005a). *Job search: Career planning guide* (5th ed.). Belmont, CA: Brooks/Cole, Cengage Learning.

*LOCK, R. D. (2005b). *Taking charge of your career direction: Career planning guide* (5th ed.). Belmont, CA: Brooks/Cole, Cengage Learning.

*LOTT, B. (1994). *Women's lives: Themes and variations in gender learning* (2nd ed.). Pacific Grove, CA: Brooks/Cole, Cengage Learning.

LOWENSTEIN, R. (2011, October 27). Occupy Wall Street: It's not a hippie thing. Bloomberg Businessweek. Retrieved from http://www.businessweek.com/magazine/occupy-wall-street-its-not-a-hippie-thing-10272011.html

MACASKILL, A. (2012). Differentiating dispositional self-forgiveness from other-forgiveness: Associations with mental health and life satisfaction. *Journal of Social and Clinical Psychology, 31*(1), 28–50.

MADDI, S. R. (2002). The story of hardiness: Twenty years of theorizing, research and practice. *Consulting Psychology Journal, 54,* 173–185.

MAHALIK, J. R. (1999a). Incorporating a gender role strain perspective in assessing and treating men's cognitive distortions. *Professional Psychology: Research and Practice, 30*(4), 333–340.

MAHALIK, J. R. (1999b). Interpersonal psychotherapy with men who experience gender role conflict. *Professional Psychology: Research and Practice, 30*(1), 5–13.

*MAIER, S. (1991). *God's love song.* Corvallis, OR: Postal Instant Press.

MALTZ, W. (2001). *The sexual healing journey: A guide for survivors of sexual abuse.* New York: HarperCollins.

*MARCUS, E. (1996). *Why suicide? Answers to 200 of the most frequently asked questions about suicide, attempted suicide, and assisted suicide.* San Francisco: HarperCollins.

*MASLACH, C. (2003). *Burnout: The cost of caring.* Cambridge: Malor Books.

MASLOW, A. (1968). *Toward a psychology of being.* New York: Van Nostrand Reinhold.

MASLOW, A. (1970). *Motivation and personality* (2nd ed.). New York: Harper & Row.

MASLOW, A. (1971). *The farther reaches of human nature.* New York: Viking.

*MATLIN, M. W. (2012). *The psychology of women* (7th ed.). Belmont, CA: Wadsworth, Cengage Learning.

McCANN, I. L., & PEARLMAN, L. A. (1990). Vicarious traumatization: A framework for understanding the psychological effects of working with victims. *Journal of Traumatic Stress, 3,* 131–149.

McCULLOUGH, M. E., & WITVLIET, C. V. (2002). The psychology of forgiveness. In C. R. Snyder, & S. J. Lopez (Eds.), *Handbook of positive psychology.* New York: Oxford University Press.

*McGOLDRICK, M. (2011). Women and the family life cycle. In M. McGoldrick, B. Carter, & N. Garcia Preto (Eds.), *The expanded family life cycle: Individual, family, and social perspectives* (4th ed., pp. 42–58). Boston: Allyn & Bacon (Pearson).

*McGOLDRICK, M., CARTER, B., & GARCIA PRETO, N. (Eds.). (2011a). *The expanded family life cycle: Individual, family, and social perspectives* (4th ed.). Boston: Allyn & Bacon (Pearson).

McGOLDRICK, M., CARTER, B., & GARCIA PRETO, N. (Eds.). (2011b). Self in context: Human development and the individual life cycle in systemic perspective. In M. McGoldrick, B. Carter, & N. Garcia Preto (Eds.), *The expanded family life cycle: Individual, family, and social perspectives* (4th ed., pp. 20–41). Boston: Allyn & Bacon.

McINTOSH, P. (1988). *White privilege and male privilege: A personal account of coming to see correspondences through work in women's studies* [Working paper #189]. Wellesley, MA: Wellesley College Center for Research on Women.

McINTOSH, P. (1998). White privilege: Unpacking the invisible knapsack. In P. S. Rothenberg (Ed.), *Race, class, and gender in the United States: An integrated study* (4th ed., pp. 165–169). New York: St. Martin's Press.

*MEICHENBAUM, D. (2007). Stress inoculation training: A preventive and treatment approach. In P. M. Lehrer, R. L. Woolfolk, & W. Sime (Eds.), *Principles and practices of stress management* (3rd ed., pp. 497–518). New York: Guilford Press.

*MEICHENBAUM, D. (2008). Stress inoculation training. In W. O'Donohue & J. E. Fisher (Eds.), *Cognitive behavior therapy: Applying empirically supported techniques in your practice* (2nd ed., pp. 529–532). Hoboken, NJ: Wiley.

MENEC, V. H. (2003). The relation between everyday activities and successful aging: A 6-year longitudinal study. *Journal and Gerontology, 58,* 74–82.

*MILLER, J., & GARRAN, A. M. (2008). *Racism in the United States: Implications for the helping professions.* Belmont, CA: Brooks/Cole, Cengage Learning.

*MILLER, J. B., & STIVER, I. P. (1997). *The healing connection: How women form relationships in therapy and in life.* Boston: Beacon Press.

MILLER, T. (1995). *How to want what you have: Discovering the magic and grandeur of ordinary existence.* New York: Avon.

MIND OVER MATTER. (2011, October). *Harvard Mental Health Letter, 28*(4), 6.

MITCHELL, J. T. (1983). When disaster strikes. . . . The Critical Incident Stress Debriefing. *Journal of Emergency Medical Services, 13*(11), 49–52.

MITCHELL, J. T., & EVERLY, G. S. (1996). *Critical incident stress debriefing: An operations manual.* Ellicott City, MD: Chevron.

MOCK, M. R. (2011). Men and the life cycle: Diversity and complexity. In M. McGoldrick, B. Carter, & N. Garcia Preto (Eds.), *The expanded family life cycle: Individual, family, and social perspectives* (4th ed., pp. 59–74). Boston: Allyn & Bacon.

*MOORE, T. (1994). *Care of the soul: A guide for cultivating depth and sacredness in everyday life.* New York: Harper (Perennial).

*MOORE, T. (1995). Embracing the everyday. In R. Carlson & B. Shield (Eds.), *Handbook for the soul* (pp. 25–31). Boston: Little, Brown.

MORENO, Z. T. (1991). *Love songs to life.* New York: Mental Health Resources. (Originally published 1970)

MORENO, Z. T., BLOMKVIST, L. D., & RUTZEL, T. (2000). *Psychodrama, surplus reality and the art of healing.* Philadelphia: Routledge (Taylor & Francis).

MORNELL, P. (1979). *Passive men, wild women.* New York: Ballantine.

MOTHER TERESA. (1999). *In the heart of the world.* New York: MJF Books.

*MOUSTAKAS, C. (1961). *Loneliness.* Englewood Cliffs, NJ: Prentice-Hall (Spectrum).

NADEAU, L., & TESSIER, R. (2011). Self-concept in children with cerebral palsy: Is there something in the wind? *Disability & Rehabilitation, 33*(10), 830–834.

NATIONAL COMMITTEE ON PAY EQUITY. (2010). *Wage gap statistically unchanged.* Retrieved from http://www.pay-equity.org/

*NAPARSTEK, B. (2006). *Invisible heroes: Survivors of trauma and how they heal.* New York: Bantam Books.

NERIA,Y., DIGRANDE, L., & ADAMS, B. G. (2011). Posttraumatic stress disorder following the September 11, 2001, terrorist attacks: A review of the literature among highly exposed populations. *American Psychologist, 66*(6), 429–446.

*NEWMAN, B. M., & NEWMAN, P. R. (2012). *Development through life: A psychosocial approach* (11th ed.). Belmont, CA: Wadsworth, Cengage Learning.

*NHAT HANH, T. (1991). *Peace is every step: The path of mindfulness in everyday life.* New York: Bantam.

NHAT HANH, T. (1992). *Touching peace: Practicing the art of mindful living.* Berkeley, CA: Parallax Press.

*NHAT HANH, T. (1997). *Teachings on love.* Berkeley, CA: Parallax Press.

NILES, S. G., JACOB, C. J., & NICHOLS, L. M. (2010). Career development and self-esteem. In M. H. Guindon (Ed.), *Self-esteem across the life span: Issues and interventions.* New York: Taylor & Francis.

NOSKO, A., TIEU, T., LAWFORD, H., & PRATT, M. W. (2011). How do I love thee? Let me count the ways: Parenting during adolescence, attachment styles, and romantic narratives in emerging adulthood. *Developmental Psychology, 47*(3), 645–657.

O'NEIL, J. M. (2008). Summarizing 25 years of research on men's gender role conflict using the Gender Role Conflict Scale: New research paradigms and clinical implications. *The Counseling Psychologist, 36*(3), 358–445.

ORR, A. J. (2011). Gendered capital: Childhood socialization and the "boy crisis" in education. *Sex Roles, 65,* 271–284.

OUELLETTE, S. C. (1993). Inquiries into hardiness. In L. Goldberger & S. Breznitz (Eds.), *Handbook of stress: Theoretical and clinical aspects* (2nd ed.). New York: Free Press.

PARDESS, E. (2005). Pride and prejudice with gay and lesbian individuals: Combining narrative and expressive practices. In C. L. Rabin (Ed.), *Understanding gender and culture in the* helping process: Practitioners' narratives from global perspectives (pp. 109–128). Belmont, CA: Wadsworth, Cengage Learning.

PARKER, S. (2011). Spirituality in counseling: A faith development perspective. *Journal of Counseling & Development, 89*, 112–119.

PATCHIN, J. W., & HINDUJA, S. (2010). Changes in adolescent online social networking behaviors from 2006 to 2009. *Computers in Human Behavior, 26*, 1818–1821.

PEHRSSON, D. E., & BOYLAN, M. (2004). Counseling suicide survivors. In D. Capuzzi, (Ed.), *Suicide across the life span: Implications for counselors* (pp. 305–324). Alexandria, VA: American Counseling Association.

PELUSO, P. R., PELUSO, J. P., WHITE, J. F., & KERN, R. M. (2004). A comparison of attachment theory and individual psychology: A review of the literature. *Journal of Counseling and Development, 82*(2), 139–145.

PETERSON, N., & GONZALEZ, R. C. (Eds.). (2000). *Career counseling models for diverse populations: Hands-on applications by practitioners.* Belmont, CA: Brooks/Cole, Cengage Learning.

*PETERSON, N., & GONZALEZ, R. C. (2005). *The role of work in people's lives: Applied career counseling and vocational psychology* (2nd ed.). Belmont, CA: Brooks/Cole, Cengage Learning.

PETERSON, C., PARK, N., & SELIGMAN, M.E.P. (2005). Orientations to happiness and life satisfaction: The full life versus the empty life. *Journal of Happiness Studies, 6*, 25–41.

*PERLS, F. S. (1969). *Gestalt therapy verbatim.* New York: Bantam.

PERLS, F. S. (1970). Four lectures. In J. Fagan & I. L. Shepherd (Eds.), *Gestalt therapy now* (pp. 14–38). New York: Harper & Row (Colophon).

PHILPOT, C. L., BROOKS, G. R., LUSTERMAN, D. D., & NUTT, R. L. (1997). *Bridging separate gender worlds: Why men and women clash and how therapists can bring them together.* Washington, DC: American Psychological Association.

PIGNOTTI, M. (2011). Reactive attachment disorder and international adoption: A systematic synthesis. *Scientific Review of Mental Health Practice, 8*(1), 30–49.

PISTOLE, C., & ARRICALE, F. (2003). Understanding attachment: Beliefs about conflict. *Journal of Counseling and Development, 81*(3), 318–328.

PLECK, J. (1995). The gender role paradigm: An update. In R. Levant & W. Pollack (Eds.), *A new psychology of men.* New York: Basic Books.

*POLLACK, W. (1998). *Real boys.* New York: Henry Holt.

POLUSNY, M. A., MEIS, L. A., MCCORMICK-DEATON, C. M., RIES, B. J.; DEGARMO, D.,THURAS, P., & ERBES, C. R. (2011). Effects of parents' experiential avoidance and PTSD on adolescent disaster-related posttraumatic stress symptomatology. *Journal of Family Psychology, 25*(2), 220–229.

POSITIVE PSYCHOLOGY CENTER. (2007). Frequently asked questions. Retrieved from http://www.ppc.sas.upenn.edu/faqs.htm

*PROCHASKA, J. O., & NORCROSS, J. C. (2010). *Systems of psychotherapy: A transtheoretical analysis* (7th ed.). Belmont, CA: Brooks/Cole, Cengage Learning.

RABINOWITZ, F. E. (2001). Group therapy for men. In G. R. Brooks & G. E. Good (Eds.), *The new handbook of psychotherapy and counseling with men, Volume 2* (pp. 603–621). San Francisco: Jossey-Bass.

*RABINOWITZ, F. E., & COCHRAN, S. V. (1994). *Man alive: A primer of men's issues.* Pacific Grove, CA: Brooks/Cole, Cengage Learning.

*RABINOWITZ, F. E., & COCHRAN, S. V. (2002). *Deepening psychotherapy with men.* Washington, DC: American Psychological Association.

*RAINWATER, J. (1979). *You're in charge! A guide to becoming your own therapist.* Los Angeles: Guild of Tutors Press.

*REAL, T. (1998). *I don't want to talk about it: Overcoming the secret legacy of male depression.* New York: Simon & Schuster (Fireside).

REIK, B. M. (2010). Transgressions, guilt, and forgiveness: A model of seeking forgiveness. *Journal of Psychology and Theology, 38*(4), 246–254.

REIVICH, K. J., SELIGMAN, M. E. P., & MCBRIDE, S. (2011). Master resilience training in the U.S. Army. *American Psychologist, 66*(1), 25–34.

REYES-RODRIGUEZ, M. L., SALA, M., VON HOLLE, A., UNIKEL, C., BULIK, C. M., CAMARA-FUENTES, L., & SUAREZ-TORRES, A. (2011). A description of disordered eating behaviors in Latino males. *Journal of American College Health, 59*(4), 266–272.

*RIDLEY, C. R. (2005). *Overcoming unintentional racism in counseling and therapy: A practitioner's guide to intentional intervention* (2nd ed.). Thousand Oaks, CA: Sage.

*RINPOCHE, S. (1994). *Meditation.* San Francisco: Harper.

ROBBINS, J. (1996). Beginning with love. In R. Carlson & B. Shield (Eds.), *Handbook for the heart: Original writings on love* (pp. 145–149). Boston: Little, Brown.

ROBINSON, E. A. (1943). *The children of the night.* New York: Scribner's. (Originally published 1897)

ROGERS, C. R. (1961). *On becoming a person: A therapist's view of psychotherapy.* Boston: Houghton Mifflin.

ROGERS, C. R. (1980). *A way of being.* Boston: Houghton Mifflin.

*ROGERS, N. (1993). *The creative connection: Expressive arts as healing.* Palo Alto, CA: Science & Behavior Books.

*ROGERS, N. (2011). *The creative connection for groups: Person-centered expressive arts for healing and social change.* Palo Alto, CA: Science and Behavior Books.

ROOT, A. K., & DENHAM, S. A. (2010). The role of gender in the socialization of emotion: Key concepts and critical issues. *New Directions for Child and Adolescent Development, 128*, 1–9.

ROPELATO, J. (2006). 2006 & 2005 US pornography industry revenue statistics. *TopTenREVIEWS.* Retrieved from http://internet-filter-review.toptenreviews.com/internet-pornography-statistics.html

ROSEN, E. J. (1999). Men in transition: The "new man." In B. Carter & M. McGoldrick (Eds.), *The expanded family life cycle: Individual, family, and social perspectives* (3rd ed., pp. 124–140). Boston: Allyn & Bacon.

RUIZ, D. M. (with MILLS, J.). (2000). *The four agreements companion book.* San Rafael, CA: Amber-Allen.

SANCHEZ, F. J., WESTEFELD, J. S., LIU, W. M., & VILAIN, E. (2010). Masculine gender role conflict and negative feelings about being gay. *Professional Psychology: Research and Practice, 41*(2), 104–111.

*SATIR, V. (1983). *Conjoint family therapy* (3rd ed.). Palo Alto, CA: Science and Behavior Books.

*SATIR, V. (1988). *The new peoplemaking.* Palo Alto, CA: Science and Behavior Books.

SATYAPRIYA, M., NAGENDRA, H. R., NAGARATHNA, R., & PADMALATHA, V. (2009). Effect of integrated yoga on stress and heart rate variability in pregnant women. *International Journal of Gynecology and Obstetrics, 104*, 218–222.

SCHAFER, W. (2000). *Stress management for wellness* (4th ed.). Belmont, CA: Wadsworth, Cengage Learning.

*SCHLOSSBERG, N. K. (2004). *Retire smart, retire happy: Finding your true path in life.* Washington, DC: American Psychological Association.

^SCHNARCH, D. (1997). *Passionate marriage.* New York: Henry Holt.

SCHUELLER, S. M., & SELIGMAN, M. E. P. (2010). Pursuit of pleasure, engagement, and meaning: Relationships to subjective and objective measures of well-being. *Journal of Positive Psychology, 5*(4), 253–263.

*SCHULTZ, D., & SCHULTZ, S. E. (2013). *Theories of personality* (10th ed.). Belmont, CA: Wadsworth, Cengage Learning.

SCHWARTZ, B., & FLOWERS, J. V. (2008). *Thoughts for therapists: Reflections on the art of healing.* Atascadero, CA: Impact.

*SCHWARTZ, M. (1996). *Morrie: In his own words.* New York: Dell (Delta Book).

SCOPELLITI, M., & TIBERIO, L. (2010). Homesickness in university students: The role of multiple place attachment. *Environment and Behavior, 42*(3), 335–350.

SEE, L. (2010). *Shanghai girls.* New York: Random House.

*SEGAL, Z. V., WILLIAMS, J. M. G., & TEASDALE, J. D. (2002). *Mindfulness-based cognitive therapy for depression: A new approach to preventing relapse.* New York: Guilford Press.

*SELIGMAN, M. E. P. (1990). *Learned optimism: How to change your mind and your life.* New York: Pocket Books.

*SELIGMAN, M. E. P. (1993). *What you can change and what you can't.* New York: Fawcett (Columbine).

*SELIGMAN, M. E. P. (2002). *Authentic happiness: Using the new positive psychology to realize your potential for lasting fulfillment.* New York: Free Press.

*SELIGMAN, M. E. P., & FOWLER, R. D. (2011). Comprehensive soldier fitness and the future of psychology. *American Psychologist, 66*(1), 82–86.

SELIGMAN, M. E. P., STEEN, T. A., PARK, N., & PETERSON, C. (2005). Positive psychology progress: Empirical validation of interventions. *American Psychologist, 60,* 410–421.

SELYE, H. (1974). *Stress without distress.* New York: Lippincott.

SETLIK, G., BOND, G. R., & HO, M. (2009). Adolescent prescription ADHD medication abuse is rising along with prescriptions for these medications. *Pediatrics, 124,* 875–880.

SHEAR, M. K., SIMON, N., WALL, M., ZISOOK, S., NEIMEYER, R., DUAN, N., . . . KESHAVIAH, A. (2011). Complicated grief and related bereavement issues for DSM-5. *Depression and Anxiety, 28,* 103–117.

SHEEHY, G. (1976). *Passages: Predictable crises of adult life.* New York: Dutton.

SHEEHY, G. (1981). *Pathfinders.* New York: Morrow.

SHEEHY, G. (1992). *The silent passage.* New York: Random House.

*SHEEHY, G. (1995). *New passages: Mapping your life across time.* New York: Random House.

*SHIELD, B., & CARLSON, R. (Eds.). (1999). *For the love of God: Handbook for the spirit.* New York: MJF Books.

SHORTER, L., BROWN, S. L., QUINTON, S. J., & HINTON, L. (2008). Relationships between body-shape discrepancies with favored celebrities and disordered eating in young women. *Journal of Applied Social Psychology, 38*(5), 1364.

SHULMAN, S., & NURMI, J. E. (2010). Understanding emerging adulthood from a goal-setting perspective. *New Directions for Child and Adolescent Development, 130,* 1–11.

*SIEGEL, B. (1988). *Love, medicine, and miracles.* New York: Harper & Row (Perennial).

*SIEGEL, B. (1989). *Peace, love, and healing. Bodymind communication and the path to self-healing: An exploration.* New York: Harper & Row.

SIEGEL, B. (1993). *How to live between office visits: A guide to life, love, and health.* New York: HarperCollins.

*SIEGEL, R. D. (2010). *The mindfulness solution: Everyday practices for everyday problems.* New York: Guilford Press.

*SIZER, F. S., & WHITNEY, E. (2011). *Nutrition: Concepts and controversies* (12th ed.). Belmont, CA: Wadsworth, Cengage Learning.

SMITH, M., & SEGAL J. (2011, December). *Signs that you're in an abusive relationship.* Retrieved from http://www.helpguide.org/mental/domestic_violence_abuse_types_signs_causes_effects.htm

SPRECHER, S., & FEHR, B. (2011). Dispositional attachment and relationship-specific attachment as predictors of compassionate love for a partner. *Journal of Social & Personal Relationships, 28*(4), 558–574.

SPRUNG, M., & HARRIS, P. L. (2010). Intrusive thoughts and young children's knowledge about thinking following a natural disaster. *Journal of Child Psychology and Psychiatry, 51*(10), 1115–1124.

REFERENCES

*STAHL, P. M. (2007). *Parenting after divorce: Resolving conflicts and meeting your children's needs* (2nd ed.). Atascadero, CA: Impact.

STEINER, C. (1975). *Scripts people live: Transactional analysis of life scripts.* New York: Bantam.

STERNBERG, R. J. (1986). A triangular theory of love. *Psychological Review, 93,* 119–135.

*STERNBERG, R. J., & BARNES, M. (Eds.). (1988). *The psychology of love.* New Haven, CT: Yale University Press.

*STERNBERG, R. J., & WEIS, K. (Eds.). (2006). *The new psychology of love.* New Haven, CT: Yale University Press.

*STONE, H., & STONE, S. (1993). *Embracing your inner critic: Turning self-criticism into a creative asset.* San Francisco: Harper.

STURGEON, M., WETTA-HALL, R., HART, T., GOOD, M., & DAKHIL, S. (2009). Effects of therapeutic massage on the quality of life among patients with breast cancer during treatment. *Journal of Alternative & Complementary Medicine, 15*(4), 373–380.

*TANNEN, D. (1987). *That's not what I meant: How conversational style makes or breaks relationships.* New York: Ballantine.

*TANNEN, D. (1991). *You just don't understand: Women and men in conversation.* New York: Ballantine.

*TATUM, B. D. (1999). *"Why are all the black kids sitting together in the cafeteria?"* New York: Basic Books.

*TAVRIS, C. (1992). *The mismeasure of women.* New York: Simon & Schuster (Touchstone).

TAYLOR, J. B. (2009). *My stroke of insight.* London: Hodder and Stoughton.

*TERKEL, S. (1975). *Working.* New York: Avon.

TIGGEMANN, M., & HOPKINS, L. A. (2011). Tattoos and piercings: Bodily expressions of uniqueness? *Body Image, 8*(3), 245–250.

TOGNOLI, J. (2003). Leaving home: Homesickness, place attachment, and transition among residential college students. *Journal of College Student Psychotherapy, 18*(1), 35–48.

TOLIN, D. F., & FOA, E. B. (2006). Sex differences in trauma and posttraumatic stress disorder: A quantitative review of 25 years of research. *Psychological Bulletin, 132*(6), 959–992.

TOP 50 THINGS TO DO TO STOP GLOBAL WARMING. (2008). Retrieved from http://globalwarming-facts .info/50-tips.html

TRACY, V. M. (1993). *The impact of childhood sexual abuse on women's sexuality.* Unpublished doctoral dissertation. La Jolla University: San Diego, CA.

TRACY-SMITH, V. (2011). *Meditation now: Your guide to building a simple practice.* Messenger Mini-Book.

*TRAVIS, J. W., & RYAN, R. S. (2004). *The wellness workbook* (3rd ed.). Berkeley, CA: Celestial Arts.

TRINKNER, R., COHN, E. S., REBELLON, C. J., & GUNDY, K. V. (2012). Don't trust anyone over 30: Parental legitimacy as a mediator between parenting style and changes in delinquent behavior over time. *Journal of Adolescence, 35*(1), 119–132.

TWENGE, J. M., & CAMPBELL, W. K. (2009). *The narcissism epidemic: Living in the age of entitlement.* New York: Free Press.

U. S. BUREAU OF THE CENSUS. (2004). *America's family and living arrangements, 2003.* Washingon, DC: U.S. Government Printing Office.

U.S. DEPARTMENT OF JUSTICE. (2011). *What is domestic violence?* Retrieved from http://www .ovw.usdoj.gov/domviolence.htm

VAN DER KOLK, B. (2008). *The body keeps the score: Memory and the evolving psychobiology of post traumatic stress.* Retrieved from http:// www.trauma-pages.com/a/vanderk4.php

VAN DER KOLK, B., MCFARLANE, A., & WEISAETH, L. (Eds.). (1996). *Traumatic stress: The effects of overwhelming experience on mind, body and society.* New York: Guilford Press.

VAN GENT, T., GOEDHART, A. W., & TREFFERS, P. D. A. (2011). Self-concept and psychopathology in deaf adolescents: Preliminary support for moderating effects of deafness-related characteristics and peer problems. *Journal of Child Psychology & Psychiatry, 52*(6), 720–728.

*VANZANT, I. (1998). *One day my soul just opened up.* New York: Simon & Schuster (Fireside).

VERGEER, G. E. (1995). Therapeutic applications of humor. *Directions in Mental Health Counseling, 5*(3), 4–11.

*VONTRESS, C. E., JOHNSON, J. A., & EPP, L. R. (1999). *Cross-cultural counseling: A casebook.* Alexandria, VA: American Counseling Association.

WAGNER, K. D., BRIEF, D. J., VIELHAUER, M. J., SUSSMAN, S., KEANE, T. M., & MALOW, R. (2009). The potential for PTSD, substance use, and HIV risk behavior among adolescents exposed to Hurricane Katrina. *Substance Use & Misuse, 44,* 1749–1767.

*WEBB, D. (1996). *Divorce and separation recovery.* Portsmouth, NH: Randall.

*WEBB, D. (2000). *50 ways to love your leaver: Getting on with your life after the breakup.* Atascadero, CA: Impact.

*WEENOLSEN, P. (1996). *The art of dying: How to leave this world with dignity and grace, at peace with yourself and your loved ones.* New York: St. Martin's Press.

*WEIL, A. (2000). *Eating well for optimum health: The essential guide to food, diet, and nutrition.* New York: Knopf.

WEINER-DAVIS, M. (1995). *Change your life and everyone in it.* New York: Simon & Schuster (Fireside).

WEIS, K., & STERNBERG, R. J. (2008). The nature of love. In S. F. Davis & W. Buskist (Eds.), *21st century psychology: A reference handbook* (Vol. 2, pp. 134–142). Thousand Oaks, CA: Sage.

WEITEN, W. (2013). *Psychology: Themes and variations* (9th ed.). Belmont, CA: Wadsworth, Cengage Learning.

*WEITEN, W., DUNN, D. S., & HAMMER, E. Y. (2012). *Psychology applied to modern life: Adjustment in the 21st century* (10th ed.). Belmont, CA: Wadsworth, Cengage Learning.

WEISS, R., & SAMENOW, C. P. (2010). Smart phones, social networking, sexting and problematic sexual behaviors—A call for research. *Sexual Addiction & Compulsivity, 17,* 241–246.

WETTERNECK, C. T., BURGESS, A. J., SHORT, M. B., SMITH, A. H., & CERVANTES, M. E. (2012). The role of sexual compulsivity, impulsivity, and experiential avoidance in Internet pornography use. *Psychological Record, 62*(1), 3–17.

WHITE, M. (1989). Saying hullo again. In M. White, *Selected papers* (pp. 29–36). Adelaide, Australia: Dulwich Centre.

WHITE, M. (2007). *Maps of narrative practice.* New York: Norton.

WHITNEY, E., DEBRUYNE, L. K., PINNA, K., & ROLFES, S. R. (2011). *Nutrition for health and health care* (4th ed.). Belmont, CA: Wadsworth, Cengage Learning.

WHITTY, M. T. (2011) Internet infidelity: A real problem. In K. S. Young & C. Nabuco de Abreu (Eds.), *Internet addiction: A handbook and guide to evaluation and treatment* (pp. 191–204). Hoboken, NJ: Wiley & Sons.

WILLARD, N. (2011). School responses to cyberbullying and sexting: The legal challenges. *Brigham Young University Education & Law Journal, 1,* 75–125.

*WILLIAMS, B., & KNIGHT, S. M. (1994). *Healthy for life: Wellness and the art of living.* Pacific Grove, CA: Brooks/Cole, Cengage Learning.

*WILLIAMS, C. (1992). *No hiding place: Empowerment and recovery for our troubled communities.* San Francisco: Harper.

WITKIN, G. (1994). *The male stress syndrome: How to survive stress in the '90s* (2nd ed.). New York: Newmarket.

*WOLFERT, A. D. (2003). *Understanding your grief: Ten essential touchstones for finding hope and healing your heart.* Fort Collins, CO: Companion Press.

WOODY, J. D. (2011). Sexual addiction/hypersexuality and the DSM: Update and practice guidance for social workers. *Journal of Social Work Practice in the Addictions, 11*(4), 301–320.

WORDEN, J. W. (2002). *Grief counseling and grief therapy: A handbook for the mental health practitioner* (3rd ed.). New York: Springer.

WORTHINGTON, E. L., Jr., & SCHERER, M. (2004). Forgiveness is an emotion-focused coping strategy that can reduce health risks and promote health resilience: Theory, review, and hypotheses. *Psychology and Health, 19*(3), 385–405.

*WUBBOLDING, R. E. (2000). *Reality therapy for the 21st century*. Muncie, IN: Accelerated Development (Taylor & Francis).

*WUBBOLDING, R. E. (2011). *Reality therapy*. Washington, DC: American Psychological Association.

WYMER, W. (2010). Consumer perceptions of prescription drug websites: A pilot study. *Health Marketing Quarterly, 27*, 173–194.

WYSOCKI, D. K., & CHILDERS, C. D. (2011). "Let my fingers do the talking"; Sexting and infidelity in cyberspace. *Sexuality & Culture, 15*(3), 217–239.

XU, Y., FARVER, J. A. M., YU, L., & ZHANG, Z. (2009). Three types of shyness in Chinese children and the relation to effortful control. *Journal of Personality and Social Psychology, 97*(6), 1061–1073.

***Y**ALOM, I. D. (1980). *Existential psychotherapy*. New York: Basic Books.

*YALOM, I. D. (2008). *Staring at the sun: Overcoming the terror of death*. San Francisco: Jossey-Bass.

***Z**IMBARDO, P. (2007). *The Lucifer Effect: Understanding how good people turn evil*. New York: Random House.

ZIMBARDO, P. G. (1987). *Shyness*. New York: Jove.

*ZIMBARDO, P. G. (1994). *Shyness*. Reading, MA: Addison- Wesley.

*ZUNKER, V. G. (2012). *Career counseling: A holistic approach* (8th ed.). Belmont, CA: Brooks/Cole, Cengage Learning.

439

REFERENCES

INDEX

Abbott, A., 141

Abbott, C., 141

A-B-C theory of personality, 81

Abeles, N., 362

Ability, 288

Abstinence, 265

Abuse, domestic, 212

Acceptance, 86, 357

Acquaintance rape, 154

Action, planning and, 21

Action stage, 6

Action, values in, 384–386

Active learner, 24

Adjustment, 8

Adler, A., 10–11, 393

Adolescence, 61–66

Adolescence, childhood and, 38–68
  adolescence, 61–66
  developing a self-concept, 57
  developmental stages, 43–44
  early childhood, 48–51
  identity versus role confusion in, 61
  impact of the first six years of life, 51–55
  infancy, 44–48
  loneliness and, 328–331
  middle childhood, 56–60
  pubescence, 60–61
  stages of personality development, 40–44

Adulthood and autonomy, 72–107
  autonomy and interdependence, 74–88
  developmental stages, 89
  early, 90–93
  emerging, 91
  entering the twenties, 91–92
  the fifties, 97–98
  generativity and stagnation, 95
  integrity versus despair, 100
  intimacy versus isolation, 90
  late adulthood, 99–104

late middle age, 97–99
  the late thirties, 94–95
  life during the forties, 95–97
  middle, 93–97
  the sixties, 98
  stages of, 88–90
  stereotypes of late, 101–102
  themes during late, 99–101
  transition from twenties to thirties, 92–93

Adulthood, stages of, 88–90

Advance directives, 352

Ageism, 101

Agency, 239

Ainsworth, M., 45–46, 185

Albom, M., 343, 357

Alcohol, drugs and, 146–149

Alcoholics Anonymous World Services, 149

American Psychiatric Association, 149

American Psychological Association (APA), 101–102

Anderson, M., 65

Anderson, S., 392

Androgyny, 252

Angelou, M., 19–20, 335, 377

Anger, 356

Anger and conflict in relationships, 209–213

Anxiety, 6

Anxious-avoidant pattern, 45

Approach-approach conflicts, 140

Approach-avoidance conflicts, 140

Aptitude tests, 288

Arbitrary inferences, 83

Armstrong, T., 27, 29, 42, 44, 48, 56, 61, 90, 94, 98, 100

Arnett, J., 91

Aronson, E., 277

Aronson, S., 350–351

Arricale, F., 45–46

Assisted suicide, 352

Attachment, 45

Attachment theory, 45

Authentic love, 181

Authoritarian parents, 51

Authoritative parents, 51

Autonomy, 11, 40, 75

Autonomy, adulthood and, 72–107
  autonomy and interdependence, 74–88
  developmental stages, 89
  early, 90–93
  emerging, 91
  entering the twenties, 91–92
  the fifties, 97–98
  generativity and stagnation, 95
  integrity versus despair, 100
  intimacy versus isolation, 90
  late adulthood, 99–104
  late middle age, 97–99
  the late thirties, 94–95
  life during the forties, 95–97
  middle, 93–97
  the sixties, 98
  stages of, 88–90
  stereotypes of late, 101–102
  themes during late, 99–101
  transition from twenties to thirties, 92–93

Autonomy and Interdependence, 74–86

Autonomy, trust and, 18

Autonomy versus shame and doubt, 48

Avoidance-avoidance conflicts, 140

Baker, R., 60

Balance, 5

Bargaining, 356–357

Barriers
  to communication, 214–218
  to loving, 187–191
  overcoming, 407–408

Basic honesty and caring, 18
Basic spiritual values, 382
Basow, S., 254
Baumrind, D., 51
Baur, K., 152, 154, 181, 221–223, 238, 253, 262, 266–268, 272
Bayes, A., 130
Beck, A., 82
Beck, J., 82, 130
Beck, R., 320
Becoming the woman or man you want to be, 234–256
  alternatives to rigid gender-role expectations, 252–254
  female roles, 244–252
  male roles, 236–244
Beisser, A., 6
Bellah, R., 377
Benjamin, J., 167
Ben-Shahar, T., 115, 118, 125, 145, 364
Benson, H., 165
Benton, S., 411
Bereavement, 360
Berman, J., 270
Berman, L., 270
Berne, E., 76
Bhatt, E., 101
Bisexual, 221
Blau, W., 351
Bly, R., 242
Bodian, S., 166
Bodily identity, 125–131
Bodily-kinesthetic learner, 28
Body and wellness, 110–133
  accepting responsibility for your body, 115–116
  body image, 127–131
  diet and nutrition, 121–123
  exercise and fitness, 119–121
  importance of touch, 127
  maintaining sound health practices, 117–124
  one man's wellness program, 114–115
  rest and sleep, 117–119
  spirituality and purpose in life, 123–124

wellness and life choices, 112–116
wellness and responsible choices, 113–114
your bodily identity, 124–131
Body image, 127–131
Boenisch, E., 383
Bok, F., 375
Bolles, R., 296
Bowlby, J., 45, 185
Boylan, M., 351
Brannon, L., 120
Brenner, P., 121, 142, 357
Brody, S., 272
Brooks, K., 178
Brundtland, G., 101
Buchanon, T., 52
Burden, R., 57
Burnout, 144
Burnstein, M., 325
Buscaglia, L., 187–188, 191

Campbell, W., 181
Canfield, J., 320
Carducci, B., 323, 325–327
Career, 285
Career decision making, 287–289
Careers, changing in midlife, 301–302
Carlson, J., 381
Carlson, R., 382
Carnes, P., 274
Carroll, J., 152–154, 156, 208, 221, 262, 269, 272, 274
Casey, L., 121
Challenge, 142
Chamberlain, L., 297
Change, 4–7, 141
  paradoxical theory of, 6
  stages of, 6–7
Chapman, G., 179
Childers, C., 220
Childhood and adolescence, 38–68
  adolescence, 61–66
  developing a self-concept, 57
  developmental stages, 43–44
  early childhood, 48–51

loneliness and, 328–331
identity versus role confusion in, 61
impact of the first six years of life, 51–55
infancy, 44–48
middle childhood, 56–60
pubescence, 60–61
stages of personality development, 40–44
Choice, 4–7
Choice theory, 20
  approach to personal growth of, 20–22
Chronic loneliness, 320
Clementi, T., 223
Cochran, S., 240, 244
Cognitive distortions, 82
Cognitive therapy, 82
Collectivism, 19
Commitment, 142
Communication barriers, 214–218
Communion, 239
Community feeling, 10
Compassion, 382
Compensation, 59
Compulsive sexual behavior, 274
Conflict, 140
  approach-approach, 140
  approach-avoidance, 140
  avoidance-avoidance, 140
  in relationships, anger and, 209–213
Connection, 75
Constructive coping, 158
Contemplation stage, 6
Corey, G., 13, 388, 391
Cornum, R., 143, 151
Corr, C., 342, 351, 358,
Corr, D., 342, 351, 358
Counseling for personal enhancement, 410
Courage, 19
Courtney-Clarke, M., 19
Creative connection, 13
Creativity, 19
Crisis, 41

Crooks, R., 152, 154, 181, 221–223, 238, 253, 262, 266–268, 272
Crosby, A., 349
Cultural perspectives on grieving, 363–364
Culture, 386
Culver, L., 157
Cutler, H., 342, 381
Cyberbullying, 65

Dalai Lama, 123, 319, 342, 378, 381–382
Danhauer, S., 167
Darcy, A., 130
Date rape, 154
Death
  fears of, 343–345
  hastened, 352
Death and loss, 340–366
  death and the meaning of life, 344–348
  freedom in dying, 352–354
  grieving over death, separation, and other losses, 360–364
  the hospice movement, 354–355
  our fears of death, 343–344
  stages of, 356–360
  suicide, 349–352
Death awareness, 345
Deep relaxation, 165–166
Defensive behavior, 146
Delany, A., 103
Delany, S., 103
Denham, S., 237
Denial, 58, 356
DePauw, S., 47
Depression, 357
Depth psychology perspective, 11
Despair, integrity versus, 100
Dibiase, R., 127
Dichotomous thinking, 83
Diet and nutrition, 121–123
DiGuiseppe, R., 82
Direction and doing, 21
Disconnection, 75

Discrimination, 389
Displacement, 58
Distress, 138
Diversity, 386–393
Divorce, separation and, 225–228
Domestic abuse, 212
Dreams, 412–414
Drugs and alcohol, 146–149
Duplex theory of love, 185
Dweck, C., 29–30
Dying, five stages of, 356
Dying, freedom in, 352–354

Early adulthood, 90–93
Early childhood, 48–50
Easwaran, E., 164
Effects of stress, 141–144
Ego defense mechanisms, 58–59
Ego integrity, 100
Eide, E., 118
Ellis, A., 81, 342
Emerging adulthood, 91
Emotional competence, 48
Emotional intelligence, 26
Emotional learner, 29
Encapsulated world, 387
Environmental sources of stress, 138–140
Epstein, M., 164
Erectile dysfunction, 270
Erikson, E., 41–42, 44, 48–49, 56, 61–62, 90, 95, 100, 202
Ethnocentric bias, 386
Eustress, 138
Evaluation, 21
Everly, G., 150
Everyday loneliness, 320
Exercise and fitness, 119–121
Existential loneliness, 320
Experiential family therapy, 15

Fantasy, 59
Fears, 31
  of death, 343–345
  of loneliness, 321–323
  of love, 190–191
Fehr, B., 186
Feist, J., 120

Female roles, 244–251
Feminist perspective, 42
Fenton, M., 148
Feuerstein, G., 166
Fields, T., 326
Fight-or-flight response, 141
Fisher, B., 227
Fitness, exercise and, 119–121
Five stages of dying, 356
Fixed mindset, 29
Flannery, T., 395
Flowers, J., 150, 164, 244, 305
Foa, E., 150–151
Fontana, D., 163–164
Forrest, A., 167
Fowler, J., 123
Fowler, R., 151
Frankl, V., 179, 334, 374
Freedom, 17–18
Freeman, S., 361, 363
Freud, S., 10, 41
Friedman, M., 149
Friend, D., 377
Fromm, E., 181
Frustration, 140
Fullerton, D., 113
Fully functioning person, 12

Ganiban, J., 47
Gardner, H., 25, 27
Garran, A., 388–390
Gay-affirmative therapy, 221
Gay and lesbian relationships, 220–221
Gay men, 221
Gender-role expectations, alternatives to, 252–254
Gender-role socialization, 236
Gender-role strain, 238
Gender-role transcendence, 253
Gender stereotypes, 238
Generativity, 95
Genevay, B., 302, 304
Germer, C., 86
Gibran, K., 187
Gilbert, E., 163, 166
Gillham, J., 5
Giving, 19

Glasser, W., 20
Glenn, D., 19–20
Glionna, J., 375
Goldberg, A., 220, 224
Goleman, D., 26, 45, 48, 56, 61
Gonzalez, R., 284, 302, 304–305
Good, M., 191
Good, P., 191
Gore, A., 395
Gottman, J., 207–208, 210, 238
Goulding, M., 76, 78
Goulding, R., 76, 78
Grief work, 360
Grieving, cultural perspectives on, 363–364
Growth mindset, 29
Growth, personal learning and, 2–35
    active learner, 24–25
    choice and change, 4–7
    choice theory approach to personal growth, 20–23
    fixed versus growth mindsets, 29–30
    humanistic approach to personal growth, 8–9
    key figures in development of humanistic approach, 9–16
    Maslow's self-actualization theory, 16–20
    models for personal growth, 7–23
    multiple intelligences and multiple learning styles, 25–29
    stages of change, 6–7
    suggestions for, 31–32
Guilt, initiative and, 49
Guindon, M., 299
Gunnoe, J., 127
Guo, Y., 139

Haldeman, D., 90–91
Hales, D., 112, 119, 123, 141, 159, 163, 167, 265–266, 270
Halligan, R., 223
Hammer, A., 377
Haney, M., 383
Hanh, T., 164

Happiness, 4–5, 10
Hardiness, 142
Harris, A., 253
Harris, K., 297
Harris, P., 149
Hate crimes, 223
Hazan, C., 185–186
Hazards of unprotected sex, 275–277
Hedtke, L., 351, 359
Helicopter parenting, 52
Henderson, L., 325–326
Here-and-now focus, 15
Heterosexism, 221
Hierarchy of needs, 16–17
Hinduja, S., 63, 65
HIV/AIDS, 275
Hodson, R., 297
Hoffman, E., 388
Holistic health, 112
Holland, J., 286, 289, 294
Holland's hexagon, 292
Hollon, S., 82
Holmes, T., 141
Homophobia, 223
Homosexuality, psychological views of, 221–222
Hopkins, L., 127
Horvatin, T., 13
Hospice movement, 354–355
Hospice program, 354
Houlihan, D., 149
Humanistic approach
    key figures in development of, 9–16
    to personal growth, 8–9
Humanistic psychology, 8–9, 15–16
Humor, 159
Hussain, A., 149
Hwang, P., 5

Identity, quest for, 372–374
Identity versus role confusion, 61
Impaired givers, 188
Inauthentic love, 184
Incest, 152
Individualism, 19

Individuation, 11, 63, 96
Industry versus inferiority, 56
Ineffective reactions to stress, 144–149
Infancy, 44–48
Initiative and guilt, 49
Injunctions, 78
    overcoming, 80
Inner critic, 84
Inner parent, 83
Insomnia, 119
Integrity versus despair, 100
Internal locus of control, 143
Internet infidelity, 219–220
Interpersonal learner, 28
Intimacy, 272
    versus isolation, 90
    types of, 202
Intimate partner violence, 212
Intrapersonal learner, 28

Jackson, M., 139
Jakupcak, M., 149
Jampolsky, G., 211–212
Jannini, E., 271
Job, 285
Jobs, S., 342
Joel, S., 186
John, E., 212
Johnson, M., 276
Jordon, J., 75
Journal, 32
Joy, 19
Julia, M., 253
Jung, C., 11, 96, 253

Kabat-Zinn, J., 85, 164, 165
Kaslow, F., 362
Kaslow, N., 350–351
Kawalla, Y., 150
Kaye, W., 131
Kiazad, K., 298
Kimmel, M., 239
King, C., 20
Kleespies, P., 352
Knight, C., 150–151
Kobasa, S., 142
Kottler, J., 381

Kubler-Ross, E., 356–358, 378
Kwok, J., 332

Labeling and mislabeling, 83
Lack of self-love, 189–190
Late adulthood, 99–104
Late middle age, 97–99
Lawyer, S., 155
Learner styles, 28–29
Learning, 19
Leisure, 305
LeMoyne, T., 52
Lenhart, A., 60, 63
Lesbian, 221
Lesbian relationships, gay and,
  220–221
Levant, R., 240
Levinson, D., 88, 90
Life choices, wellness and,
  112–117
Life, philosophy of, 378
Life script, 77
Lincoln, A., 48
Listening, 32
Living will, 352
Lock, R., 285
Logical-mathematical learner, 27
Logotherapy, 374
Loneliness, 318
  and adolescence, 329–331
  and childhood, 328–329
  chronic, 320
  creating our own through shy-
    ness, 323–327
  everyday, 320
  existential, 320
  experience of, 320–321
  and later years, 333–335
  fear of, 321–323
  and life stages, 328–335
  and middle age, 332–333
  and our life stages, 328–335
  and solitude, 316–336
  time alone as a source of
    strength, 335
  transient, 320
  and young adulthood, 331–332
Loss, death and, 340–366

death and the meaning of life,
  344–348
freedom in dying, 352–354
grieving over death, separation, and other losses,
  360–364
the hospice movement,
  354–355
our fears of death, 343–344
stages of, 356–360
suicide, 349–352
Love, 20, 91, 176–196
  in a changing world, 192–193
  authentic and inauthentic,
    181–184
  duplex theory of, 185
  fear of, 189–190
  makes a difference, 178–180
  myths and misconceptions
    about, 187–189
  self-, 180–181
  theories of, 185–186
Loving, barriers to, 187–191
Lowenstein, R., 299
Lucifer effect, 375–376

Macaskill, A., 212
Machel, G., 101
Machiavellianism, 298
Madden, S., 130
Maddi, S., 143
Magnification and minimization, 83
Mahalik, J., 238
Maier, S., 183, 384
Maintaining sound health prac-
  tices, 117–125
Maintenance stage, 6
Male roles, 236–244
Maltz, W., 154
Managing stress, 136–172
  constructive responses to
    stress, 158–160
  deep relaxation, 165–166
  effects of stress, 141–144
  environmental sources of
    stress, 138–140
  ineffective reactions to stress,
    144–149

meditation, 162–164
mindfulness, 164–165
posttraumatic stress disorder,
  149–151
psychological sources of
  stress, 140–141
resilience in coping with
  stress, 142–143
sexual exploitation, 151–156
sources of stress, 138–141
therapeutic massage, 168–169
time management, 160–162
vicarious traumatization, 157
yoga, 166–167
Mandela, N., 100–101
Mankiller, W., 377
Martin, B., 121
Maslach, C., 144
Maslow, A., 15–17
Massage therapy, 168
Masterbation, 267
Matlin, M., 221–222, 236, 239,
  245, 247–249, 253, 389
McCann, I., 157
McCullough, M., 211
McGoldrick, M., 41–42, 49, 56,
  64, 75, 90, 94, 98, 100, 245,
  247, 252
McIntosh, P., 390–391
Meaning and purpose, search for,
  377–380
Meaning and values, 370–398
  embracing diversity, 386–393
  the Lucifer effect, 375–376
  making a difference, 393–396
  people who live with passion
    and purpose, 374–375
  quest for identity, 372–374
  religion/spirituality and mean-
    ing, 381–383
  search for meaning and pur-
    pose, 377–380
  values in action, 384–386
  when ordinary people do ex-
    traordinary things, 376–377
Meaning of life, 377
Meaningful relationships,
  204–208

Meditation, 162–164
Meichenbaum, D., 81
Meir, G., 125
Menec, V., 305
Meriwether, L., 19
Mervielde, I., 47
Middle adulthood, 93–97
Middle childhood, 56–60
Middleton, V., 392
Miller, J., 388–390
Miller, J. B., 42, 64, 66, 75
Mindfulness, 85, 164–165
Minimization, magnification and, 83
Mislabeling, labeling and, 83
Mitchell, J, 150
Moore, T., 181, 189, 318
Morelock, J., 352
Moreno, J., 14
Moreno, Z., 13–14
Mourning, 361
Multilevel recovery, 145
Multiple intelligences, 25–29
Multiple learning styles, 25–29
Musical-rhythmic learner, 27
Mutual empathy, 262
Myths and misconceptions about love, 187–189

Nadeau, L., 57
Naparstek, B., 149, 151
National Committee on Pay Equity, 248
Naturalist learner, 28
Needs, wants and, 21
Neglectful parents, 51
Neria, Y., 149
Newman, B., 56, 61, 94, 97, 99
Newman, P., 56, 61, 94, 97, 99
Nhat Hanh, T., 180
Niles, S., 299
Norcross, J., 6
Nosko, A., 186
Nurmi, J., 92
Nutrition, diet and, 121–123

Obama, M., 114
Objective well-being, 9

Occupation, 285
O'Connor, T., 377
O'Neil, J., 238
Online dating, 218–219
Open attitude, 32
Opportunity, windows of, 45
Orgasm, 269
Orr, A., 237
Other-esteem, 5
Overcoming injunctions, 80
Overgeneralization, 83

Paradoxical theory of change, 6
Pardess, E., 221–222
Parker, S., 123
Patchin, J., 63, 65
Pathways to personal growth, 402–416
    counseling as a path to self-understanding, 409–412
    dreams as a path to self-understanding, 412–414
    overcoming barriers, 407–408
    pathways for continued self-exploration, 409
    self-assessment as a key to personal growth, 404–407
Pearlman, L., 157
Pehrsson, D., 351
Peluso, P., 45–46
Perls, F., 413
Permissive parents, 51
Perseverance, 19
Person-centered approach, 11–12
Person-centered expressive arts therapy, 12–13
Personal growth
    humanistic approach to, 8–9
    pathways to, 402–416
Personal learning and growth, 2–35
    active learner, 24–25
    choice and change, 4–7
    choice theory approach to personal growth, 20–23

fixed versus growth mindsets, 29–30
humanistic approach to personal growth, 8–9
key figures in development of humanistic approach, 9–16
Maslow's self-actualization theory, 16–20
models for personal growth, 7–23
multiple intelligences and multiple learning styles, 25–29
stages of change, 6–7
suggestions for, 31–32
Personality development, stages of, 40–44
Personality types, 289–296
Personalization, 83
Peterson, N., 284, 302, 304–305
Philosophy of life, 378
Physical tasks, 358
Piaff, E., 14
Pignotti, M., 47
Pistole, C., 45–46
Planning and action, 21
Playfulness, 48
Pleck, J., 238, 240
Pollack, W., 237, 239
Polusny, M., 149
Positive psychology, 9
Posttraumatic stress disorders, 149–151
Practicing self-disclosure, 32
Prayer of Saint Francis of Assisi, 183
Precontemplation stage, 6
Prejudice, 389
Preparation stage, 6
Preparing, 31
Pressure, 141
Prochaska, J., 6
Progressive muscle relaxation, 165
Projection, 58–59
Psychoanalysis, 41
Psychodrama, 13–14
Psychological maturity, 75

Psychological moratorium, 62
Psychological sources of stress, 140–141
Psychological tasks, 358
Psychological views of homo-sexuality, 221–222
Psychology, positive, 9
Psychosocial theory, 41
Psychosomatic illnesses, 141
Pubescence, 60–61
Purpose, search for meaning and, 377–380

Rabinowitz, F., 240, 244
Rahe, R., 141
Rainwater, J., 413
Rape, 154
Rational emotive behavior therapy, 81
Rationalization, 59
Reaction formation, 59
Real, T., 237, 240
Reality therapy, 20
Recreation, 284, 305–308
Recreation, work and, 282–312
    changing careers in midlife, 301–302
    choices at work, 297–301
    choosing an occupation or career, 286–293
    higher education as your work, 285–286
    place of recreation in your life, 305–309
    process of deciding on a career, 294–297
    retirement, 302–305
Reflections. See also Self-inventories.
    adulthood and autonomy, 73, 86–88, 93, 99, 104
    becoming the woman or man you want to be, 235, 243, 251–252, 254
    body and wellness, 111, 116–117, 124–125, 131
    childhood and adolescence, 39, 55, 60, 66

death and loss, 341, 348, 354, 364
loneliness and solitude, 317, 324–325, 327, 329
love, 177, 184, 193
managing stress, 137, 143–144, 157, 168–169
meaning and values, 371, 373–374, 380, 386, 396
pathways to personal growth, 403
personal learning and growth, 3, 22–25, 30
relationships, 201, 203–204, 208–209, 213–214, 220, 225, 228–229
sexuality, 261, 266, 269, 274, 277
work and recreation, 283, 293, 296–297, 308–309
Regression, 59
Reik, B., 212
Reivich, K., 143
Relational model of death and grieving, 358
Relationships, 200–231
    in a changing world, 218–220
    anger and conflict in, 209–214
    dealing with communication barriers, 214–218
    gay and lesbian, 220–225
    meaningful, 204–209
    separation and divorce, 225–229
    and social networking, 218
    types of intimacy, 202–204
Relaxation response, 165
Religion, 123
Re-membering, 359
Repression, 58
Resilience, 47–48, 142
Responsibility, 115
Responsible choices, wellness and, 113–114
Rest and sleep, 117–119
Retirement, 302–305
Reyes-Rodriguez, M., 130
"Richard Cory" poem, 323

Ridley, C., 389
Rinpoche, S., 164
Robbins, J., 178
Robinson, E., 323
Rogers, C., 11–12, 15, 214–215
Rogers, N., 12–13
Root, A., 237
Ropelato, J., 274
Ryan, R., 113

Saint Francis of Assisi, prayer of, 183
Samenow, C., 275
SAMIC³, 22
Sanchez, F., 238
Satir, V., 15
Satyapriya, M., 166
Schafer, W., 123
Scherer, M., 211
Schlossberg, N., 304–305
Schueller, S., 9
Schultz, D., 9, 11, 16, 96–97
Schultz, S., 9, 11, 16, 96–97
Schreiber, E., 13
Schwartz, B., 150, 164, 244, 305
Scopelliti, M., 320
Scott, W., 103
Search for meaning and purpose, 377–380
Secure pattern, 45
See, L., 332
Segal, J., 213
Segal, Z., 85
Selective abstraction, 83
Self-actualization, 8–10, 16, 19, 25
Self-actualization theory, 16–20
Self-actualizing person, 16
Self-assessment, 404–407
Self-authorship, 61
Self-awareness, 17
Self-concept, 57
Self-defeating thinking, 81
Self-determination, 10–11
Self-disclosure, practicing, 32
Self-doubt, 189–190

Self-efficacy, 61
Self-esteem, 5, 15, 299–300
Self-exploration, 7, 409
Self-fulfilling prophecies, 32
Self-healing, 13
Self-in-context, 41
Self-instructional training, 81
Self-inventories. *See also*
Reflections.
  adulthood and autonomy, 73,
    86–88, 93, 99, 104
  becoming the woman or man
    you want to be, 235, 243,
    251–252, 254
  body and wellness, 111,
    116–117, 124–125, 131
  childhood and adolescence,
    39, 55, 60, 66
  death and loss, 341, 348, 354,
    364
  loneliness and solitude, 317,
    324–325, 327, 329
  love, 177, 184, 193
  managing stress, 137, 143–144,
    157, 168–169
  meaning and values, 371,
    373–374, 380, 386, 396
  pathways to personal growth,
    403
  personal learning and growth,
    3, 22–25, 30
  relationships, 201, 203–204,
    208–209, 213–214, 220, 225,
    228–229
  sexuality, 261, 266, 269,
    274, 277
  work and recreation, 283, 293,
    296–297, 308–309
Self–love, 180–181
  lack of, 189–190
Self-realization, 377
Self-respect, 19
Self-sufficiency, 61
Self-understanding, 409–414
Seligman, M., 9, 143, 151
Sensuality, 269
Separation and divorce,
  225–228

Serenity prayer, 6, 411
Setlik, G., 148
Sex, guilt and misconceptions
  about, 267–269
Sexism, 236
Sexting, 65
Sexual abstinence, 265
Sexual addiction, 274–275
Sexual exploitation, 151–152
Sexual harassment, 155–156
Sexual orientation, 221
Sexual values, 264–266
Sexuality, 260–279
  controversy over sexual
    addiction, 274–275
  developing your sexual values,
    264–266
  guilt and misconceptions
    about sex, 267–269
  hazards of unprotected sex,
    275–277
  healthy dimensions of,
    271–272
  learning to enjoy, 269–271
  sex and intimacy, 272–274
Selye, H., 138
Shadow side, 11
Shaver, P., 185–186
Shear, M., 361
Sheehy, G., 90
Shield, B., 382
Shorter, L., 130
Showalter, M., 118
Shulman, S., 92
Shyness, 323–327
Siegel, B., 113
Siegel, R., 164–165
Silver, N., 208, 210
Sleep deprivation, 117
Sleep, rest and, 117–119
Smith, J., 220, 224
Smith, M., 213
Social interest, 10
Social networking, relationships
  and, 218
Social orientation, 10
Social tasks, 358
Solitude, 318

Solitude, loneliness and, 316–336
  creating our own loneliness
    through shyness, 323–327
  experience of loneliness,
    320–321
  learning to confront the fear of
    loneliness, 321–323
  loneliness and our life stages,
    328–335
  time alone as a source of
    strength, 335
  value of solitude, 318–320
Sources of stress, 138–141
  environmental, 138–140
  psychological, 140–141
Spiritual tasks, 358
Spiritual values, basic, 382
Spirituality, 19, 123, 381
Sprecher, S., 186
Sprung, M., 149
Stages of adulthood, 88–90
Stages of change, 6–7
Stages of personality develop-
  ment, 40–44
Stagnation, 95
Stahl, P., 227
Steiner, C., 76
Stereotypes, 101–104, 388
Sternberg, R., 185
Stiver, I., 42, 64, 66, 75
Stone, H., 84
Stone, S., 84
Stress
  constructive responses to,
    158–160
  effects of, 141–144
  ineffective reactions to,
    144–149
Stress, managing, 136–172
  constructive responses to
    stress, 158–160
  deep relaxation, 165–166
  effects of stress, 141–144
  environmental sources of
    stress, 138–140
  ineffective reactions to stress,
    144–149
  meditation, 162–164

mindfulness, 164–165
posttraumatic stress disorder, 149–151
psychological sources of stress, 140–141
resilience in coping with stress, 142–143
sexual exploitation, 151–156
sources of stress, 138–141
therapeutic massage, 168–169
time management, 160–162
vicarious traumatization, 157
yoga, 166–167
Sturgeon, M., 168
Subjective well-being, 9
Suicide, 349–352
assisted, 352
rational, 351
Sutton, C., 19
Sweeten, K., 48
Systemic perspective, 41

Taking risks, 20
Task-based model for coping with dying, 358
physical tasks, 358
psychological tasks, 358
social tasks, 358
spiritual tasks, 358
Tatum, B., 65, 330
Temperament, 47
Tessier, R., 57
Theories of love, 185–186
Therapeutic massage, 168–169
Tiberio, L., 320
Tiggemann, M., 127
Time management, 160–162
Tognoli, J., 320
Tolin, D., 150–151
Total behavior, 20
Touch, 127
Tracy, V., 153
Transactional analysis, 76
Travis, J., 113
Trinkner, R., 52
Trust, 31

Trust and autonomy, 18
Trust versus mistrust, 44
Tutu, D., 101, 378
Twenge, J., 181

Unfinished business, 351
Unintentional racism, 389
Unprotected sex, hazards of, 275–277
U. S. Department of Justice, 212

Values, 372, 384–386
Values, basic spiritual, 382
Values, meaning and, 370–398
embracing diversity, 386–393
the Lucifer effect, 375–376
making a difference, 393–396
people who live with passion and purpose, 374–375
quest for identity, 372–374
religion/spirituality and meaning, 381–383
search for meaning and purpose, 377–380
values in action, 384–386
when ordinary people do extraordinary things, 376–377
van der Kolk, B., 151
Van Gent, T., 57
Varra, E., 149
Verbal-linguistic learner, 27
Very old age, 99
Vicarious traumatization, 157
Views of homosexuality, psychological, 221–222
Visual-spatial learner, 27

Wagner, K., 149
Wants and needs, 21
Watts, V., 19
WDEP, 21
Weil, A., 122
Weis, K., 185
Weishaar, M., 82
Weiss, R., 275

Weiten, W., 5, 9, 117–118, 140, 154, 158, 218, 239, 241–242, 245–246, 253–254, 320, 349
Wellness, 112
Wellness and life choices, 112–117
Wellness and responsible choices, 113–114
Wellness, body and, 110–133
accepting responsibility for your body, 115–116
body image, 127–131
diet and nutrition, 121–123
exercise and fitness, 119–121
importance of touch, 127
maintaining sound health practices, 117–124
one man's wellness program, 114–115
rest and sleep, 117–119
spirituality and purpose in life, 123–124
wellness and life choices, 112–116
wellness and responsible choices, 113–114
your bodily identity, 124–131
Wellness program, 114–115
Wetterneck, C., 275
White, K., 60
White, M., 359–360
White privilege, 390
Whitney, E., 119, 122
Whitty, M., 219
Willard, N., 65
Williams, C., 20, 394
Windows of opportunity, 45
Winslade, J., 351, 359
Witvliet, C., 211
Wolfert, A., 360
Woody, J., 274
Worden, J., 362
Work, 91, 285
Work and recreation, 282–312
changing careers in midlife, 301–302
choices at work, 297–301
choosing an occupation or career, 286–293

Work and recreation (continued)
  higher education as your work, 285–286
  place of recreation in your life, 305–309
  process of deciding on a career, 294–297
  retirement, 302–305
Work values, 289

Worldview, 91
Worthington, E., 211
Wubbolding, R., 21–22
Wymer, W., 115
Wysocki, D., 220

Xu, Y., 324

Yalom, I., 320, 343–344

Yard, M., 377
Yoga, 166–167
Young, A., 19

Zimbardo, P., 325–327, 375–376
Zunker, V., 240, 245, 284, 288–289, 294

INDEX